The Executive Nurse

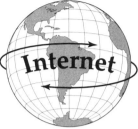

THE EXECUTIVE NURSE

Leadership for New Health Care Transitions

Sandra R. Byers

Ph.D, R.N., C.N.A.A.

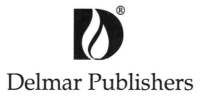

Delmar Publishers

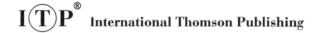 International Thomson Publishing

Albany • Bonn • Boston • Cincinnati • Detroit • London • Madrid
Melbourne • Mexico City • New York • Pacific Grove • Paris • San Francisco
Singapore • Tokyo • Toronto • Washington

Cover design: Brucie Rosch

Delmar Staff
Senior Acquisitions Editor: Bill Burgower
Assistant Editor: Hilary Schrauf
Senior Project Editor: Judith Boyd Nelson
Production Coordinator: Sandra Woods
Art and Design Coordinator: Carol D. Keohane

Copyright © 1997
By Delmar Publishers
a division of International Thomson Publishing Inc.

I(T)P The ITP logo is a registered trademark under license.

Printed in the United States of America

For more information, contact:

Delmar Publishers
3 Columbia Circle, Box 15015
Albany, New York 12212-5015

International Thomson Publishing Europe
Berkshire House 168–173
High Holborn
London, WC1V 7AA
England

Thomas Nelson Australia
102 Dodds Street
South Melbourne, 3205
Victoria, Australia

Nelson Canada
1120 Birchmount Road
Scarborough, Ontario
Canada, M1K 5G4

International Thomson Editores
Campos Eliseos 385, Piso 7
Col Polanco
11560 Mexico D F Mexico

International Thomson Publishing GmbH
Konigswinterer Strasse 418
53227 Bonn
Germany

International Thomson Publishing Asia
221 Henderson Road
#05–10 Henderson Building
Singapore 0315

International Thomson Publishing—Japan
Hirakawacho Kyowa Building, 3F
2-2-1 Hirakawacho
Chiyoda-ku, tokyo 102
Japan

1 2 3 4 5 6 7 8 9 10 XXX 02 01 00 99 98 97 96

Library of Congress Cataloging-in-Publication Data
The executive nurse : Leadership for new health care transitions / Sandra R. Byers.
    p.   cm.
    Includes bibliographical references and index.
    ISBN 0–8273–6272–2
    1. Nursing services—Administration. 2. Leadership. 3. Nurse administrators.
I. Byers, Sandra R.
    [DNLM: 1. Nursing Services—organization & administration. 2. Nurse Administrators.
3. Leadership—nurses' instruction. WY 105 E96   1997]
RT89.E96   1997
362.1'73'068—dc20
DNLM/DLC   96–12779
for Library of Congress   CIP

*To the dedicated nurses
who are the visionary leaders
implementing professional nursing
in new health care paradigms*

*To my husband, Tom,
and our children and grandchildren,
Linda, Forrest, Sara, Brianna, Alli, Stephen and Stacy*

CONTRIBUTORS

Sharon Aadalen, Ph.D., R.N.
Consortium Project Director, Health
  Bond
Immanuel–St. Joseph's Hospital
Mankato, Minnesota

Arlene Austinson, R.N., M.N.
Assistant Administrator
Nursing and Patient Care
Providence Portland Medical Center
Portland, Oregon

Marjorie Beyers, Ph.D., R.N., F.A.A.N.
Executive Director
American Organization of Nurse
  Executives
Chicago, Illinois

Julie M. Brightwell, J.D., B.S.N., R.N.
Attorney at Law
Schottenstein, Zox & Dunn
Columbus, Ohio

Gail Bromley, M.S.N., R.N.
Vice President
Clinical Services
Lakewood Hospital
Lakewood, Ohio

Donna K. Brown, Ph.D.
Oak Wood Associates
Grand Rapids, Ohio

Harriet V. Coeling, Ph.D., R.N.
Associate Professor
Kent State University
School of Nursing
Kent, Ohio

Marie J. Driever, Ph.D., R.N.
Assistant Director of Nursing
Quality Assessment/Research
Providence Portland Medical Center
Portland, Oregon

Kathleen M. Driscoll, JD., M.S., R.N.
Associate Professor
University of Cincinnati
College of Nursing and Health
Cincinnati, Ohio

Sue Fitzsimons, Ph.D., R.N.
Senior Vice President, Hospital
  Operations
Miami Valley Hospital
Dayton, Ohio

Lynette Froehlich, R.N., P.C.A.
Administrator
Health Bond Project Director
Arlington Municipal Hospital
Arlington, Minnesota

Susan R. Goldsmith, M.S.
Project Coordinator
Community Design Model
Harbor–UCLA Medical Center
Torrance, California

Mary Kay Hohenstein, M.Ed., R.N.
Instructional Dean
Health and Safety Division
South Central Technical College
Mankato, Minnesota

Lauren Jones, Ph.D., R.N.
Principal
Organizational Learning Group
Mt. Pleasant, South Carolina

Maryalice Jordan-Marsh, Ph.D., R.N.
Assistant Chair, Baccalaureate and
  Master Program
USC Nursing Department
Los Angeles, California
Co-Project Director
Community Design Model
Harbor–UCLA Medical Center
Torrance, California

Annette McBeth, M.S., R.N.
Vice President
Immanuel–St. Joseph's Hospital
Mankato, Minnesota

Mary R. McClelland, R.N., M.A., M.S., F.A.O.N.E.
Port Huron, Michigan

Peggy J. Nazarey, M.S.N., R.N.
Director of Nursing
Project Director
Community Design Model
Harbor–UCLA Medical Center
Torrance, California

Rita E. Numerof, Ph.D.
President
Numerof & Associates, Inc.
St. Louis, Missouri

Darren Pennington, Ph.D.
Research Data Manager/Analyst
Providence Portland Medical Center
Portland, Oregon

Shirley Raetz, R.N., P.C.A.
Director of Nursing
Health Bond Project Director
Waseca Area Memorial Hospital
Waseca, Minnesota

Mary Jane Reinhart, D.N.S., R.N.
Visiting Assistant Professor
Miami University
Department of Nursing
Oxford, Ohio
Nurse Researcher at Hospice
Dayton, Ohio

Elisa Sanchez
Staff Assistant
Community Design Model
Harbor–UCLA Medical Center
Torrance, California

Linda D. Schaffner, M.S., R.N.
Senior Vice President
Health Services/Physician Services
Bethesda, Inc.
Cincinnati, Ohio

Mary Schoessler, Ed.D., R.N.
Assistant Director of Nursing Education
Providence Portland Medical Center
Portland, Oregon

Kathryn Schweer, Ph.D., R.N.
Dean, School of Nursing
Mankato State University
Mankato, Minnesota

Paula V. Siler, M.S., R.N.
Director, Professional Practice Affairs,
    Nursing
Co-Project Director
Community Design Model
Harbor–UCLA Medical Center
Torrance, California

Susan Hoefflinger Taft, Ph.D., M.S.N., R.N.
Associate Professor
Kent State University
Director MSN-MBA/MPA Dual Degree
    Programs
Kent, Ohio

Janice Voukidis, B.S.N., R.N.
Coordinator
Quality Assessment/Improvement
Providence Portland Medical Center
Portland, Oregon

CONTENTS

FOREWORD

A new wind is blowing in health care and the journey to patient-first care is reaching its destination. Nurses have witnessed this revolution in a way that other health professionals have not had easy access to, and in this book Byers has captured the essence of both the changing and the already changed role of the executive nurse in a corporate position. Truly a participatory text, Byers has drawn together a group of expert executives to share their wisdom. This book will be a hallmark in the field and an excellent sequel to *The Professional Practice of Nursing Administration, Second Edition,* by Simms, Price, and Ervin. It truly merges executive practice and clinical thinking. Further, it lays the groundwork for understanding the modern organizational environment. Leadership is at all levels in organizations but it is the executive nurse at the corporate level who can stimulate and orchestrate the transformation of visions to action. The modern executive nurse is expected to function in a world in which all people think—not just corporate executives.

Today, executive nurses are defining their roles as they work. Their work is a school, and every day there is something new to learn. Some talk about servant leadership. Others talk about a world of shared power and continuous quality and process improvement. The bottom line is the shift in concept of power and the evolution of nursing's contract with the public, rather than with physicians or institutions. The other shift is from organizational to a national and even international mentality, with full respect for cultures and human diversity.

The executive nurse can lead the way to understanding the rapidly changing cultural environments in health care. Participants in the organizational culture are as important as co-workers in the executive wing. Understanding what people do, not just what they say they should do, has become of paramount importance in understanding work environments. One of the major goals of the executive nurse is to create participatory environments in which individuals see themselves as partners with a common vision, mission, and goals. Nursing has come of age and the essentials of nursing include both business and clinical knowledge and skills. Market culture, indeed culture beyond patient/family culture, was unknown in earlier nursing texts. Byers' text provides important chapters on culture—for without understanding culture, the corporate executive nurse is not apt to survive in the reengineered health care environments of the twenty-first century.

Ambulatory care expands while inpatient care shrinks; so too does the idea of one institution, the hospital, delivering health care. The customer base has expanded to include patient families, insurance groups, large corporations, other members of health networks, contracting businesses or cooperative purchasing groups, and even the U.S. government. There will be fewer hospitals in the year 2000, and more community and home-based methods of caring for society's health needs will be in place. Patient-centered rather than physician- or nurse-centered care will be the unifying theme for quality care. Clinical and management values will be maintained concurrently; the teacher/coach role has never had more opportunity for development than in the executive role.

The executive nurse will be expected to be able to reframe and entertain bold new creations and have the ability to see around corners and through the fog of ambiguity. These nurses must see leadership as a lifelong learning process and must be willing to take a new view of the future with its machinery and abundance of technology. Technology will not only be comprised of equipment but also include knowledge and skills, which will require a readiness for learning and the application of research. Therefore, executive nurses must be learners, users, and teachers of new technology, and boldly go where no nurse has gone before. Strategic planning will involve participatory thinking and shared visions. Team learning will be a must. A different kind of executive nurse will be needed, one who values people and who has a clear concept of non-zero-sum based power in which the amount of power in an organization is not finite but is an ever-evolving sum as people become empowered through their own learning and self-development.

There is a creative tension today between current reality and vision. The ability to understand this tension is essential to developing practices that nurture patient-centered outcomes. Preparing for these roles will involve deans of schools of nursing as executive nurses in their enterprises as well as executive nurses in practice settings. Cross-fertilization of ideas and integrating research and clinical practice are essential in the new "health for all" world. Executive nurses in both environments must be ready to serve as cross-cultural consultants and must be willing and ready to learn new sophisticated planning systems and advanced management tools. The ability to assume broader roles will be nurtured through multidisciplinary work and interaction.

Mission, not financial crisis, will be the driving force behind productivity gains. Byers and her uniquely qualified authors offer numerous approaches to excellent executive practice based on literature from the fields of administration and organizational studies and on the authors' corporate experience. A total quality management (TQM) environment, which provides multiple opportunities for nursing, allows and expects that nurses will move away from a "silo" mentality, in which nurses remain in their own realm and do not understand the big picture of the health care system. Silo mentality does not promote horizontal communication and the silo structure creates an unwritten law that thinking only occurs at the top of the pyramid. Productive health care organizations are thinking/learning enterprises, the opposite of stagnant organizations, in which the number of policies and procedures is inversely proportional to the amount of thinking expected.

All of these new ideas are introduced in Byers' book. The new executive nurse has a coaching role, a teaching role, and a totally different level of integrated thinking. Redesigning care delivery will emerge from the mingling of disciplines—physics, engineering, the traditional biochemistry, medical, and health sciences—and will be responsive to societal needs. There will be a different definition of power and an appreciation of the expansion of power. The inclusion of an ever-increasing number of nurse scientists in the health care culture will bring in people who are individualistic, self-empowered, and less group oriented. This will be a challenge for the executive nurse who seeks to balance human resources in a meaningful and productive way while enriching the workforce with quality researchers.

The new executive nurse will have a clearer understanding of the differences between technical nurse assistants and graduate prepared nurses whose preparation in schools of nursing administration will be an integration of executive leadership, clinical education, and research. Nursing may no longer be the largest area in health care institutions and this will create the need for executive nurses who are prepared to work with people from a variety of health-related disciplines who are self-starters and independent thinkers, who may wish to plan care modalities that include nontraditional care methods. In a world in which power no longer resides at the top of the organization or silo, a radically different approach is proposed in which everyone counts and the total amount of power is always expanding. Within the learning organization, workers are empowered to use their intellectual abilities. The whole of any organization is greater than the sum of its parts; thus the concept of non-summativity prevails, as is so well described in Byers' text.

Yes, indeed, the concept of leadership is changing and the idea that the corporate executive nurse is the only one who thinks in the organization is out of fashion. Every nurse is a potential leader and creative thinking is important to the acceptance of innovation at all levels of work in any institution. Byers' book has captured the essence of these ideas in multiple ways, demonstrating appreciation for linkages between practice and education, multidisciplinary approaches to care, lifelong learning, and continuing education. The importance of the teaching/coaching role is ably and masterfully emphasized in this challenging text. Written by excellent executives in the field, it is a must for the practicing or learning-to-practice corporate executive nurse. It will also be a valued text for any health care executive because the concepts presented are not limited to nursing.

Lillian M. Simms, Ph.D., R.N., F.A.A.N.
The University of Michigan

PREFACE

The Executive Nurse is intended to be futuristic. The book is built on current health care system realities and clearly looks forward to new health care system paradigms where the executive nurse will play a key leadership role as fundamental rules change. Executive nurse leadership is a critical component in all health care delivery settings: ambulatory, acute, occupational, home health, rehabilitation, and long term care. The book is written primarily for the executive nurse or chief nursing officer and for aspiring nurse leaders. Although most of the scenarios come from acute care settings, the content is readily adaptable to all settings, wherever nursing care is given. The book's dominant focus on nursing leadership allows reasonable application of the content to all types of health care delivery systems.

This book is a practical presentation of the essential new areas of expertise required of the executive nurse for the decade and century ahead. Most of the contributions in this book are drawn from practical experience and years of trial and error by leaders in their unique environments. It is not intended to be inclusive. Dedicated chapters on health information, computerization, and managed care are purposely omitted because they require extensive treatment. Chapters do refer to the impact of computerization and managed care on the role of the executive nurse and the leadership skills needed for new health care systems. The book is a valuable reference for executive nurses who aspire to excellence and are in the process of self-assessment and growth. The Executive Nurse can serve as a catalyst and resource for nurse managers.

This book is intended to be enlightening for educators and researchers—to help them view the health care system from the perspectives of executive nurses. Education, research, and clinical practice are interdependent and must be integrated in health care delivery to produce positive outcomes for consumers, students, and all clinicians. The executive nurse plays an important role in promoting integration and interdependency in the health care system and in the larger community. *The Executive Nurse* provides information to assist educators and researchers in understanding the nursing leadership challenges in the health care delivery system and to facilitate collegial dialogue, understanding, and mutual solutions. It is hoped that *The Executive Nurse* will stimulate discussion and further research in masters and doctoral programs. It can be an important tool for continuing education opportunities.

The book is divided into three sections: the new leadership roles and the challenge of organizational culture, the executive nurse as an innovator and evaluator of new organizational models, and the changes in critical role responsibilities in new organizations as the executive nurse anticipates and prepares for the future. The chapters represent a mix of scholarly and research-based analyses and practical and "real-life" examples of current and future role requirements. A few themes are evident throughout all chapters. These themes reinforce and demonstrate the complex relationships within the entire system and the application of the essential skills and knowledge at many different points in the enactment of the executive nurses' role. Such themes as culture, transformation, learning, continual improvement, legal, and ethical accountability, innovation and teamwork are conspicuous throughout the book and demonstrate the need for excellence and competitive creativity.

The editor wishes to acknowledge individuals who were critical in the evolution of this book. First, Thomas J. Byers, husband, friend, and constant optimist. Second, Lillian Simms, who was my inspiration with this new endeavor. Her wisdom, advice, and encouragement were authentic and a sincere testimony to the meaning of professional mentoring. Next, two competent editors and willing coworkers, Lisa Meyer and Erin Petersen. Their assistance was invaluable just when it was needed most. Five colleagues reviewed the manuscript at various developmental phases: Beryl Chickerella, Elaine Lakin, Gay Lindsay, Mary R. McClelland, Linda Rossi, and Geraldine Vogel. Three colleagues stepped in at the last moment to write two chapters—a real test of nursing collegial relationships! Mary K. Kohles, Deputy Director of "Strengthening Hospital Nursing: A Program To Improve Patient Care," was an invaluable resource. She recommended three of the chapters contained in this book and gave me thoughtful insights and support. A special acknowledgement to the many wonderful nurses who have been the silent inspiration for the ideas in this book. Debra Flis and Hilary Schrauf, assistant editors at Delmar Publishers, and Judith Johnstone, book producer, were helpful, responsive and encouraging. Thank you all.

Sandra R. Byers

INTRODUCTION

> And it ought to be remembered that there is nothing more diffi-
> cult to take in hand, more perilous to conduct, or more uncertain
> in its success, than to take the lead in the introduction of a new
> order of things.
>
> N. Machiavelli, *The Prince,* 1513

The position of the executive nurse or the chief nurse officer in the larger and more diverse acute-care delivery system has achieved a new level of recognition and accountability. The position has new risks and excitement. Many executive nurses are not prepared to lead at this new level and to impact the health care system as empowered leaders. They are trapped in old paradigms and models and are trying to lead effectively and creatively in a health care system demanding something different of leadership. The chapters in this book present the dynamic position of the executive nurse and many of the skills needed for nurses to be leaders in all types of health care environments.

The Executive Nurse: Leadership for New Health Care Transitions is organized around position requirements of the executive nurse as the chief nurse officer in a variety of health care facilities. The book discusses how this position has been evolving and hypothesizes what it will be in the future. It emphasizes the knowledge and skill needed to be a proactive force in health care decision making.

Part I focuses on the role of the executive nurse in the corporate position and the impact of organizational culture. Chapter 1 explores the role in terms of organizational structure and identifies phases in role implementation. Then the historical evolution of this position, in keeping with hospitals' moves to more corporate type structures, is presented. The chapter emphasizes the importance of the executive nurse's knowledge, skills, values, and experiences at this corporate level, as well as the critical need for the nurses's voice to be heard and understood in the long-term strategic planning for the corporation. The stresses and challenges of the position are discussed, along with the survival strategies and strengths needed by the executive nurse.

Leadership strategies applicable to the corporation and to the nursing department are presented in Chapter 2. It identifies "leadership equilibrium," proactive functioning, and "bombardment" along with ways to lead in these circumstances.

Chapter 3 addresses external opportunities in the political arena and the responsibilities of the executive nurse to influence health care policy based on expertise and experience in the acute-care environment. Options for active involvement and the knowledge needed to function are presented.

Chapter 4 presents organizational culture and survival issues as the setting for Part II. It defines the origin of hospital culture: culture is rooted in the fundamental survival strategy of the organization. It gives examples of how a community hospital's culture might differ from that of a teaching hospital, a county hospital, or a research center. To work effectively within any given culture, the nurse executive must understand the origins of that culture or the core organizational values. Chapter 4 reviews the components of organizational culture: the notions of homogeneity (hospital culture), heterogeneity (subculture), and the common components of culture (e.g. values, symbols, stories). Understanding where culture comes from and how it is manifested, the nurse executive is urged to use cultural knowledge to set expectations and to plan meaningful change.

Part II addresses innovative models of nursing care delivery and an evaluation approach to assist the executive nurse with the tools to redirect or reinforce change. Transformation and transition (for example, resizing and reengineering) are the ends and the means of new models and each phase requires unique executive nurse expertise. The models identify a new and different executive nurse position and demonstrate the importance of all providers, their work, and their level of performance. Mary K. Kohles, R.N., M.S.W., deputy director of the Strengthening Nursing Project, shared the following introduction to Chapters 5 and 6.

> Health care organizations are dominated by the tensions among the forces of competition and conflict, and power and influence. How the tension from those forces is played out in the organization is largely determined by the influencing behaviors employed by the management/leadership team. Influence and influencing are integral departments of the innovative, futuristic health care leader, whether it be the executive nurse or other executives, physicians, trustees, or other organizational leaders. It is an expectation, not a choice, that the new generation executive nurse demonstrate behaviors to influence transitional strategies for building innovative models for the organization's future. The Strengthening Hospital Nursing Program (SHNP) was conceived by The Robert Wood Johnson Foundation and The Pew Charitable Trusts in the 1980s. It demonstrates that institutionwide restructuring can assist in the development of models for meeting patient and family needs by all health care providers working together.
>
> The executive nurse must influence innovation while at the same time preserving day-to-day operations. How influence happens is largely up to the executive nurse—frequently through collaboration with a core team. The core team consists of individuals, often multidisciplinary, who are dedicated full- or part-time to institutionwide improvements such as restructuring, redesigning, reengineering, or reinventing efforts. The core team's director (project) or coordinator is often in a staff position versus a line position, reporting directly to the executive nurse or the organization's executive team. The director and the team are facilitators of the process rather than decision-makers or approvers of the interventions. The core team, working collaboratively with the executive nurse, provides a visible, interactive link with grassroots stakeholders and with middle and line management. The director

and core team are conduits through which new ideas can be formed, nurtured, tested, and implemented. The driving force behind the restructuring successes of SHNP is the participating organization's core team. The core team's ability to influence change is strengthened by endorsement from executive leadership and alignment with the leadership's shared vision. The collaborative relationship among the team members is established and identified as credible institutionwide. The organizational leaders recognize that each core team member plays a unique role, not only in his or her daily administration and clinical responsibilities, but also in restructuring-related efforts. Each brings support from a different sector of the health care system. Each brings distinct skills and knowledge to the restructuring effort. And each, more than likely, envisions "success" in slightly different terms, yet together they influence change by influencing key care providers, including nurses, physicians, support staff, and other health care professionals.

Chapters 5 and 6 present two different approaches by core teams working together to achieve (influence) a common goal: improvement of patient care services. One approach is presented by the core team (design team) from Harbor–UCLA Medical Center. Their efforts focus on strategies for managing transitions at the organizational, team, and individual levels. Specific attention is given to structural innovations that can be initiated by the executive nurse in concert with an interdisciplinary team. These strategies and innovations are described in the context of the Community Design Model (CDM). The CDM is an organizational design developed at Harbor–UCLA Medical Center that serves as a framework for broad-scale organizational change.

The second approach is by a consortium of three Minnesota Hospitals and two Minnesota higher educational institutions; Immanuel–St. Joseph Hospital, Arlington Memorial Hospital, and Waseca Area Memorial Hospital; and Mankato State University, and Mankato Technical College. The consortium is known as Health Bond, which means building opportunities and new directions through a service and education partnership. The focus by the Health Bond authors is on collaborative relationships between the executive nurses and faculty who make up the partnership. The authors discuss their transition from traditional power to emergent sources of power. Emergent sources of power are a shared vision, principled actions, decentralized decisionmaking, reflection skills, focus on patient care outcomes, and generalist competencies. The Health Bond partners then discuss their roles as internal and external consultants. They view themselves as external consultants to each other and internal consultants as they carry out redesign efforts within their individual organizations.

Although the approaches presented by the authors are different, they use similar influencing behaviors. They act as influencer, persuader, integrator, and coach, bringing the redesign effort to their colleagues in a form that is personal, understandable, and pertinent. They use skills of persuasion, negotiation, and communication. They recognize that it is important to present information clearly and concisely, make complicated things sound simple. They have learned to involve executive leadership and other key stakeholders at all levels of the organization, valuing everyone's opinions and perceptions. They have learned to respect differences, making differences an opportunity for innovation. They have learned to pay particular attention to middle managers. SHNP experiences have demonstrated that middle managers are the most vulnerable in the change process. The authors have capitalized on the evolving role of the executive nurse as a change agent, influencing change through collaboration and partnerships.

Along with the authors, other SHNP nurse leaders acknowledge that asking for help is a powerful influencing behavior. Nurse leaders have learned that asking for help gives the person who is being asked a sense of value and worth for their real and potential contribution to the organization's mission. Another influencing behavior, used by SHNP nurse leaders, is to give recognition to the contribution made by a person or team for a specific performance. The leaders understand that recognition gets to the person's self-esteem and sense of satisfaction and accomplishment. SHNP nurse leaders use affiliation as an influencing behavior. Affiliation gets at the person's need to belong and desire to help others. Other influencing behaviors employed by SHNP nurse leaders are listening to care providers at the unit level and using what they have heard, keeping affected stakeholders informed, and knowing what stakeholders do at all levels of the organization.

Because of the dynamics and complexities of restructuring processes, the executive nurse can no longer influence as a single leader. The executive nurse must look to such approaches as developing and evolving a core team. Together they will influence others, cascading the change process through the organization and out to the community for an improved health care delivery system, a system that can contend with the forces of competition and conflict, and power and influence.

Total quality management (TQM) is defined and the role of the executive nurse presented in Chapter 7. The chapter emphasizes what an executive nurse needs to know about TQM, how to best implement TQM, what the executive nurse brings to the institution's development of TQM, and how TQM can be used in strategic planning. Chapter 7 addresses the myths, rhetoric, and corporate culture surrounding TQM.

The "learning organization," another approach to system change, is presented in Chapter 8. It describes the "bridging" that needs to occur internally and externally for the organization to prosper and respond to all customers. This is a paradigm shift. The chapter reviews guidelines to pinpoint areas for examination, change, follow-up, and evaluation. It focuses on how this paradigm can support the need for health care to be open and responsive to changes in the larger system using practical examples.

New organizational approaches frequently do not include the rigor of evaluation concurrent with implementation. This is a difficult task. Chapter 9 presents the stance that new organizational models of care delivery and the process by which they are created demand a rethinking of the approach to evaluation. The process of developing new organizational models brings about innovation and learning, which in turn promotes further innovation and understanding necessary to initiate new ways to deliver care. This new evaluation approach has two core purposes: to generate quality data and to promote continual learning.

In preparing the executive nurse for the future, Part III begins by presenting organizational culture and the critical and distinct nursing unit subculture. Organizational culture changes present a different set of challenges at different levels of the organization, and consequently the hiring and empowering of unit managers must be an integral component of system transformation. Chapter 10 explains the different types of organizational culture (corporate, professional, organizational level, and work group). It includes unit-culture content areas: physical/psychosocial focus, large/small power distance, individualism/collectivism, criticism/approval and strong/weak uncertainty avoidance. Organizational phenomenon are described as different from organizational culture and the reasons for differences between the levels of culture within the organization are presented. The chapter describes how to use the information about unit culture to hire nursing unit managers for any given group, promote unit team building, bring about change on a unit, hire employees that will fit in and stay, manage the implementation of innovations, and assist in creatively solving organizational problems.

Chapter 11 is based on the author's current research in the power of decision making by executive nurses. The research categorized decisions as central, formal, or stratified. Power is defined as the potential to achieve desired outcomes. The power shifts and decision-making roles of the executive nurse, with the constant dilemma of profit versus altruism in a service profession, heighten the need to be aware and learn how to implement power. Power is present in all settings and exerting this power via critical decisions influences patient and work group outcomes.

Chapter 12 presents the important roles and functions of a consultant. Most executive nurses do not interact with consultants until the institution's board of trustees or chief executive officer decide the institution needs a "consultant." This chapter presents the consultant role as a positive way to help achieve the executive nurse's agenda to benefit nursing, nurses, and the consumer. The consultant can facilitate and help to manage the many changes occurring within systems. This chapter explains what the nurse executives needs to know to hire and work effectively with a consultant (i.e., need for and type of consultant, credentials, process of selection, and how to use a consultant to accomplish the goals).

Chapter 13 is pivotal for the nursing leader. It identifies and explores the legal and ethical concerns in the changing health care environment from the perspective of executive nurse, nurse manager, and staff. An overview of law and ethics is provided that includes areas of consumer and total-societal health care needs, professional commitment to societal needs versus facility loyalty, redesigned nursing care delivery, labor law responses to consumer and staff, health providers' health, employee rights versus consumer rights, and computerizing patient data versus the patient's right to confidentiality.

Chapter 14, the final chapter, addresses lifelong learning and educating nurses for the future. It describes what that future might be like. This chapter introduces the importance of caregiver education in the hospital setting and relates education and competencies to quality of care. It discusses the relationships with schools of nursing as competencies are identified, developed and change over time, what the nurse needs to function now and in the future in terms of competencies, the role of continuing education, assessment techniques, justification for education in the nursing budget, and how nursing education relates to national health care. It identifies the role of the executive nurse in the educational arena, looks at mentoring and the importance of research, which links education and quality of care. Knowledge evolves so rapidly with the use of computers and communication technology that the value of professional nursing in the acute-care environment will be dependent on the executive nurse's being able to integrate nursing research and knowledge into the everyday work of the professional nurse. The author launches the reader into the future with scenarios that are becoming reality.

The discussion questions at the end of each chapter are designed to encourage readers to think progressively and proactively and to apply the chapter's contents to their own life experiences and unique health care setting. The Appendix presents NUCAT–3, a Nursing Unit Cultural Assessment Tool that can be applied by the executive nurse in the initial stage of determining where we can begin.

This book presents interesting and complex role changes in the executive nurse position. The position is full of opportunity and adventure in all settings. It has rewards and value within the health care system. The nursing profession must support and recognize this position wholeheartedly. These individuals daily venture into uncharted waters as professional nursing leaders striving toward service excellence in a challenging health care system.

Leadership Roles and the Challenge of Organizational Culture

PART I

CHAPTER 1

Marjorie Beyers

The Executive Nurse in a Corporate Structure

Introduction

The future for the executive nurse's role is very bright because nursing services are part of health care's core business. This chapter describes executive nurse roles and functions as they are evolving in the current health care system. The position of executive nurse will continue to evolve with changes in health care delivery.

EVOLVING ROLES

Today, executive nurses are defining their new roles as they work. Executive nurse roles, although in existence for dozens of years in some settings, are just now becoming mainstream in health care services. One example of a longstanding executive nurse role can be found in the Veterans Administration, which is one of the largest health care systems in the United States. The executive nurse role was more recently developed in multi-institutional systems, which have been growing in number since the 1970s. Most of the ten top multi-institutional health care systems in the United States have included the functions of executive nurses in one form or another. Nurses in these roles were responsible for nursing services in two or more institutions, usually hospitals.

Even more recently, the executive nurse role is being developed in vertically integrated networks for health care delivery and within single-purpose or multi-institutional settings that are "behaving" like corporations.

The role and functions of executive nurses have not been extensively studied and therefore information presented in this chapter was developed from observation, personal experience, discussion, and selected interviews with individuals in these roles. To narrow the range of variation in executive nurse roles, this chapter is written from the perspective of the executive nurse in a network or in a multi-institutional setting.

EXECUTIVE NURSE ROLES

Role is often defined by relationships in the corporation. Who one reports to and who one's peers are define the level and scope of the role. In the corporation, the executive nurse relates to a boss and peers within the corporate structure. The executive nurse represents the nursing component of health care at the corporate level and also provides input to corporate-level activities such as quality improvement programs, strategic planning, finance, risk management, human resources, and other areas. In addition, the purpose of the role is to develop and deliver programs or projects having to do with clinical care. The executive nurse has a constituency throughout the corporation of those persons who will be the ultimate users of the programs or project services or products, that is, the caregivers.

Therefore, two key role relationships for the executive nurse are those with other corporate staff in both reports and peers, and those with the constituency of nurses and others in divisions of the corporation known as entities or components. These relationships are necessary to accomplish the objectives of the role. The corporate staff is involved in corporate-wide initiatives and activities and is key to the executive nurse role because plans, expectations, and perceptions are established at that level. At the same time, the constituency of executive nurses and managers in the corporation's entities is the end user of programs and services, and this constituency determines the purposes and effectiveness of the functions.

EXECUTIVE NURSE IDENTITY

Although variation prevails, some common themes emerge in the core identity of the executive nurse in almost all settings. These themes provide insight into the complexity of the role and allow comparison of the executive nurse role with top nurse administrator roles throughout the corporation. This comparison is essential because executive nurse identity depends on clear understanding of the differences between the executive nurse role and the roles of nurses in agencies or institutions within the corporation. Executive nurse identity themes are accountability and stewardship.

Accountability

Accountability is a mainstream theme in corporate nursing roles. In a corporation, people depend on one another; one person's behavior affects another's well-being in unique ways. The executive nurse's actions greatly affect others' welfare. How nursing care and nursing services are interpreted by the executive nurse influences how nursing care and nursing services are delivered throughout the corporation.

Accountable behavior is defined differently according to how relationships are developed or designed for the executive nurse role. In all corporations the role is viewed as contributing to the corporate mission, vision, goals, and key concepts about health care adopted by the corporation. There is a commonly understood expectation that corporate staff is committed to the mission and all it implies in developing services and programs. Accountable behaviors are developed from the mission and vision and applied to the functions. For example, an expectation to improve the quality of care delivered has to be developed within the organizational structure and context to be meaningful. In corporations, the accountability may be negotiated by the principles in any activity, as in work plans or contracts. Such is the case when the executive nurse fulfills a staff role.

Stewardship

Stewardship is a corollary of the concept of accountability and is a central theme in the executive nurse role. Stewardship of resources is a prevailing management theme for all nurse administrators, and one major resource is people. Former bureaucratic methods have given way to involving people in the work, with accountability for decision making related to design of care delivery and to selection and use of resources for patient care delivery. In a corporation, individuals accountable for nursing services in each and every corporate entity have power and control in that entity. Power thus distributed requires an appropriate participative management approach by the executive nurse in which leadership development is a priority.

Stewardship in executive nursing roles is effectively used in the context of shared or self-governance. Understanding accountability from the corporate perspective is difficult because there is a distributed accountability for corporate-wide initiatives and a local or organization-specific accountability for each corporate entity. Accountability thus distributed from one organization to many implies complexity that the executive nurse must respect and manage in the stewardship aspects of the role. This understanding is leading to new approaches to forming partnerships in nursing services, and to new approaches to leadership development.

CAUSES FOR ROLE VARIATION

Features of corporations are reflected in the variation of roles and functions of executive nurses. Two major corporate features that influence the role are (a) the corporate culture, and (b) the corporation's context and structural variables within the corporate organization. The executive nurse role is interdependent with the culture, the context, and the nature of the organizational relationships. Each of these aspects is discussed briefly in this section.

Culture

Corporate culture is expressed in values and attitudes about health care, about work, and about the relationships between the staffs of the corporate office and those of corporate components or divisions. Appropriate and acceptable behaviors are judged against the corporate culture in various ways. A state of corporate well-being is experienced when there is consistency in the values and attitudes of staff throughout the corporation. Confusion and discordance emerge when there is inconsistency. How nursing is viewed and supported in the corporate culture is a product of the values and attitudes of the diverse leadership groups, corporately and within individual divisions; these two cultures must strive for constancy between them for nursing to be supported and valued.

How patients or clients are viewed and cared for is also a product of values and attitudes.

Behaviors relating to how work is managed, how people are employed, and how the corporation relates to its publics are all products of the corporate culture. The strength of a corporate culture is measured by the consistency in which persons internal and external to the corporation describe it. Strong cultures are like strong personalities. The traits and capabilities are visible and known to others. At the same time culture can be subtle, in the sense that one must be part of the culture to truly understand its nuances. In corporate cultures, the value system is probably easiest to discern initially. Nuances of that system are learned over time, and through relationships.

Context

Corporate context describes the situation within, and external to, the corporation. Context in this usage goes beyond the external environment of an organization. A corporation has several environments (e.g., the "global" environment, the local environment) surrounding each of its organizations. The corporation relates to its surroundings in various ways. The corporate services influence the extent and nature of the environmental relationship as well. Corporations with a variety of services (e.g., long-term care, hospitals, managed care, hospice, home care) penetrate the community more deeply than corporations with a single service.

Another way of describing context is the position of the health care business in relation to the industry. In today's world of mergers, affiliations, and a myriad of agreements, the context must be described for the particular situation.

Organizational Structures

There are several ways to describe corporations from the organizational perspective. The most clearly defining terms for health organizations today are vertical and horizontal integration, centralization, and decentralization. Factors that influence structure, and therefore executive nurse roles, are related to the type of organization. These factors include scope of services offered and size. All of these organizational aspects impact the executive nurse role; each is described separately in this section.

Vertical and Horizontal Integration

Health care organizations may be structured as vertically integrated or horizontally integrated. **Vertically integrated** health care systems refer to those with a spectrum of health care services along the continuum of care for wellness, prevention, acute and chronic care, disease management and rehabilitation, ambulatory care, long-term and home care, and hospice care. **Horizontally integrated** systems contain organizations of one type, such as hospitals.

Centralization or Decentralization

The terms **centralization** and **decentralization** describe how power, authority, and control are distributed throughout the organization. Executive nurse roles may be structured as centralized or decentralized. The terms *centralized* and *decentralized* have special meaning for the nature of the relationships between the corporate executive nurse and executive nurses located in organizational components of the corporation. In centralized structures, line authority usually prevails, whereas staff authority is predominant in decentralized structures.

In today's fluid organizational structures, which value continuous learning and process improvement, most organizations are combinations of centralized and decentralized forms. Executive nurses must design programs and projects according to the type of organizational structure, because the structure influences not only authority and operational policies but also the critical communication patterns of relationships in the workplace.

Size and Scope

Two other organizational structural features that influence the executive nurse role and functions are the size of the corporation and the scope of services. Nursing is part of the core business of the health care organization and thus is influenced by these organizational variables. **Size** relates to the number of units or organizational divisions and geographic settings in which people work and the capacity of each, such as number of beds or volume of services. **Scope** of service relates to the complexity of services (from a single entity to a community health network in one or more geographic settings) or to the number of different services offered in any one location.

Widespread distribution of corporate organizations over multiple geographic areas requires the executive nurse to relate to people in ways that support successful services where they live. One size definitely does not fit all, because community expectations relate to unique community mores and ideas about health care, specific population groups, and local opportunities for employment. The economic resources in a community also influence the community relationships with health care organizations, as well as their expectations for health care services. The executive nurse must understand and relate to these variations to be successful in designing corporate-wide programs and services.

EXECUTIVE NURSE RESOURCES

Resources vary for the executive nurse position. The budget for the position may be a line item in the corporate budget, or the activities of the executive nurse may be developed and budgeted on a programmatic, or project, basis. Needless to say, resources are scarce and creativity in resource use and allocation is essential.

CORPORATE ROLE EXPECTATIONS

The investment in the executive nurse position is predicated on expectations of the role. One expectation, not related to resources, is that of presence or leadership. Another expectation is communication expertise.

Presence

Although the value of presence is not widely written about in the literature, having a leader at the corporate level who has presence is important to nurses throughout the corporation. How one establishes **presence** is related to the capability to communicate with both corporate staff and the constituencies. Communication is a high priority to effective executive nurses.

Communication

How effectively the corporate executive nurse communicates is related to the support the corporate role will receive. Communication helps to build corporate and constituent relationships, which are essential to fulfilling the mission and goals. Because communication is so important, some thoughts about the nature and resources for communication are included here.

The executive nurse plans communication in relation to the resources for technologic support of communications. Because communication influences the quality of relationships, attention to uses of technology to improve the quality of communications is a priority for the executive nurse. Communication flows from and influences relationships.

In today's world, timeliness and quality of communications are two important attributes. If a corporation has on-line communications capability, people in geographically distant locations can communicate in a timely manner, thus reducing the distance factor in corporate relationships. Interactive video is another medium that enhances communication and reduces the distance factor. Electronic mail, computer software programs for network conversations, and other media also enhance communications. However, using these resources requires that time be allocated for learning and becoming comfortable with the technology.

In addition to the timeliness of communications, the nature of information transmitted from the corporate office to the entities is a factor in success. Perceptions of how meaningful the communication is to the end users, the degree of participation in both needs assessment and development of communications, and the expectations established in the communication for feedback or follow-through are aspects of communication that influence the relationship. The way policies and procedures are formulated and transmitted, the way data about performance is collected and shared, and the way information about the corporation is evolved are products of culture and context that influence the organizational structure in both formal and informal behaviors.

EXECUTIVE NURSE PERFORMANCE

Little is written about the expected behaviors, or benchmarks for performance, for the executive nurse. In practice, there are several similar features, despite variations in the corporation and corporate structures.

Corporate Behaviors

As a corporate staff person, the executive nurse usually works with an executive team and with executive-level nurses. Most executive nurses work with organizations within the corporation to participate in the search and selection of key nursing staff, to interpret nursing to other corporate staff such as human resources and legal staff, to serve as a resource for clinical nursing inputs in the corporate decision making and policy-formation processes, and to work with corporate staff to shape vision, mission, and goals. In some corporations, the executive nurse works with quality management staff to develop guidelines and standards of nursing care and of patient care services.

Participation by executive nurses in examining issues and in shaping and implementing policies is also related to the culture and structure of the corporation. In centralized structures, there may be one approach and commonly used methods for nursing service delivery, nursing quality management, and quality improvement. In some centralized systems, the executive nurse may be expected to develop policies, take them through an approval process, and then promulgate them throughout the corporation. In decentralized structures, the executive nurse may plan for involvement of all executive nurses in decision making about policies and performance expectations.

Corporate Interdependence

Some of the most crucial functions of any society must be carried out collectively. This statement is certainly true within corporations. Because of the intimate nature of nursing care and the interdependence of nursing care with that provided by other types of health professionals, not only the executive nurse but also the corporate staff must be sensitive to local needs and demands both in the care situations and in the supporting organizations. As mentioned previously, communications technology is lessening the distance between the corporate office and the entity where care is provided. Likewise, the power in decision making is being distributed more evenly throughout the corporation because of developments in information technology.

Information technology has allowed common definition of data elements, formats for collecting data, and ways to transmit reports about data and information throughout a corporation. Practices of benchmarking, norming, and developing ranges of performance indicators relate to the new information technology, which has brought to life methods that can improve processes and allow continual learning. Application of policies and procedures in a local entity is now a function that can be implemented across categories of clients receiving care in geographically distant locations. This information technology has decreased the inherent vulnerability of executive nurse roles as they relate to the priority of local functions over corporate dictums; local functions always take precedence in care delivery. For example, a care plan can be formatted and used throughout a corporation, but the care decisions and substance of the care plan are a local accountability.

RELATING TO THE CONSTITUENCY

The executive nurse should focus on the community of nurse leaders in the corporation as the primary constituency. One of the potential roles of the executive nurse relates to how the nursing leadership define themselves as a community. In most health care multisystem organizations, the executive nurse role grew from realization of collective interests among the nurse leaders.

Scope and Scale

The value of the executive nurse role lies in the gains to be made through economies of scope and scale. All executive nurses deal with designing nursing care delivery, with standards of staffing and care planning, and with interdisciplinary team development in caring for patients of different populations. The economies of scale and scope are realized in corporations in several ways.

An **economy of scale** is employing one consultant to work with all of the nurses to examine an aspect of nursing services, such as what to do with the patient classification system. An **economy of scope** is relating nursing care standards to all entities and in all locations where nursing care is provided. The measures of value of mutual undertakings are not limited to deliverables—agreement on a patient classification system or on a commonly used philosophy. They are also measured by the value of sharing ideas, continually learning from one another, and relating to persons who are from different organizations, in different locations, with different management teams. A degree of objectivity is realized when one compares information and impressions. In some cases, what seems to be situational is in reality an industry phenomenon. For example, downsizing is not happening in one location exclusively; it is being planned and implemented throughout the world, in health care corporations and in all types of businesses. Separating what is happening overall from one's own work situation is very important in maintaining the objectivity and rationality needed in today's health care environment.

ROLE FORMATION PHASES

Whatever the predominant reason for formation of the executive nurse role and functions, developmental phases usually occur. One might also consider formation as the beginning of a new position in a corporation in which the expectations are more general than specific. Although presented in sequence in the following section, the phases of formation may occur in different combinations and in varying order.

Phase I

This phase involves building relationships among top nurse administrators in all corporate entities. Bringing together nurses accountable for care in ambulatory, acute, long-term, home care, and hospice settings facilitates learning about how nursing care is delivered in each of the corporate components, in both vertically integrated and horizontally integrated systems.

Phase II

This phase begins with making agreements and authorizing some or all of the members to act as a group, or on the group's behalf. In this phase, members seek common ground for developing policy and look for approaches both for the work and for working together. Policy emanates from the fundamentals of nursing care delivery and management. Activities for this second phase of development include:

- Shaping a common vision of what the executive nurse group should be—for example, the vision of uninterrupted nursing services across settings.
- Developing a common philosophy that reflects beliefs about meeting patient needs, individually and collectively.
- Identifying means to achieve the vision and the driving forces, constraining forces, strengths, and barriers.
- Affirming values related to human dignity, access to care, ethics, professional behavior, and servant leadership.

Phase III

Readiness for working together is developed in Phases I and II. The objective of the executive nurse is to have the participating individuals see themselves as partners with a common vision, mission, and goals. Phase III focuses on design of care delivery in the corporation. Certain fundamental aspects essential to efficacious nursing services are addressed. Activities must be developed with active participation and with multidisciplinary clinical teams, clinical nurse experts, and persons who speak clinical language and financial language about patient care. Key aspects are to:

- Identify key providers of services in the corporation, including community agencies and partners.
- Engage members in definition and planning.
- Predict the continuum of services a given patient/client population will require.
- Agree on corporate-wide programs that unify all entities, such as standards of patient care, the nursing care component, and practice applicable in all settings. Standards should ensure consistency in care in all settings, the appropri-

ate utilization of services in each setting, and that relationships promote continuity between and among settings.

- Apply nursing process consistently and appropriately in all corporate settings to promote continuity, reduce redundancy, and facilitate efficient use of resources for a constant level of quality.

- Develop communications, including needs assessment and commensurate planning, that incorporate the resources and planning required to achieve goals. The group's resources may have to be mediated and, in many instances, variations in resource accounting may have to be reconciled.

- Agree on definition of terms for activities, for data and for formats used to transmit information between and among settings. Ideally, a common format for communication is used. Records and written communication usually imply a certain regulatory requirement to which individuals in different settings may react. The executive nurse has to use the culture to interpret, as well as to help the group form, such communications. To be useful in a variety of settings, common definitions and sequential plans must be applicable to the varying circumstances.

- Identify indicators of progress, appropriate for the work and for each setting.

By the time the group has agreed on principles of design, communications, and ways to discuss and measure the process and outcomes, there should be a level of trust generated that serves the group well in its work.

Phase IV

Phase IV is the working experience, planned and developed in earlier phases. This phase is best entered from a base of trust but may be driven by economic necessity, sponsorship, or other factors. Centering on increasing efficacy in both clinical and financial aspects of nursing services is encouraged by trust. The community of nursing leaders may contain a variety of views, in some instances necessitating conflict resolution. In phases of working together, there is the danger of strong perceptions of intrusion on territory, real and perceived, and vested interests that must be satisfied. Power and control issues usually enter at this point.

Forming a community of nursing leaders to accomplish the corporate business is challenging. Working together allows the opportunity to join clinical and economic elements of patient care services and resources. The corporate services for nurse leaders should improve the processes and quality of care, reduce costs, and reduce duplication of efforts. Further improvements result from learning, adapting, and continuing to develop new approaches and programs. Using technology and research is important to continuing growth and development.

Nursing service leaders spend considerable time procuring and allocating resources. Developing executive nurse groups can realize the potentials for easing some of the challenges of cost constraints and staffing enigmas through sharing program approaches and resources. At the resource level, the leaders come together to accomplish the following:

- Examine resources required for projects and determine ways to work together to maximize the resources.
- Assess aspects of nursing services that can be shared across settings, such as continuing nursing education, process improvement programs, and business plans for patient care services.
- Design communication formats that facilitate effective sharing and development.
- Agree on performance targets to meet service goals.

Phase V

Continued development of cohesive focus is emphasized in this phase. Governance and executive level functions at the corporate and entity levels need to be considered in this ongoing phase of working together. Marketing programs, and projects to demonstrate how they fit into the strategic plans in each entity, are important for continued support of the effort.

Arrangements that enforce accountability on those who act on behalf of their fellows requires an organizational architecture and the measure of how well it promotes performance. Types of arrangements commonly found include:

- A nurses' council of executives, managers, and others who decide policy and operating approaches to corporate-wide projects and programs.
- Established key programmatic areas for making the community of nurse leaders effective with agreed-on shared accountability.

One of the most important considerations is how to deter opportunism and promote faithful stewardship among leaders. Common mission, vision, and similarity in purpose comprise the pathway to more lasting relationships and to change. Even as problems are solved and progress is made, new issues and problems arise. The continuity of research and development that will enhance continual learning over time is a primary challenge for the executive nurse.

Summary

The executive nurse in a corporate structure has an evolving role, dependent on corporate culture, that is expressed in values, attitudes and relationships, and corporate structural variables such as centralization versus decentralization, vertical and horizontal organization, and the size and scope of the corporation. The executive nurse develops an identity within this corporate structure via accountability and stewardship. The nurse discusses corporate role expectations such as leadership presence and communication as well as specific executive nurse behaviors including interdependency, relating to the nursing constituencies, and economies of scope and scale. This chapter described five phases of role and behavior development: building relationships, vision agreements and policy development, care delivery design, working relationships, and cohesive governance and accountability.

Discussion Questions

1. What are the specific skills needed by the executive nurse in each of the five formation phases?
2. Identify and describe the structural features and the organizational processes that impact the executive nurse's position in your health care facility.

References

Beyers, M. (1984). Getting on top of organizational change. *Journal of Nursing Administration, 14* (10), 32–39; (11), 31–37;(12), 32–37.

Block, P. (1993). *Stewardship: Choosing service over self-interest.* San Francisco: Berrett-Koehler Publishers.

Land, G., Jarman, B. (1992). Break-point and beyond: Mastering the future—today. New York: Harper Business, 173–188.

Bennis, W. (1993). *An invented life: Reflections on leadership and change.* Reading, MA: Addison-Wesley.

Berwick, D. M., Godfrey, A. B., Roessner, J. (1990). *Curing health care: New strategies for quality improvement.* San Francisco: Jossey-Bass.

Evashwick, C. J., Weiss, L. J. (1987). *Managing the continuum of care.* Rockville, MD: Aspen Publishers.

Katzenback, J. R., Smith, D. K. (1993). The wisdom of teams: Creating the high-performance organization. New York: Harper Business, 87–109.

CHAPTER 2

Gail E. Bromley

An Executive Nurse in Action

Introduction

Reflect for a moment on how you, a nurse executive, were socialized and mentored by individuals in your personal and professional lives. Experiences influence how each of us practices nursing and how we as nursing leaders, in all care settings, influence the professional growth of our staff members. Corporate leadership requires strength and vision, strategies, and a sense of equilibrium. These areas are critical to the success of executive nurses in all health care systems and within the nursing service organization.

LEADERSHIP STRENGTH AND VISION

Executive nurses' personal and professional strengths set the tone and the direction of the nursing service organizations for which they have administrative responsibility. The executive nurse who has high standards, a positive mind set, a sense of humor, and a focus on success with both patient outcome indicators and professional staff development will create a work environment that is energizing and growth producing.

A global view and knowledge of the health care environment provide the foundation for the vision, strategic planning, and goals of the nursing service organization. The executive nurse is the professional who blends the patient and professional nursing focus with the corporate goals. Each of these plans and goals must provide a road map for both leading and facilitating the patient care delivery process.

The rapid pace of the health care environment, the constant demand to respond to organizational change, alternatives to patient care delivery, and external regional and national factors impacting on health care constantly challenge the strongest executive nurse. The nursing leadership position has a primary responsibility to be focused and to function in an assertive and highly motivated manner.

LEADERSHIP STRATEGIES

Corporate Strategies

The executive nurse works within a corporate structure to provide nursing data, information, and analysis to support the board of trustees' global direction and policy and the corporate team's implementation of those directions and policies. Corporate strategies usually include areas such as marketing issues; patient, physician and employee satisfaction; quality of care; and economic standing of the organization. The executive nurse–corporate interface is best served when sound clinical, professional, business, political, and ethical leadership is demonstrated as the priority patient-care delivery issues are addressed openly and the resulting decisions are implemented. The executive nurse integrates the information needed to provide the patient service vision within the financial, operational, and professional corporate-planning and implementation phases. For example, with every budget developed, the following factors are considered: patient care outcomes, patient/staff/physician satisfaction, patient care services provided, program implementation, and patient care costs.

Quality Patient Care
The organizational support and, typically, the board of trustees and CEO support, for providing high-quality, cost-effective patient care has definite impact on the success or failure of the nurse leader's performance and influence. When the patient is the focus, and corporate and interdisciplinary teams understand and agree to the patient focus as a priority, then the health care organization's mission can be accomplished. The health care environment and the actual organizational commitment to a project or change are significant factors in successfully implementing all patient care delivery programs.

Marketing and Advertising
In the past, emphasis on the marketing and advertising of health care involved persuasive techniques designed to attract patients and families to the health care product that hospitals provided, namely inpatient care provided by an interdisciplinary team of professionals. That health care product has a very different appearance now. Patient care includes pre-admission assessment, patient and family teaching, hospitalization, discharge planning and home health care, skilled nursing care, rehabilitation, hospice, and respite care. At approximately the same time as the health care product is changing, coalitions of hospital associations and businesses are using consumer-report methods to evaluate individual hospitals and to provide comparative data. One example is the Cleveland Health Quality Choice Project of Cleveland, Ohio. This coalition provides a means to evaluate specific patient-care delivery indicators, morbidity, mortality, length of stay, and patient satisfaction data. In the Greater Cleveland area, the cost data by hospital was published in a local newspaper and useful decision-making information was provided for consumers. This data, combined with internal data, could then be used by hospi-

tals and nursing service organizations to identify areas that would benefit from additional (or new) focused goals. Nursing service organizations in health care settings and clinical services departments can use this data to plan improved patient care.

The clinical components, such as process improvement monitoring, patient functional status, and patient satisfaction components are now part of most trend data reports and support patient-focused care models. Patients are best cared for when they are provided state-of-the-art, clinically sound care, when they are informed of their care in a clear and consistent manner by knowledgeable professionals, and when they feel that they are in a safe, clean, and supportive environment. Efforts to improve care by most providers center around these expectations. Dialogue between the executive nurse and the board of trustees' patient-care committee—as well as dialogue between the executive nurse and the nursing standards committee, quality assessment and improvement committee, and peer review committee—increase the likelihood that care is properly delivered to each patient.

Nursing Organization Strategies

Communicating the Vision

Executive nurses provide the link between staff nurses, nurse leaders, and the corporate leadership staff. Corporate strategic planning determines the nursing service organization's priorities. Joint goals between the corporation and the nursing service organization tend to focus on quality and cost goals during this era of managed health care. Corporations try to assure that these goals are implemented while still maintaining health care standards. The professional nurses' goals must include sound clinical knowledge and practice as well as an appreciation for patient, family, and colleague satisfaction.

The executive nurse works within the professional nursing team to communicate clearly and to implement the nursing service organization's philosophy, professional expectations, standards of care, and fiscal responsibility. Clear philosophical and pragmatic visions for care and professionalism, when established by consensus, enable the professional staff to share and internalize the nursing and corporate vision. Through communication, collaboration, and consensus, the executive nurse and the nursing service organization staff plan and implement those patient-focused care projects and professional practice programs that will meet patient needs in a cost-effective manner.

Environmental and Situational Issues

The environmental and situational issues in health care delivery are many and varied. For example, hospital mergers, department consolidations, and professional nurse–unlicensed personnel partnership models are having a powerful and challenging impact on how staff function day to day. They impact the delegation of care and potential outcomes. These changes influence the way care is delivered and require constant explanations and clarifications to assure effective implementation. Confusion may result as staff responsibilities are reassigned. Staff may feel very insecure because of the potential that their jobs could be eliminated. The environment is volatile, and promises cannot be made. This impacts all health care providers, but especially the staff in a setting with high longevity and a tendency to resist change. The emotional intensity can be felt by staff and by patients.

Executive nurses have a powerful role in the design and implementation of patient-care delivery models. Strategic planning and budgeting must include nurse staffing patterns that meet patient care needs and are not driven by cost alone. Nursing staff must be appropriately educated and trained in order to achieve the measurable and realistic outcomes desired by payors, providers, and consumers.

Case managers and clinical nurse specialists provide clinical expertise, reinforce standards, and educate the nursing staff. The case managers and clinical specialists in a nursing organization monitor and coordinate patient care to promote continuity, improve quality, and assure hospital stays that meet patient and family needs as well as third-party payer requirements. Patient and family education, effectively provided, helps ease the hospital-to home transition. Both patients and families are then able to continue to meet the health care needs of the patient and know when to ask for additional clinical assistance or advice.

Clinical Pathways
The clinical pathways being developed in institutions are daily road maps that include standards of care, care processes, and treatments for clinical diagnosis. The interdisciplinary professional team uses the clinical pathways based on patients' diagnoses and unique needs. The pathways assist staff, patients, and families to utilize the hospital experience in a more effective way. Executive nurses need to use these clinical pathways as tools for planning and evaluating care, as well as for meeting staffing needs.

Maintaining a Learning Environment
Each of the health care organizations in which an executive nurse works is a learning environment. Peter Senge, in *The Fifth Discipline Field Book* (1994), provides pragmatic examples to help leaders better understand and improve the ways in which their organizations function. A powerful message Senge conveys is the importance of the leader's articulating a vision and building staff consensus with that shared vision.

Consensus Building and Growth
The nursing service organization functions at an optimal level when there is consensus building and staff growth. Nursing staff members who have planned and developed standards of care and a peer-review monitoring system are in a position to evaluate both practice patterns and patient outcomes. When staff caring for a consumer, in any setting, are informed and educated about the quality and cost of the patient care being provided, the accountability for outcomes is placed where there can be the greatest impact on both the cost and the quality. The executive nurse's role involves constant communication about the improvements in patient care as well as the identification of staff educational needs or system changes that will help to improve care. Examples of components that must be in place to support patient care improvement by staff include: a credentialing process to support, recognize, and increase the number of competent providers; an accurate cost-information process that provides one basis for selecting a particular drug or treatment as related to the potential long- and short-term consequences for the

patient; and patient-satisfaction survey data that can sensitize staff to the special needs of any given population and provide guidance for patient and family education programs.

LEADERSHIP EQUILIBRIUM

Coping with the frequency and types of changes is a major issue in the current health care environment. The fast pace, and the constant internal and external changes influencing not only the hospital but also the entire health care system, place pressure on the nurse leader to develop confidence in the agreed-upon corporate visions for patient care delivery. Stamina and an ability to create a balance in one's professional life makes a difference in how a nursing leader functions. Professional demands include program development, problem solving, employee and staff concerns, adjustments to regulatory changes, and lots of paper work. Collegial relationships, networking, and participation in professional organizations facilitate successful function. These contacts inform the executive nurse about critical issues in the profession outside of the organization, concerns of staff in other areas of practice, and what changes are anticipated externally.

Patient Care Priority

The demands on the executive nurse in a corporate setting necessitate a focus on priority issues that will enhance patient care delivery. There are numerous distractions, ranging from minor crises (e.g., not having enough chart packets) to major crises (e.g., high patient volume that coincides with a high incidence of staff illness owing to flu or a community disaster).

Patients expect the same kind of care that we ourselves would expect as patients. Regardless of the health care setting and its unique culture, respecting the staff, cultivating an environment that assures patients have their needs met, and providing education to staff and patients to promote health and wellness are essential functions that the executive nurse must support and implement.

Bombardment

Bombardment is the most frequently experienced challenge in a nurse leader's professional life. Some executive nurses experience constant bombardment as a stress, others as a challenge. Every event, interruption, or crisis that distracts an executive nurse from the leadership, planning, and implementation of projects and programs needed to sustain the nursing service organization and the health care organization, must be critiqued and managed. A positive mind set and positive attitude can combat these challenges and make for a tolerable leadership experience despite the bombardment by stressors. The nurse leader's mind set, combined with an ability to listen to others and work collaboratively, plays a decisive role in what can be accomplished within a nursing service organization.

The stressors and the tension from bombardment dissipate when staff are reenergized. The executive nurse can encourage staff creatively and acknowledge their accomplishments. Also, an ample dose of laughter makes each day and each interaction more enjoyable.

Proactive Functioning

Health care remains a service industry, nursing remains a service profession, and both are provided in the context of a business environment. The patient care delivery must be patient focused. It is most beneficial when the executive nurse communicates, and role models, positive and sensitive professional interactions. Expecting honesty and integrity in dealing with people may sound old-fashioned but these virtues still provide enhanced credibility to the leader in both corporate and staff interactions.

The executive nurse is accountable for setting the tone and the pace for clinical service standards. This individual's values and expectations are paramount to establishing a high-functioning nursing service organization within a corporate setting. Nursing leaders who enjoy a strong political base and who can communicate the rationale for projects and programs are more likely to gain support and credibility from staff and corporate members.

The leader's humanitarian treatment of the staff directly affects how well the staff delivers patient care. A healthy, high-functioning staff, supported by the leader, is able to focus their efforts on patient and organizational objectives and provide important services to patients, families, and colleagues both efficiently and effectively.

A TYPICAL DAY

Scenario 2.1

A typical day begins by planning for an "average" day. This means approaching the day with flexibility, a sense of humor, and a firm resolve to handle problems as they arise. For example, in the past there was a more constant patient flow and a predictability to patient census. Now, with a change in focus, from inpatient care to home care, health and wellness, and reducing lengths of stay, staff scheduling has greater variability because of the disincentives to admit patients to the hospital. Cost-per-case monitoring requires specific patient tracking systems and the personnel to gather, enter, retrieve, and interpret the data generated and then apply the analysis to the patient's therapeutic needs and total care. Managed care necessitates a patient care delivery perspective that includes a patient and family assessment before admission, with patient and family education begun during the pre-admission phase. The executive nurse is required to establish a plan to provide continuity of patient care beginning at pre-admission. The continuum of patient care, which includes hospitalization and posthospitalization, requires planning and staff scheduling that will build rapport and confidence.

This typical day also requires confidence and rapid decision making by the executive nurse. This person must make rapid, prioritized decisions about situations as they present, based on the data available and what is deemed to be in the best interests of patient care and in the best interests of the nursing organization and hospital.

A day in the life of an executive nurse is a unique and fascinating blend of team building and speed reading, combining theoretical nursing concepts and assuring patient satisfaction, while maintaining quality patient care. No day is complete without some interruptions, positive patient and family comments, and a nursing staff and clinical nurse manager gratified by their having successfully implemented a patient-focused project. The following scenario illustrates these points.

Typical Day Schedule

Early morning board meeting was preceded by a middle-of-the-night phone call about a patient mishap.

A nurse-physician conflict ensued during the patient incident.

- Difficulties resulted that generated staff morale problems.

- Subsequently, it was necessary to document perceptions and practice issues affecting patient care.

- Risk management investigation resulted.

- Identification and investigation of nurse misconduct followed.

- Identification and investigation of physician misconduct involved members of the medical staff.

- Mechanisms were established to assure safe patient care.

The board meeting's agenda included the presentation of patient satisfaction data and analysis. Recommended ways to improve patient and staff satisfaction were discussed, and proposals made.

A series of staff meetings followed.

- Quality improvement and assessment, peer review, and patient-outcome indicator data were reviewed to better understand how to implement concurrent quality improvement.

- This required staff inservice and education to support the staff's knowledge and use their expertise to improve care.

Nursing staff meetings were held to re-establish standards of care using clinical pathways.

A patient-care redesign committee included the reworking and consideration of patient chart forms. The goal was to have a patient chart be the chronological database for patient information, including medical and wellness history. (When, or if, one does not have computerization, a clear, concise patient-care record is needed. It must display readily accessible data/trends to provide useful information for patient care.) An interdisciplinary focus is required to provide the best care for the patient.

A family member of one of the patients called to explain, rather emphatically, that she did not feel patient-care needs had been met.

A family member expressed concern that a patient is not ready to be discharged from the hospital. (These patient and family situations require immediate attention and concurrent quality assessment, planning, implementation and evaluation).

A staff member had a personal crisis. The situation, as it presented, suggests that the nurse may be an impaired nurse.

- Fact finding, investigation, and intervention may take place.
- Intervention with some variation of a peer assistance program for nurses may be initiated to obtain an assessment and intervention for the nurse.

A decision to postpone the implementation of a software computer program may be necessary because the hospital system requires more preparation time. Calming staff members who anticipated a "quick fix" was needed.

Preparation for an external accreditation survey demanded review, rewriting, modifications, and streamlining of paperwork. This process required organizing information and educating staff about their patient care delivery documentation and the agency's expectations.

Positive comments about staff who have provided care and compassion required immediate acknowledgments and letters commending them for continuing the tradition of empathy and quality care for all patients.

Reevaluation of patient-focused care and a staff with new responsibilities required constant support and listening. Facilitating the project meant supporting the staff to do the right thing, the first time and every time.

Typical Day Summary

The typical-day scenario illustrates the varied and complex activities and decisions required of the executive nurse. Each day requires an outlook that involves consensus building and healthy professional dialogue. The nursing leader must view each situation as an opportunity to grow and to build in fairness, trust and respect. A balance between personal and professional life is essential. A time to think and reflect, alone and with others, is imperative. The thinking process instills strength in the leader.

Summary

The executive nurse has a leadership role in health care organizations that is challenging and complex. It is not a position for every nurse leader. It is influenced by personal characteristics and qualities as well as by environmental and situational issues. Success requires leadership strength and vision, strategies at the corporate and nursing organization levels, and leadership equilibrium with proactive functioning.

Discussion Questions

1. What unique personal characteristics and qualities do you bring to the nursing leadership role?

2. How would you use these characteristics to lead a nursing organization into the future?

References

Curtin, L. L. (1994). Ethics for, in, and about nursing administration. *Nursing Management,* December: 25–28.

Flarey, D. L. (1991). Health care managers in transition. *Journal of Nursing Administration,* December: 8–10.

Frangos, S. J., Bennett, S. J. (1993). *Team zebra.* Essex Junction, VT: Oliver Wright Publications.

Munn, E. M., Saulsbery, P. H. (1992). Facility planning: A blueprint for nurse executives. *Journal of Nursing Administration,* January, 13–17.

Sovie, M. D. (1995). Tailoring hospitals for managed care and integrated health systems. *Nursing Economics,* April, 77–83.

Senge, P. M. (1990). *The fifth discipline: The art and practice of the learning organization.* New York: Doubleday.

Senge, P. M., Roberts, C., Ross, R. B., et al. (1994). *The fifth discipline fieldbook.* New York: Doubleday.

Sandra R. Byers

CHAPTER **3**

Leadership in Health Care Policy

Introduction

The executive nurse plays a leadership role in health care policy development at the local, state, and national level. It is an essential component of the position, particularly in the leadership of organizations as they transform, merge, and re-engineer, creating new paradigms, for ". . . the secret to the new governance lies in policy-making" (Carver, 1990, p. 25). For many executive nurses, health care policy involvement, external to the facility, may be a new arena. Mason states ". . . nurses' voices have been absent from the policy tables in their places of work, as well as in government"(1993, p. 3).

This chapter provides a rationale for executive nurse involvement in health care policy and then describes health care policy, the process of policy development, the executive nurses' unique contributions, competencies and activities, and policy evaluation suggestions. It is intended to create enthusiasm and awareness about health care policy among executive nurses and to encourage their active participation in health care policy making.

INVOLVEMENT

Why should the executive nurse be involved in health care policy? Health care policy determines the services many patients will receive, who provides it (Hanley, 1987), and who pays for it. It impacts nursing's core—nursing care to consumers.

Patient Services

Executive nurses have the knowledge and practical experience to help policy makers understand consumers' needs and to help consumers make decisions about their "health future." Nurses are needed as the link between health care, the values and needs of citizens as individuals and in community, and health policy development at state and local levels.

> The experience that nurses bring to policy serves as a bridge between what is needed and realistic in the health care system, and the laws and regulations that govern that system. Because of their education and experiences, nurses are well equipped to speak to services needed for populations such as the uninsured, the handicapped, and the sick, as well as those who desire to stay healthy. (Sharp, Biggs, & Wakefield, 1991, p. 17)

Who Provides Nursing Services

Policy impacts the allocation of nursing resources through nurse licensure and regulation of nurses' scope of practice and through institutional hiring and utilization policies. The executive nurse is the key individual accountable for the allocation and utilization of human resources providing nursing care. Because of this particular accountability, there are opportunities and responsibilities to identify potential consequences of resource decisions to health care. For example: What are the patient outcomes with inappropriate restriction or extension of nursing's scope of practice? What is the need for nurse-managed community centers to help educate consumers about healthy behaviors and provide primary prevention services? What is the impact of financial barriers for consumers and what does that mean in terms of health care being provided or eliminated? The executive nurse's involvement in external policy development can promote the recognition that nurses control nursing practice and are focused on consumer wellness, health and caring, quality, and cost throughout the continuum of care.

Who Pays

A significant source of health care reimbursement is the federal government. The role of government in the structure, financing, and delivery of health care services in the United States has evolved from that of a constricted provider of services and protector of public health to that of a major financial sponsor, whose policies and procedures have increasingly intruded on the autonomy and prerogatives of the providers of care (Litman & Robins, 1991, p. 15).

Buerhaus (1994, p. 458) emphasizes the importance of nursing's involvement at the state level as more of the financing for health care is shifted to states from the federal government. The shift includes such issues as: day care, time off for childbirth and adoption, and time off to care for ill parents, abortion, the homeless, and HIV-positive clients. As the role of government and managed-care organizations has become more pronounced in directing care choices, executive nurses must interpret what are efficient and effective health services from a quality and cost perspective to many audiences.

HEALTH CARE POLICY

Definitions

Policy is defined by Webster as "prudence or wisdom in the management of affairs; management or procedure based primarily on material interest; a definite course or method of action selected from among alternatives and in light of given conditions to guide and determine present and future decisions"(1988, p. 910). In the nursing literature, policy is defined as "authoritative decision making" (Stimpson & Hanley, 1991, p. 12) and encompassing "authoritative guidelines that direct human behavior toward specific goals in either the private or public sector" (Hanley, 1993, p. 71). According to Abdellah,

> Policy is referred to as a plan of action, a way of management, practical wisdom and prudence, and political skill. Politics are often referred to as the art and science of government concerned with guiding or influencing health policy. (1991, p. 2).

Policy related to health care service delivery is referred to as health care policy.

Managing Health Care Policy

The process of health care policy development occurs within the broader policy environment and is influenced by planning, implementing, and evaluating activities.

Planning

Health care policy has not been rational in terms of health planning. There has been no overall health plan, so legislation is strongly influenced by those who are organized, act in their own self-interest, and provide political support to receive legislative benefits (Feldstein, 1988, p. 16). Policies, in the form of legislation, are developed by lawmakers at the request of constituencies or interest groups. Policies surface as government mandates such as Medicare and Medicaid. In these instances, health care policies have significantly influenced the services offered as they have come to be based on government reimbursements rather than on consumer needs.

Policies are rooted in the self-interests of those who have the most to gain or lose in the process of controlling, redistributing, or eliminating a particular resource (Feldstein, 1988). Stakeholders with health care resources will probably be affected by any health care policy. The affected individual or organization, whether truly affected or perceived by them to be affected, may then decide to influence or control that resource by public policy. This point is supported by Kalisch and Kalisch, who define policy "as a consciously chosen course of action (or inaction) toward some end" (1982, p. 61).

Implementing

There are many social, economic, legal, and ethical forces in society interacting and influencing the policies and the process. This dynamic process creates new and complex issues. For example, the competition for control, power, and leadership occurs within a particular context and within organizations, especially during implementation. Bargaining, negotiation, coercion, and compromise are daily activities throughout the policy process (Simms, 1994, p. 47). Bolman and Deal (1991) describe organizations in terms of four frames: structure, human resource, symbolic, and political. Their political frame views organizations as arenas where interest groups compete for power and scarce resources.

According to Bryson (1992, p. 14), power and control generates from technology, public policy, interconnectiveness, and population growth. "Because policies permeate and dominate all aspects of organizational life, they present the most powerful lever for the exercise of leadership" (Carver, 1990, p. 28). The executive nurse, accountable for the delivery of nursing services, influences large networks, human and material resources, and the technology applied to care needs. Key facts such as demographics about network clients are available to the executive nurse for resource-allocation decisions and planning programs.

Evaluation

Many policies have not been thoroughly analyzed prior to implementation for possible quality, access, or cost/benefit consequences to consumers, payers, or providers. The evaluation of the results of public policy is an area in need of research, especially at this time when accountability and outcomes of interventions are so important to strategic planning and reform.

Policies express a perspective, a way of viewing the world, and can represent specific values. Values, particularly in times of change, come under scrutiny. Policies have no inherent good or bad value. The "goodness" of a policy rests with the interpretation, implementation, and short- and long-term evaluation of the policy and what a particular stakeholder views as winning or losing. It is generally assumed that state and community policies are aimed at achieving the greatest good for the greatest number of people. Policy, according to Abdellah (1991, p. 2), implies "for the public good." However, with the increase in the number and influence of special-interest groups and paid lobbyists, media attention, money available to influence voters and lawmakers, and the appearance of more government involvement in public and private institutions, it is frequently difficult to evaluate the effects on the public good. The results of health care policy are evident in areas such as health care services received or not received by consumers, and regulations about who can provide what services and who receives pay for particular services rendered. Reviewing the work of Aaron Wildavsky, a renowned political scientist, Jones (1995) writes,". . . he [Wildavsky] was convinced that, for understandable but incorrect reasons, as a culture we were rushing to control before we evaluated the evidence" (p. 14). He (Wildavsky) was interested in the basis for health, safety, and environmental policy not because of his views on the overestimation of, and overreaction to, risks, but

> . . . his goal was to demonstrate that average citizens, faced with a bewildering and often conflicting body of evidence and recommendations, could gather information, analyze it, and draw conclusions for themselves about what was right. As a result, they could then participate in the debate over risk and safety and attempt to influence decisions as they should in a truly democratic

society. The alternative was to be dominated by special interests
and radicals and the politicians and scientists who serve them.
(Jones, 1995, p. 14)

An interesting scenario highlights the critical importance of policy evaluation
and input before passage. A state law was passed (in Ohio) that mandated hospitals to find out from an unwed Medicaid mother during her hospitalization the
name of the biological father and to "counsel" the mother and if possible the biological father on the importance to the child of this information for future social
security and medical insurance purposes. The paternity acknowledgement was
stated as voluntary on the part of the unwed mother and biological father. At the
same time, there was a Medicaid application to be filled in that did ask for the
name of the biological father, but no other information. The Medicaid application
was for those unwed mothers who were not already on Medicaid. In addition, it
was believed by lawmakers that the name of the biological father should be on the
birth certificate to avoid legal issues and possibly genetic testing at a later time; but
the new legislation did not consider existing laws, which did not provide for this
use of the birth certificate, and did not clarify "paternity." The hospitals would receive a minimal fee for performing this "secretarial" function that was believed by
a legislator to require only that information be placed on the dietary tray. The
mother was not mandated to provide the information, but she was to be made
aware of its importance by hospital staff, who were to explain the forms and their
importance, and to witness the signatures. The legislation did not deal with the
issue of minors and the legal validity of their signatures. The legislation placed the
implementation responsibility on two different state agencies. One for the education of the providers, Medicaid agencies, and courts, and the other for the payment to hospitals. This legislation was very difficult and costly to implement. A few
examples follow.

The state agency, based on administrative rules, could not pay any outside
group without a contract with that group. This resulted in individual contracts
with every hospital in the state that were long and involved. The law had no
penalty for noncompliance (not signing the contract) so, although hospitals might
agree with the need and the concept, it was viewed as performing the "state's
work" and not the responsibility of hospital staff who cared for a mother and baby
during a critical life experience. The hospitals were not impressed with the small
fee, which did not begin to cover the staffing costs needed to implement the law.
The courts did not recognize the birth certificate as the legal document for establishing paternity according to other existing laws. And, the paternity forms were to
be sent to the mother's county Medicaid agency, which meant establishing linkages with many counties for most hospitals. The birth certificate went to the health
department and the Medicaid forms were to be sent to the state agency. Hospitals
and health care providers found that this activity imposed on their relationships
with consumers and a difficult task, given the length of hospitalization. Hospital
employees also questioned their liability because they were to witness signatures
on the forms that might be used later in court. The hospital was put in a position
of deciding whether to pursue the insurance company, if there was one, of the biological father.

The implementation required six monthly meetings of hospital representatives, including executive nurses and the two state agencies involved, to resolve contract issues and the reporting mechanisms for payments. There were two additional task forces. One task force developed the educational materials, and a maternal/child health nursing director was very influential in this process. The other task force dealt with the integration and impact on all the other Medicaid agencies and the legal system involved with unwed mothers and babies. Hospitals had to educate separately the majority of their obstetrical staff because of shifts and weekends. The legislators and governor were seen as fighting the abuse of Medicaid dollars and protecting the child's future. This legislative effort would have benefited from open and honest dialogue with all constituencies and an understanding of social agencies and hospital care. It was an enormous challenge to enact and was amended after additional legislative debates.

POLICY DEVELOPMENT

Historically, most policy has developed through the political process, or "politics." Politics is the " art or science of government: the art or science concerned with guiding or influencing governmental policy; the art or science concerned with winning and holding control over a government; political actions, practices, or policies; . . .competition between competing interest groups or individuals for power and leadership (as in a government)" (Webster, 1988, p. 911).

The political process is becoming recognized and accepted as a learned activity and not a "back room" mystery; a democratic right to be exercised.

> In a free society, public policies come about through the action of
> the peoples. These public policies influence individual lives at
> every stage; financing of prenatal care, state aid to school districts,
> job training and placement, law enforcement, and determining
> retirement benefits. (Duncan, Jabine, & de Wolf, 1993, p. 15)

Policy Process Characteristics

Public policy development takes place in an environment that is "dynamic, complicated and often murky" (Bocchino & Wakefield, 1992, p. 53). It is incremental change and primarily deals with issues applicable to the larger public. Policy making is a rational and continuing process (Feldstein, 1988). It is not static, but is "continuously shaped by the social and political processes that form it, from initiation through adoption, implementation, assessment and reformulation" (Milio, 1984, p. 317). The process is slow and deliberate, requiring patience, optimism, and the ability to integrate and welcome changing faces at the table. The changing faces frequently represent special groups with varying levels of interest and understanding, as well as multiple values. All perspectives help to define the problem and the results. The process is designed to be participatory so as to facilitate hearing all perspectives and facts.

Public Policy Issues

As mentioned previously, public policies come about because of the self-interests of people. Self-interest and values produce tensions that trigger change. Public problems become policy issues when conflicts in values arise over options for solving the problem.

The decision to use the policy process on any given topic is a conscious one and implies a course of action with a consequence; it is dependent on what issue is thought to benefit and be affected by the political process. Also the decision is influenced by the strength and conviction of personal and societal values. Engaging in critical reflection of values and reviewing the background of an issue contributes to framing a particular political initiative and enables a more accurate assessment of the political agenda. "Public health policy formulation is viewed as the way issues are raised on the public agenda; the process by which laws are passed committing resources to programs that affect people; the development or withdrawal of rules and regulations that interpret laws, the process of program implementation; and the evaluation of the usefulness of the program" (Abdellah, 1991, p. 2).

Policy Process

Stimpson and Hanley (1991) identified a structure to the policy process by defining four phases:

1. Identification of the problem
2. Formulation of policy options through the legislative process
3. Implementation after policy adoption through program design and administration through the regulatory process
4. Evaluation and collection of data to determine program effectiveness in resolving the original issues

The process encompasses the formal and informal strategies of authorities as they interact with concerned individuals and organized interest groups following the prescribed steps of the process (Stimpson and Hanley, 1991).

Backer (1991) supports the importance of problem identification and parallels the policy development process to the nursing process and the development of a care plan. She suggests that nurses can use their assessment skills in defining a problem, identifying the issues, discussing and framing the issues, analyzing data and resources, and deciding on the problem definition. Each step of problem identification is influenced by the parties for whom it is a problem, the interested constituencies.

EXECUTIVE NURSES' COMPETENCIES

The executive nurse offers a unique combination of values, knowledge, skills, and attitudes to the content and process of health care policy. This combination has been forged through generic and continuing education and administrative, managerial, and clinical experiences in a variety of delivery settings. All these attributes, when joined with political knowledge and experience, equip and empower the executive nurse to be a major force in health care policy development, implementation, and evaluation. This section discusses skills particularly important to involvement with health care policy: communication, consumer advocacy, power, risk-taking, coalition-building, quality of care evaluation, and consumer-focused decision-making skills.

Communication Skills

Written and verbal communication skills are critical for the success of an executive nurse. Effective methods arise out of practical testing of ways to communicate the essence of a message and adapting that message to all educational levels and cultures. The executive nurse knows the importance of clarity in communications because poorly communicated directions can result in devastating results for patient care. It is necessary to relate the nursing perspective to many audiences, including chief executive officers, boards of trustees, and external support groups. Presentations must be vivid and accurate so that others fully grasp the message and its context. How a particular event is described influences how others perceive it. The ideas of others must be synthesized and presented accurately to help maintain the credibility and the support of staff and colleagues. Nurses have been taught to document details about patients' reactions to treatments and procedures, communicate them to others, and integrate patients' and families' needs into intervention plans. The position requires that results are measured and communicated.

Consumer Advocate

The executive nurse is called upon to identify the essential components that contribute to the health and well-being of consumers and employees. This critical information should be shared and utilized as policies are developed in other arenas. Important problems are identified daily and assessed as to scope and complexity. Because of the number of important issues at any given time, the executive nurse quickly learns to prioritize. Facts and applicable research are analyzed to assist in this process and the findings applied to the policy issue. Active involvement at the highest administrative level means deciding what policies are critical to patient care and speaking out for what is most important to positive patient results.

Power

The executive nurse understands the uses and abuses of power, the types of power, and how and when to use power appropriately. Physicians, the chief executive officer, the board, unions, and nurses also have degrees of power and control within the facility. Today, leadership based on power is being replaced by a management philosophy of continual process improvement, team empowerment, and decision-making as close to the problem as possible. Bryson and Crosby (1992) describe an approach that helps to explain the dynamics of continual quality management: a "shared-power" world where no one is "in charge" and where objectives, activities, resources, power, or authority must be shared to achieve collective gains or minimize losses. There are essential public leadership skills in a shared-power framework:

> . . . understanding the social, political and economic "givens," understanding the people involved, especially oneself, building teams, nurturing effective and humane organizations, interorganizational networks and communities, creating and communicating meaning, making and implementing legislative, executive, and administrative policy decisions, sanctioning conduct that is enforcing constitutions, laws, and norms and resolving residual conflicts, and putting it all together. (Bryson, 1992, p. 33)

A "shared-power" approach is important because current issues facing policy makers are complex and pervasive and no single group can solve all the economic and social issues. Teenage pregnancy, violence and abuse, and drug and alcohol addiction are examples of complex societal issues that cannot be resolved by one institution. In the health care system, the formation of networks, alliances, affiliations, foundations, and forums point to shared power, shared risk, and shared resources to minimize loses and demonstrate positive results. This approach encourages a new perspective in dealing with complex issues, internal and external to the facility, and promotes both appropriate independence and interdependence of the organization's human expertise and resources.

The executive nurse learns how to use power in positive ways to promote and implement change. Mason and colleagues (1991) write about the importance of integration into the system to influence and alter the power structure and the values and priorities of the system. Organizational power comes from three sources: "information (data, technical knowledge, political intelligence, expertise); resources (funds, materials, space, staff, time); and support (endorsement, backing, approval, legitimacy)" (Kantor, 1983, p. 216). The political process requires an understanding of organizational power sources and an appreciation for power centers (e.g., the chairperson of the state finance committee) and an understanding of what that position means when moving policy through government bodies. The executive nurse "moves" many policies through the hospital structure before implementation and can transfer that skill to the health care policy process.

Risk-Taking

The executive nurse lives the meaning of risk-taking. This means learning when the risk is essential to quality patient care and when, with retrospective evaluation and feedback, a different solution, timing, or action might have produced a more desirable outcome. The "hill to die on" is a metaphor used to raise the question of whether this particular issue is "the" one that will lead to dire consequences and if this is "the" one to risk personal and professional values. In the policy arena risk-taking, or when to continue or when to retreat, may be critical, and the ability to judge the strengths and weaknesses of a position is very important to policy success.

Coalition Building

The ability to build and develop coalitions is a strength of the executive nurse. The position requires an appreciation and understanding of many viewpoints internal and external to the facility: consumers, employees, various departments, communities, and payers. Frequently, innovations and support come from coalitions thought of as "outside" the health care community.

The consumer is in the acute-care setting temporarily and is a part of the larger community. Therefore an integrated system of care and support should be identified and implemented. Nursing personnel are qualified to be the link. Discharge planning, home care support, physician offices, and ambulatory services are being brought closer together via computer technology. Coalitions, representing these various functions, locations, and activities working together may provide a seamless service system. The "management of critical boundary-spanning issues is the task of the top: developing strategies, tactics, and structural mechanisms for functioning and triumphing in a turbulent and highly politicized environment" (Kantor, p. 49). The successful nurse executive learns how to span boundaries and build coalitions and can apply these skills to the public policy process.

Quality of Care

A major concern in health care policy is "quality": quality of life, quality of care, quality of the service, quality measurement. Although difficult to define, the executive nurse knows the importance of quality as defined by both patients and expert clinicians because of the day-to-day, 24-hour accountability for nursing services. As facilities adjust to decreasing resources, unnecessary services that decrease productivity and increase cost are routinely debated as to what they will or will not do for the patient in terms of results, care received or not received, or quality of patient care. Needed services are identified that, given at the right time and place, will assure positive patient outcomes. Evaluating the results of care and identifying what appears to be effective is a normal part of the nursing care process. Facilities implement systemwide "patient critical paths" and "care maps" based on patient diagnoses and the diagnostic and therapeutic processes medically appropriate. This approach promotes more objective evaluation of quality patient care and encourages an environment of collaboration and continual improvement.

Consumer Focus

The nurse is "patient-dependent" (i.e., a nurse needs a patient, a consumer) and a patient needs the expertise of a nurse. This is nursing's professional contract with society, as well as nursing's image, and the basis of nursing's credibility.

> . . . professional practice requires knowledge and skill essential to the public welfare; therefore it is a public good. Public goods nourish and preserve public welfare. A just public policy requires the delivery of such essential public goods to the whole community. In return, society bestows upon those who serve the public good power, status and privileges to the extent that they help meet the public's needs. (Curtin, 1992, p. 8)

The executive nurse, as a professional practitioner, is grounded in the public-good perspective. The clinical nature of nursing, in any setting, means that it is the work of and for professional nurses with the assistance of others. As a function of this obligation to the public, nurses evaluate the outcomes of their work and improve their contributions to the public. The role of the advanced practice nurse, clinical nurse specialist, nurse midwife, and nurse anesthetist are examples of the evolution of nursing's contract with the public, rather than with physicians or institutions.

Nurses' intimate and confidential relationship with patients gives them the opportunity to witness the results of the health care system: the results of patient education or lack of education on patients' decision making, the ability of some patients to care for themselves and be independent of numerous office visits, the lack of support systems to overcome an addiction problem requiring more than what the payers are willing to support, the refusal of some physicians to support the immunization of selected medicare patients in the hospital environment (probably requiring the patient to have an office visit at a later time or go without). The nurse is the health care professional who provides the empathetic, caring, and knowledgeable link between the confusing language and culture of "health care," the high-tech answers to life and death, and the consumer's need and desire for a quality life. Health care policy and legislation must accurately represent the public's views.

The executive nurse asks the hard questions and constructs concerns from the consumer's perspective (i.e.,how will this test help me make a decision about my future or current behavior?). The executive nurse is a patient-advocate when patients are unable to advocate for themselves and can frame the policy issue from the patient's perspective. Ideas and projects must be tested, analyzed, and evaluated and the executive nurse has that knowledge and skill.

COMPETENCIES APPLIED TO HEALTH CARE POLICY

The competencies of the executive nurse discussed above are valuable assets to the nursing profession in health policy development and implementation. The health care policy arena also has unique characteristics, and the two need to be integrated for best results. This section attempts to integrate executive nurse competencies within the structure and process of the policy arena. Generally, the ideas are applicable to involvement in public or private governing boards as well.

Interaction with Legislators

The executive nurse has many opportunities to be involved with the public policy process. The decision to become active and the level of activity is dependent on the amount of time and energy available and committed. In addition to assessing personal time, energy, and commitment levels, there are other decisions to be made when the executive nurse enters the political arena. These decisions may change as the nurse becomes more active and involved. It is critical, once the decision to be involved is made, that the executive nurse learn the political process. A few basic points are briefly explained here; in general, they reflect the process used by most state legislatures. But, it is important to learn the structure of your own state.

Bill Process

Draft legislation is introduced into the House or the Senate by a legislator, or sponsor, and becomes a bill when assigned a number specific to the legislative body of origin. The process of selecting and securing a sponsor is very important to the success of draft legislation, as is the selection of the body (House or Senate) in which to introduce the proposed bill. Once introduced into one of the bodies, it is assigned to an appropriate committee for hearings and debate and is referred back to the same legislative body for a vote. If the draft bill passes, it is introduced in the other body with a new number and sponsor, plus committee assignment for hearings and debate. Following approval by both houses, it is sent to the governor for signature. There are numerous stops along the way: conference committees debate a bill when there are conflicting changes between the two bodies; a committee checks for compliance with existing rules and regulations; someone schedules the draft bills into each of the bodies; and people review the bill from other state departments. There is a period of time after the governor signs the bill before it takes effect. The committee chairperson has control over the committee agenda, although for some of these activities specific time frames are spelled out in rules and regulations. There are opportunities for tactical delays and for constructive input.

The executive nurse may decide to be involved with a particular piece of legislation and then become disappointed when it either gets "lost in committee," is "dead" due to lack of interest, support or consensus, or is gone when a session ends. (It may be reintroduced next session with new numbers and new legislative sponsors.)

In the assessment of the political environment there are "cycles" and "personalities" of each cycle that are similar to the cycles experienced in other administrative arenas: election, budget, session, and vacation cycles. These cycles impact the prioritization of issues. In addition to the overall structure and flow, there are nuances in the legislative process of writing and drafting bills that involve other parts of the government. A commission or department may be responsible for writing, analyzing, and codifying bills and reporting the status of legislation for standing, conference, and interim committees. There may be a budget office or a joint committee of the House and Senate responsible for fiscal information. These special services are usually accessible only through the request of a legislator. Although the names of these functions may vary from state to state, the process is the same. There are many parts to the process of enacting a law and timing is important.

Elected Representatives

The elected representatives are key to the process; know who they are, ways to access them, their political agenda and potential aspirations, their special interests and background, what committees they serve on, whether they are decision-makers influential with your issues, and their voting record. A consistent, visible, and dependable participant is recognized. The dynamics involved in dealing with legislators is important.

> Public policies must usually be endorsed by politicians—those most directly involved in policy decisions—before they can be implemented, and politicians are likely to move cautiously, and often

> reluctantly, up the steps toward new policies. Their caution stems
> from three interconnected needs: the need to be sure the move is
> politically acceptable, technically workable and legally and ethi-
> cally defensible; the need to have the move endorsed by a coali-
> tion large enough to support and protect it; and the desire to
> keep as many options as possible open as long as possible.
> (Bryson, 1992, p. 9)

Legislators usually want to be elected again and so need votes, money, and volunteers who will campaign for their point of view and have access to networks of
other voters. The executive nurse has access to many health care groups and
providers and can help to inform them. In the beginning, it is helpful to arrange
personal visits or invite legislators to your facility at key times to educate and inform them. The executive nurse can provide content for speeches or volunteer to
help design the health care agenda for a legislator. All forms of communication
are valuable; they should all be based on facts. Facts associated with positive and
negative outcomes are powerful, and life examples explain health care needs simply and dynamically. Life examples influence decision making when presented sin-
cerely and with a strong consumer focus. Legislators represent the public, and
they want to stay in touch. The executive nurse has the opportunity to act as a con-
duit and to express the health care concerns of the public.

There are additional ways to be involved in the public policy process. If the executive nurse is viewed as an expert in a particular area, then the role of expert
witness or consultant to a committee or legislator is possible. It is important to
write and let your interest and expertise be known.

Committees are frequently appointed by the governor or by groups of legislators. A way to get appointed is to know who is making the assignments and then
demonstrate knowledge about the issue. You must tell them that you are willing to
work and will be available. You must state whether you represent a particular constituency or yourself as a voter and citizen, as well as applicable employment positions.

When the executive nurse is involved with the political process, the issue of
party alliances may be raised. If the intent is to stay issue-focused by representing
the consumer, you will need to remain party neutral. However, the party makeup
of the legislators and the governor will influence strategies, contacts back home,
and the overall process, formal and informal. It is important, when representing
and speaking for a given constituency, that allegiance is clearly presented. This
helps to position and focus the alliances of the speaker and the issue in a certain
way to achieve the desired goals.

Attitude

To be actively involved, the executive nurse needs a positive attitude and the belief
that what is offered is important, valuable, and essential to the policy process.
Executive nurses are an effective and efficient voice for nursing and can gather,
analyze, and present nursing care from the vantage point of many patient–health
service contacts: acute care, ambulatory, home health, long-term care, emergency

room, and more. This does not mean other types of nurses are not important to the political process, but the executive nurse, based on leadership experience and wide clinical exposure, can address the interests of a large number of providers and consumers.

Self-Presentation

The executive nurse establishes and maintains credibility by presenting relevant facts and contributing to constructive solutions. Credibility is built and maintained with consistent and persistent actions. It is a function of open and honest communications with no hidden agendas. It is critical to walk the talk and be able to acknowledge ones' realistic contributions. Particularly in the complex, deliberate policy process, credibility, consistency, and facts are critical to positive outcomes.

The executive nurse must present as knowledgeable about the formal legislative process: the way a bill becomes a law, parliamentary procedure, and the channels to be followed for communications. The formal democratic system has a structure and flow by virtue of governing bodies, committees, and public hearings. At the same time, the informal system is important. These informal contacts may be accomplished when there is acknowledgement by the informal leaders that the executive nurse's contributions are important to their agenda, or a powerful interest group with certain resources is represented, or simply as one who has information important to the discussion. The informal system is influenced by "back home contacts," who you meet to have coffee, who is included at "brainstorm sessions" before hearings, and who receives a copy of draft legislation before others. The informal process is also influenced by legislators who request to talk with certain individuals and exclude others, with the intent of negotiating a compromise or evaluating the bottom line of a given interest group. But the informal dialogue is framed by the formal structure and the process of public policy development. There is a delicate balance between formal and informal interactions.

Consumer Perspective

The focus of the executive nurse's contributions to the policy process is the knowledge and information about consumers of health care services and the way to encourage efficiencies and positive consumer outcomes in the delivery of those services. The consumers' point of view, not self-interests, will advance health care.

Frequently, the executive nurse is not designated to be involved in representing nursing to legislators. In many states the professional organization is the collective bargaining unit for the profession and hires lobbyists to represent nursing so as to ensure consistent contact with legislators. Nurse members may give testimony, meet with their district representatives, or write letters to influence the process. Nurses who work in the federal government must abide by the regulations of the Hatch Act (see Mason, et al., 1993, pp. 702–703). But, for some professional associations, the involvement of executive nurses presents concerns about loyalties, fear that management views will dominate the results of policies, and that nurse job security, wages and hours, or clinical-practice parameters will suffer. Facts, and open dialogue from all of nursing's perspectives, must be utilized when discussing and acting on potentially divisive issues. If nursing is perceived as looking out for itself, not considerate of other points of view and uncompromising, nursing will not be included at the decision-making table. Mutual goals, clearly understood and articulated, will assist in this endeavor. The ability to work with a team of players and recognize the contributions of other health care providers is important. A consumer-issue focus helps create a more compatible framework for the entire team. It is politically astute to check out the perceptions being created with someone who gives honest, accurate feedback and is peripheral to the immediate discussion. In the heat of debate, emotions can take control and blur the consumer focus.

Specific Policy Activities

The executive nurse must be competent and committed to perform specific activities throughout the involvement with the public policy process. These activities require involvement, time, and energy. Being "political" requires "campaigning, lobbying, bargaining, negotiating, caucusing, collaborating and winning votes"(Kantor, 1983, p. 216).

Stakeholder Identification

The executive nurse should assess and identify, in general, four main types of potential stakeholders: those who will advocate for the issue, those who will oppose the issue, those who are neutral and might go either way, and those who choose to stay out of the debate. "Understandings" are discussed between groups, and it is a complex environment in which to function. Therefore, it is important to bring some predictability into this process with the identification of potential stakeholders and their positions. This identification applies to legislators too. A key question is, Who will be affected, negatively or positively, by the policy? This inquiry may uncover the unexpected opposition of an interest group whose concerns were not considered. It is helpful to enlist the support of a large group on an issue of importance to you even if the issue may not be as important to them. It is coalition building that will be remembered by the group when an issue of importance comes along for them. Some people in the field refer to this as knowing what "chits" you have with groups and knowing when and how to use them. It may also be "cross-lobbying," which is increasingly common and influences the debate from behind the scenes (Weisskopf, 1994). Knowing and understanding power, formal and informal relationships, and the history of those relationships is very helpful.

Sometimes the best strategy is to discourage a powerful lobbying group from adopting your issue. An example is the importance of advanced practice nurses' limited prescriptive authority in the hospital. Does the nursing profession want the hospital advocacy group to be involved with this issue or to remain neutral? When hospital admissions require a physician order by law and hospitalization is for the severely ill person, limited prescriptive authority in the hospital may not be as important as in other health care settings. So the strategy may be to not engage the hospital advocacy group in this debate. However, it may be an issue for nurse-managed centers and ambulatory environments, which could be viewed very differently by the parties involved.

Communications

As discussed earlier, communication skills are important, and in the public policy process many methods are effective. Letters, face-to-face meetings, telephone calls, and telegrams—all have merit based on the issue and the time frame. In whatever method, identify who you represent and establish an appropriate level of rapport, presenting clear and objective information and the outcomes desired. Data, analyzed and presented informatively, is essential. Busy lawmakers do not appreciate smoke screens or exaggerations. Whatever the method, carefully explain the issues and use simple, yet strong, examples. Your presentation will influence the perception of the issues by the recipient of the communication. The executive nurse contributes in a special way: evaluating the larger impact of policy changes on consumers, providers, and payers in the employing facility and bringing this experience to the public policy process. The executive nurse is expected to evaluate change, what works and what does not work, in practice and for consumers.

Testifying   A special communication skill is testifying, or presenting testimony. It sounds rather legal and frightening, but it is a benign process as long as you are aware of the protocols and have time to plan. Time permitting, what appears most effective is to prepare written testimony for the committee members, and especially for the committee recorder and the various legislative assistants. Based on the number of hearings, the number slated to give testimony, and the potential for controversy, the verbal presentation should be a topical review of the information with reference to the written detail. Highlighting important points, issues of importance to all constituents, and a willingness to work with others in achieving a good law is favorably received. It is very effective to speak without reading the script and to give examples from experiences.

It is helpful if the person giving testimony for an organization or involved in draft bill discussions with other interest groups has a set of principles or guidelines endorsed by the group. This permits the person testifying or negotiating to know how much compromise is acceptable or how to respond to questions from the legislators. It is a process of give and take.

The formal acknowledgement of the chairperson and the committee is a part of the initial opening and, if there is dialogue between the committee and the person giving the testimony, the person giving the testimony replies to questions only through the chairperson and then to the questioning legislator. It is a protocol that recognizes the power and status of the chairperson. The committee chairperson may relax this formality, depending on the nature of the committee, the issue at hand, the participants, and "who is there." When media representatives are in the room, chances are the proceedings will be more formal. Usually there is a speaker form to be filled out before the meeting that indicates your desire to give testimony, your name, and whether you represent an organization. The chairperson will call your name and identify the organization when it is your turn to give testimony. Kantor (1983, p. 179) offers additional suggestions in preparing and giving testimony. She suggests translating concerns into specific criticisms and counter questions with data and well-mounted arguments. An open and public approach to issues versus secrecy will prevent being cut off from the real core issue. Possible solutions and a willingness to be involved with correcting the problem indicates the commitment lawmakers are seeking in order to support and pass a proposed law.

Lobbying A lobbyist hired for a particular interest group must be registered at state or national level, and has special regulations relative to expenses and appropriate behavior. However, informally the notion of lobbying is, in broad terms, any communication designed to influence another person to act according to your interests. Broadly, any type of communication could be lobbying if the main purpose is to influence behavior. Educational lobbying emphasizes the informative aspects of communication and is seen as a strong way to influence legislators, who have an overwhelming number of issues that they must be informed about and act on. Legislators will want to know if your organization has a position or policy on the issue, your membership composition and numbers, why this issue is of concern to them, and if they are willing to assist in implementation. It is important, when representing a constituency, that their position be stated first and that the connection with other groups be stated second. It is "politically astute" to indicate the support of other groups collaborating with you; you should identify and know the health care issues in your community because legislators may ask about broader issues as an indicator of your involvement and influence.

Interdependency and Interaction

The public policy process, or the political process, is based on the notions of participatory democracy and representative government (Litman, 1991, p. 8). These two processes can create conflict points, and interactions and interdependencies within the entire health care system should be recognized when engaged in the making of public policy. Public policies will have a better chance of positive outcomes and implementation if all stakeholders are included in the process. At the same time, the reality is that in a democracy there may be strongly diverse views and opinions, all with good intent. Again, a balance between a special interest groups' position and what is good for society as a whole is a challenge for lawmakers and those involved with the process.

Here is a scenario that illustrates these points. An attempt was made by the governor and a state legislator to pass an AIDS bill that included mandatory disclosure of health providers' HIV status. There was significant opposition to this proposal and concern by many groups about the impact on health care consumers and providers. This was an emotional and complex issue. The governor was willing to delay the proposed bill for one year. However, during that time a task force had to arrive at a solution. A group of individuals representing nursing, medicine, dentistry, occupational health, community health, consumers, infection control, licensing boards, and hospitals was convened by the health department. This group had to draft guidelines to be enacted into law. Together the group educated one another about the issues for their constituencies and then educated the legislators. They were able to design a system that addressed the needs of all involved. They were able to influence and change the proposed bill significantly and at the same time protect the public and health care providers.

The executive nurse must be aware that support for or opposition to a particular policy may come from unexpected organizations and individuals. It is important to know who the stakeholders are or who might be concerned about the particular issue, as well as who is not concerned, and why, and who they represent and network with. Most organized groups or associations have their own agenda, which is a part of their mission and is what focuses and holds their group together; it is what drives their political agenda, and can be teased out of most position statements. This is their self-interest agenda and in many cases their self-preservation. It will be protected. It is important to know the organizations' positions, the underlying motives of the position, and the underlying motives of the public policy in development. What will the policy, if enacted, do for or against the stakeholders' agenda? Frequently, there is more than one driving agenda item in an organization, but the core will be self-preservation. This is evident in the many health care providers who are concerned about public health and well-being and member competency, but are also motivated to protect self-interests and market niche.

The executive nurse is experienced in collecting, analyzing, and combining the ideas and positions of many types of health care providers. These ideas are "reality checked" by others to see whether they are true to the intent and to make sure their ideas are included. This expertise is valuable in working with other groups during the policy process.

The executive nurse functions more comfortably if relationships with other groups and the public develop both formally and informally. This facilitates a better understanding of various points of view and the compromises that might be needed. It is important to raise a broad range of factors that might shape the policy outcome(s) because of the groups involved and then develop ways to capitalize on those factors and neutralize those that cannot be capitalized on (Bocchino & Wakefield, 1992, p. 55).

Individuals representing the media are effective in feedback and in helping others develop networks. For example, laws on advance directives require a great deal of legislator, consumer, health care provider, health facility, and lawyer education, and an informed media can be very helpful. A nurse lawyer in one state was instrumental in bringing together all these constituencies to look at ways to inform and increase the number of consumers with advance directives. The laws were passed but implementation was slow. This group met and brainstormed what they could do to impact and implement the law. They volunteered to implement various approaches, such as news spots about where consumers could obtain information, education courses for health care providers, and a simple but complete pamphlet to be distributed at senior centers and drug stores. The media were especially helpful and knowledgeable on how to reach the most consumers and very willing to help the group deliver the message.

Talbott (1993, p. 138) summarizes political action with ten principles:

1. Look at the big picture

2. Do your homework

3. Nothing ventured, nothing gained

4. Get a toe in the door

5. Quid pro quo

    6. Walk a mile in another's moccasins

    7. Strike while the iron is hot

    8. Read between the lines

    9. Half a loaf is better than none

   10. Rome was not built in a day

HEALTH CARE POLICY MODELS

Most health care consumers, providers, and payers believe the United States is in the midst of a paradigm shift in health care. So how does the executive nurse evaluate the impact of health care policy on the organization and know what involvement will benefit the consumer and the nursing profession?

A number of helpful models for involvement and for understanding public policy and "politics" exist in the nursing literature. Stimpson and Hanley's (1991) model suggests: identifying core issues, deciding jurisdiction, performing background checks; then, setting objectives with criteria to assess objectives; proposing alternative solutions and formulating criteria to evaluate their effects on desired outcomes, political feasibility, time constraints, and manpower resources. The positive and negative consequences are identified, and alternatives prioritized and scored based on qualitative and quantitative factors. Backer's model (1991) is designed to guide problem definition in policy development and is based on nursing process assessment skills. A feminist model for political empowerment is presented by Mason, Backer and Georges (1991) and emphasizes respect for others and for self, power-sharing, and equality. Theresa Chalich and Lorraine Smith (1992) discuss the political involvement of nurses as grassroots involvement and then movement up a ladder with four rungs from civic involvement to long-term power wielding and partisan politics. These are all important contributions to nursing's search for knowledge and will assist in furthering and encouraging nursing policy research.

Scalzi and Wilson (1990) surveyed 184 top-level, U.S. nurse executives in home health, acute care, long-term care, and occupational health settings. They found that law and health care policy were ranked as the most time consuming and most important by nurse executives regardless of the practice setting. The role of education and socialization in health policy and politics was deemed essential for future nurse administrators (Hall-Long, 1995, p. 27).

A research model in the policy area is proposed by Nagelkerk and Henry (1991). They suggest leadership through policy research by supporting and collaborating with policy researchers around significant social problems. Nurse executives and policy researchers could collect and analyze pertinent data and suggest alternative solutions to put forward to policy makers. The policy research is evaluated based on importance, feasibility, validity, and originality. "Leading through policy research requires that we understand policy making, anticipate competing views, and communicate throughout a project with those who will use our work" (Nagelkerk & Henry, 1991, p. 22).

There is a need for models to assess or evaluate health care policy, whether it is a potential, proposed, or implemented policy. Policies that impact the facility and patient care originate both internally and externally. The impact on the facility and consumers of new and different policies, in many different spheres, is critical and exponential. For example, the overall impact of the federally mandated OSHA requirements is difficult to quantify. A law mandating patient and family hospital-based education concerning child support is causing impact on hospital resources and information systems. A health care policy model, particularly for acute care, would help in planning and evaluating, and in being proactive rather than reactive to changes in public policy. Predictive and program evaluation models may be a source for future exploration (see Chapter 9).

A starting point for the executive nurse in developing a useful model is to explore and present policy issues to colleagues and the nursing staff. This also allows the opportunity for educating others about the political process and for serving as a mentor. The result will probably be more questions than answers. It is important to document these questions because, for that facility, they point to the critical factors that impact its operations and outcomes, and suggest a model on how to evaluate policies impacting your facility. Employees and consumers are excellent sources for keeping in touch with the community and for how major policies are affecting them. For example, a current issue is the use of unlicensed personnel in hospitals. This is a policy issue that has internal and external implications and should be addressed with broad representation from all levels of health care providers and consumers.

The community has a distinct culture: in its language, religions, media, education, legal affairs, and the arts. The impact of policies on these institutions in society will also assist in the overall assessment. By networking and learning the local political structure, it will become easier to prioritize what is important to the external constituencies.

A conversation with Joel Barker, in Flower (1991), contributes an interesting approach to progressive policy model development. Barker says we should look for and recognize new patterns of behavior and discover the future by asking the following questions: What are the problems I wish I could solve and don't know how? What are the intractable problems? If I could break any rules I wanted, what would I do to solve these problems? What's our cost per problem and what's our time between problems solved? This kind of questioning points to the important policy issues and helps eliminate the policies which hinder and halt change and progress. The responses to these and other questions are what policy makers are concerned about: being on the up-side of change. The executive nurse is the catalyst, the collaborator,and the consumer-focused person to help make positive health care policies.

Summary

The executive nurse is a valuable asset in the development and implementation of public policy at community, state, and federal levels. Practical experience and a strong knowledge of health and illness care is a dynamic combination. The ability and skill to understand and clearly articulate the health needs of consumers can improve health policy. The political environment and the way to assist politicians in their tasks relative to health policy can be learned. The decision to act is the most important decision and "the most important factor in learning political skill is finding mentors and friends who are politically involved and will believe in us, support us, teach us, critique us, and then celebrate with us" (Leavitt & Barry, 1993, p. 47). There is a role for every executive nurse in health care policy, and the time to come forward is now.

Discussion Questions

1. In your practice setting, what policies positively impact patient care and what policies negatively impact patient care?

2. What action could you take to correct a negative policy?

3. If you chaired a committee to revise your state's nurse practice act, discuss steps and the plan for reaching a successful conclusion.

References

Abdellah, F. G. (1991). *Nursing's role in the future. A case for health policy decision making.* Center Nursing Press, Sigma Theta Tau International, Monograph Series 91.

Bocchino, C. A., Wakefield, M. K. (1992). Perspectives forces influencing public policy. *Nursing Economics, 10,*(1), 53–55.

Backer, B. A. (1991). You can get there from here: Guide to problem definition in policy development. *Journal of Psychosocial Nursing, 29*(10), 24–28.

Bryson, J. M., Crosby, B. B. (1992). *Leadership for the common good.* San Francisco: Jossey-Bass.

Buerhaus, P. I. (1994). Nursing economics and politics in a global economy. In L. Simms, et al. *The professional practice of nursing administration.* 2nd ed. Albany, New York: Delmar.

Carver, J. (1990). Boards that make a difference. San Francisco: Jossey-Bass.

Chalich, T., Smith, L. (1992). Nursing at the grassroots. *Nursing and Health Care, 13*(5), 242–244.

Curtin, L. L. (1992). For sale to the highest bidder? *Nursing Management, 23*(6),7–8.

Duncan, G. T., Jabine, T. B., de Wolf, V. A., eds. (1993). *Private lives and public policies.* Washington: National Academy Press.

Feldstein, P. J. (1988). *The politics of health legislation.* Ann Arbor: Health Administration Press.

Flower, J. (1991). Don't wait for the crisis: Finding the paradigm in the pattern. A conversation with Joel Barker. *Healthcare Forum Journal,* November/December, 29–31.

Hall-Long, B. A. (1995). Nursing's past, present, and future political experiences. *Nursing and Health Care, 16*(1), 24–28.

Hanley, B. (1987). Political participation: How do nurses compare with other professional women? *Nursing Economics, 5*(4), 179–186.

Hanley, B. E. (1993). Policy development and analysis. In D. J. Mason, et al. *Policy and politics for nurses.* Philadelphia: WB Saunders, 71–87.

Jones, L. R. (1995). Aaron Wildavsky: A man and scholar for all seasons. *Public Administration Review, 55*(1), 3–16.

Kalisch, B. J., Kalisch, P. A. (1982). *Politics of nursing.* Philadelphia: Lippincott.

Kantor, R. M. (1983). *The change masters.* New York: Simon & Schuster.

Kuehnert, P. L. (1991). The public health policy advocate: Fostering the health of communities. *Clinical Nurse Specialist, 5*(1), 5–10.

Leavitt, J. K., Barry, C. T. (1993). Learning the ropes. In D. J. Mason, et al. *Policy and politics for nurses.* Philadelphia: WB Saunders, 47–67.

Litman, T. J., Robins, L. S. (1991). *Health politics and policy.* Albany: Delmar.

Mason, D. J., Backer, B. A., Georges, C. A. (1991). Toward a feminist model for the political empowerment of nurses. *Image: Journal of Nursing Scholarship, 23*(2),72–77.

Mason, D. J., Talbott, S. W., Leavitt, J. K. (1993). *Policy and politics for nurses.* Philadelphia: WB Saunders.

Milio, N. (1984). Nursing research and the study of health policy. *Annual Review of Nursing Research, 2,* 317.

Nagelkerk, J. M. and Nenry, B. (1991). Leadership through policy research. *Journal of Nursing Administration, 21*(5), 20–24.

Sharp, N., Biggs, S., Wakefield, M. (1991). Public policy: New opportunities for nurses. *Nursing and Health Care, 12,*(1), 16–22.

Simms, L. M., Price, S. A., Ervin, N. E. (1994). *The professional practice of nursing administration.* 2nd ed. Albany: Delmar.

Stimpson, M., Hanley, B. (1991). Nurse policy analyst. *Nursing and Health Care, 10,*(12:1), 10–15.

Talbott, S. W. (1993). Political analysis: Structure and process. In D. J. Mason, et al. *Policy and politics for nurses.* Philadelphia: WB Saunders. 129–148.

Webster's Ninth New Collegiate Dictionary. (1988). Springfield, MA: Merriam-Webster.

Weisskopf, M. Health care lobbies lobby each other. *The Washington Post,* March 1, 1994.

Susan Hoefflinger Taft

CHAPTER 4

Paradoxical Challenge
Preserve and Transform the Organizational Culture

Introduction

Culture is to humans as water is to fish. It is the context of any social gathering—the atmosphere, everywhere, present in everything we do, think, feel, sense, and express. We create it, and then culture comes back to control us with its considerable social authority. It is subjective reality, collectively shared. The metaphors describing culture reflect its protean and ubiquitous nature. It is: "a distinct way of life," "community glue," "social fiber," "social tissue," a "bubble of meaning." Culture is both cause and effect—derivative of human experience, creator of meaning, and producer of future behavior.

On many of the attributes of culture there is virtually universal agreement. Culture is:

- Learned
- Shared by social groups
- A source of meaning
- Neutral (neither "good" nor "bad")
- Adaptive
- Persistent, pervasive, and dynamic
- Reoccurring, repetitive
- Symbolic
- Cumulative and transgenerational
- A relatively stable but complex pattern open to subjective and diverse interpretations. (Barley, 1991; Bartunek & Moch, 1991; Morey & Luthans, 1985; Schein, 1991b; Taft, 1988; Young, 1991)

Beyond these identified attributes of culture, which are widely shared across disciplines and practice sites, agreement begins to thin out regarding what culture is. There are varied definitions of the components of culture. When culture as a concept is compared across the literatures of different disciplines, the relationships between the components of culture shift like weather vanes in a gusty wind. Many conceptual contradictions and instances of circular logic are present. For example, is a sign a type of symbol, or are symbols and signs synonyms? How are rites and rituals different? Does one lead to the other? Do rites create traditions? If so, then are rites the building blocks of customs? Cause-and-effect relationships here are unclear. There is no conceptual framework of cultural components on which experts can agree. Large gulfs in definitions are particularly evident between anthropologists and organizational scientists. (Look ahead to Table 4.2 for an attempt to integrate these definitions.)

Although fine distinctions among the concepts of culture have yet to be developed, the executive in any health care setting often has acquired, through experience, considerable practical understanding of organizational cultures. Having command of that knowledge can significantly enhance the executive nurse's managerial facility and leadership. The decisions, policies, or practices of a particular executive nurse that are relatively consistent with the organizational culture are apt to be successful. Those that are inconsistent, counter-cultural, or perceived to be of limited relevance to the existing culture are less apt to succeed—unless they offer promise of future directions critical for agency survival.

If the executive fathoms the form and function of the workplace culture, then the entire structure of meaning in that setting is understandable. While this structure of meaning may not be so tangible as would be, for example, the weight-bearing beams of a new building, it is nonetheless the stable and enduring foundation underlying any social setting. Culture provides the deep structure of meaning of communal organization life.

Many articles written about organizational cultures describe in detail the manifestations of a culture (e.g., stories and legends, traditions, heroes and heroines, any symbols of a way of life. But exploration of the deep structural origins of culture is often lacking. It is the purpose of this chapter to help executive nurses in all settings connect those visible cultural manifestations to the subterranean stream of meaning from which they spring—or, more simply, to provide an understanding of both the superficial and deep principles of organizational culture. Because the scope of executive nurses' work extends across the entire health organization, and because nurse leaders occupy major roles in shaping the strategies that secure the future survival of their institutions, they are both creators of and players in their workplace cultures. Knowledge of organizational culture is important to executives because understanding it will aid in accomplishing what they believe to be important.

This chapter is organized into five major sections that identify the manifestations of cultures within all health agencies. The sections address values as the heart of culture, multicultural organizations, hospital culture types, cultural understanding important to nurse leaders, and the identification of how culture can be effective.

VALUES—THE HEART OF CULTURE

Values are the very heart of a culture. They are initially established by the founders of an organization, and they evolve and transform over time. Values are the foundation of all outward manifestations of culture.

But values are not the central core of culture, nor are they the seed that brings forth new organizational life. They are not the original energy source for a culture. A more fundamental need sparks new cultural life: the human drive to survive.

All living creatures, and hence their cultures, begin with a single pre-eminent task—to ensure survival. Hunting-and-gathering tribes worshipped the spirits of nature, developing cultures which held the sun, rain, animals, and stars in high regard. Native Americans of the Western plains used the buffalo—their source of food, clothing, shelter, and tools—as their cultural symbol. Theistic religions worship God. Manifested outwardly through numerous rites and ceremonies, they place their destiny in God's hands: the cross symbolizes the ultimate promise of eternal life. Maritime cultures, which excelled in navigation and shipbuilding, developed the tools of navigation and astronomy to guide and protect them on the seas. Tough young men from impoverished urban ghettos present themselves with a display of machismo. They value guns and knives and methods of force as the tools of their cultural survival.

Capitalist societies such as the United States or Japan value goods and services, materials and consumption. In America, Wall Street serves as the economic barometer of the nation. Popular magazines create heroes and icons of the wealthiest business leaders or the highest-paid sports figures. In hospitals, status has been accorded to the heavy admitters and to the high-output surgeons. These are the currencies of survival. In a capitalist society, the producers of material value receive the highest forms of cultural approval. It is a social exchange between survival agents and the beneficiaries (Blau, 1986). While the currencies vary across cultures—from the agility and strength of the hunter to the financial successes of the stockbroker, from the power of prayer to the precision of navigational tools—the fundamental task is always the same: Survive!

Living organizations therefore have survival as their first concern. To ensure survival is the single most important job a culture has to perform. Cultural values form directly from this pre-eminent task. In capitalist societies, economic activities are the subterranean lifestream of those cultures. Figure 4.1 depicts this relationship for an organization.

Spark of Life

At the inner core of an organizational culture is the spark of life: the creation of a new enterprise. Once in existence, it seeks to continue living. If an enterprise becomes secure in its prospects for survival, then it will seek to thrive. In the United States, to maintain survival generally means to make money, while to thrive requires making more money! Surrounding the spark of life, the inner core, are the organization's mission, vision, and strategy, which were originally designed and are continuously reshaped to ensure a favorable competitive position (i.e., success in

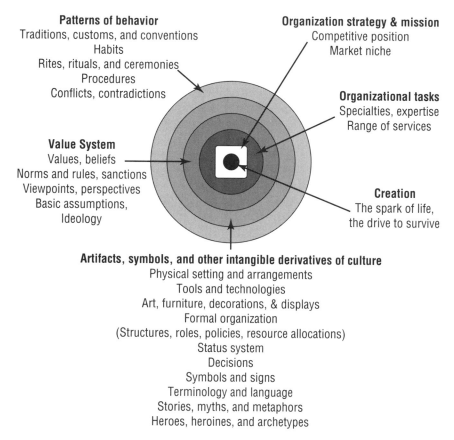

Patterns of behavior
Traditions, customs, and conventions
Habits
Rites, rituals, and ceremonies
Procedures
Conflicts, contradictions

Organization strategy & mission
Competitive position
Market niche

Organizational tasks
Specialties, expertise
Range of services

Value System
Values, beliefs
Norms and rules, sanctions
Viewpoints, perspectives
Basic assumptions,
Ideology

Creation
The spark of life,
the drive to survive

Artifacts, symbols, and other intangible derivatives of culture
Physical setting and arrangements
Tools and technologies
Art, furniture, decorations, & displays
Formal organization
(Structures, roles, policies, resource allocations)
Status system
Decisions
Symbols and signs
Terminology and language
Stories, myths, and metaphors
Heroes, heroines, and archetypes

Figure 4.1 *Layers of organizational culture.*

the marketplace). The quality of the services an organization delivers, both actual and perceived, is an important component of its competitive strength. A continuing adaptation to the environment and its needs will lead to evolutionary change in the culture. Continuing effectiveness for an organization is a complex and not entirely rational matter. It results from the dynamic interrelationships of such factors as consumer demand, leadership, resource availability, key cultural values, management policies and practices, the perceived quality of the goods and services, and the business environment of the enterprise. Any generalizations one might make about an organization's culture and its effectiveness must, to be complete, incorporate the relation of that culture to its surrounding social and economic context (Denison, 1990; Sackman, 1991; Wiener, 1988).

The organizational tasks, or specialties, the third ring out from the center in Figure 4.1, are those services provided by the enterprise for their strategic likelihood of ensuring viability. They match a perceived need in the environment with what the organization offers as its technical expertise.

Values, which appeared as the fourth ring in Figure 4.1, derive from these fundamental choices of survival strategy and task specialties. Values are formed at the inception of an enterprise, when the founder or founding group establishes a way to run the new business. Over time, founders, partners, and employees build a common history. They develop shared assumptions about their business, its environment, and what they should do to survive and grow. An accumulation of experiences builds a tacit "theory" about success and survival. Experience with external adaptation (i.e., redefining the mission and/or markets) and internal integration (i.e., restructuring to respond to a new mission or markets) enable organizational learning and change to occur. The approaches that solve the group's problems repeatedly, and that reduce anxieties about threats to survival, will come to be accepted as critical values (Schein, 1991a). Thus performance that is consistent with effective strategic choices will establish what is important.

Transmitting Values

Values become a shorthand method of transmitting these messages of "what's important." Human beings find appeal and meaning in values—more so than in giving conscious attention to the unsettling notion of surviving or not surviving—and so they tend to identify with values, gradually absorbing them into their consciousness and employing them as the internal gyroscope for the culture. Values become the heart of culture because they are what stir human beings, they are what they feel. Because values can become deeply embedded within the consciousness of organizational members, they are notoriously difficult to change. It is important for leaders to understand that values derive from the survival strategy of the organization, as was portrayed in Figure 4.1, and not vice versa. The key to changing values is to make explicit their link to strategic imperatives.

The patterns of basic assumptions and values will tend to determine organizational behavior (Hatch, 1993; Schein, 1991a, 1991b, 1987). Basic assumptions are fundamental beliefs that are below conscious awareness, whereas values may be consciously known, or at least accessible to awareness. For example, a hospital culture's basic assumptions may be identified in part by looking at the board of trustees. What is the composition of the board? What types of people serve? Considering the nature of board membership, what can be inferred about the organization's values? What types of people are viewed as links to survival? A board consisting of community members, local leaders, and consumers implies a very different set of values than does a board comprised of corporate CEOs, political insiders, and members of wealthy families. Or, look at the powerful committees of an organization. Who serves on them, and who doesn't? How is the chair determined? Who votes? Can meetings be observed by outsiders? The underlying assumptions and a hierarchy of values are often revealed in the exclusive boundaries, membership, and privileges of governing bodies.

The environment changes continually, at varying degrees of magnitude and at different rates of speed. However, when an organization's environment changes significantly, pre-existing assumptions may continue to drive behavior, unquestioned and taken for granted as "the way we do things around here," even when those ways are no longer current and adaptive (Shafritz & Ott, 1987). If outdated assumptions continue to drive behavior, organizational survival will be threatened.

Since values reflect the collective beliefs held by members about how their organization survives, they also provide recognition of who or what is to be credited for their relative success. Value is attached to different kinds of work based on its perceived contribution to organizational survival. This is the source of the hierarchical order of the power structure. Salesmen in corporations, "rainmakers" in accounting or law firms, or top researchers in universities are accorded superior status because they bring in lifegiving resources.

While survival strategy is the core of culture, cultures develop, grow, and evolve in unique and idiosyncratic ways. Thus, organizations with nearly identical strategies will not manifest wholly interchangeable cultures. Although many similarities may be present, the variability inherent in life itself will shape any two organizational cultures differently. Additionally, even the most consistent of cultures (perhaps IBM or AT&T in bygone days) contain ambiguities, contradictions, and volatility (Meyerson, 1991). Today's hyperkinetic environments exaggerate these tendencies.

In Figure 4.1, the external two layers were the outward manifestations of culture. These include the tangible artifacts, which are physical items or other concrete manifestations of culture accessible to the five senses, and the intangible symbolic meanings, such as interpretations of the language or the organizational status system, or inferences regarding stories and heroes/heroines. of the past. The formal structure is a semitangible artifact of the culture, while a myth from the agency's history is a more symbolic than concrete artifact. Finally, the outermost layer of a culture is formed from the pattern of behavior exhibited by members. Behavior may be prescribed or proscribed, as by procedures and custom, or naturally and informally developed from within the cultural context. Human behavior both derives from and gives form to the culture.

All of this may seem quite abstract and rather academic. What is its practical relevance? Of what value is this to nursing or patient care? Let us look at a few scenarios.

Scenario 4.1   **New Marketing Emphases**

For many years, hospitals have advertised and promoted their medical expertise: the latest surgery techniques, the world-renowned cardiology service, the most advanced obstetrical care. This practice is consistent with a strategy centered around an institution's outstanding medical accomplishments. Conventional marketing wisdom assumed that medicine was the critical market draw. The internal hospital culture reflected these "survival" beliefs in its status system; that is, physicians held the lion's share of the power, particularly those practitioners with the "big names."

In the past decade, marketing initiatives (which reflect the underlying survival strategy) have shifted noticeably. Glossy hospital marketing brochures still promote big name or innovative physicians, which continues to be good marketing. But now they commonly feature articles on the contributions of other members of a medical team as well: advances in physical therapy treatments that restore patients to functional well-being; home-care nursing programs that enable the chronically or terminally ill to remain at home; health promotion groups run by advanced practice nurses for midlife women; social-work facilitation of support groups for the mentally ill; or reports of a patient's own hospitalization story showing how he is a critical member of the team. More often today, many participants are credited with creating a hospital's success stories. There is a "whole" which is valued as the reason for being of the "parts." This shift represents a change in survival strategy and, therefore, organizational culture.

Nurses On Call

Scenario 4.2

In the urban area where I live, "nurse on call" phone services have been provided by several competing hospitals. Specially trained nurses talk with members of the public about a broad array of individual health problems. These nurse services may receive hundreds of calls in a 24-hour period; some result in new patient referrals to the sponsoring hospital and/or to affiliated physicians. Hospital administrators in the participating institutions track the direct and indirect positive results of nurse on call services. Some of the physicians—those who have benefitted by the referral of new patients into their practices—also support the service. From the perspective of the hospital administrator or physician, the image of nursing is enhanced in this strategically valuable role. However this enhancement may not occur within HMO or PPO settings in which nursing services of this type bear no direct relation to "bringing in business." The perceived value of nursing gets a boost when it contributes to patient referrals. The nurse's role in securing resources for the hospital will directly affect both her short- and long-term centrality in the culture.

Exploring Case Management

Scenario 4.3

As an executive nurse, you would like to institute, on a trial basis, either primary nursing or case management on half of your nursing units. You think that either model could offer improvements in the quality of patient care while concurrently, through more timely patient care management and discharge processes, saving the hospital money. The enhancement of quality in patient care and improvement in efficiencies are of equal importance in nursing case management. In addition, your long-term goal is to move toward adding nursing care of patients pre- and post-hospitalization, deploying your inpatient staff to expand patient contact over the continuum of care. You see a major restructuring of patient care in this direction as consistent with the hospital's survival strategy. What approach would you need to take to sell your ideas, either to hospital administrators or to physicians? What about the nursing staff? What data do you have or might you collect to strengthen your case? Economic benefits of change, if demonstrable, typically speak the loudest. For example, a comparison of cost benefits and care quality between trial and traditional units could provide a powerful and persuasive lever. Linking your ideas to the hospital's strategic plan may enhance support. In addition, deep understanding of your hospital culture will enable you to anticipate which elements of the models might find acceptance. In settings where leaders hold fast to the traditional values of the medical model (and all that implies), or where patient and family satisfaction levels are not critical factors in maintaining a stable market share, it may be that the potential benefits of either primary nursing or case management, or of restructuring nursing care delivery, are difficult to sell. Change may be moot, however, since these agencies are unlikely to survive the decade.

Scenario 4.4   Matching Nurses to Patients

Your patient mix stretches across a broad spectrum—from oncology patients undergoing experimental drug protocols, to acutely ill postoperative patients undergoing innovative surgical techniques, to nursing home patients admitted for treatment of urinary track infections or pneumonia. The hospital's strategy (i.e., its "external adaptation") is to provide a full continuum of care from the most advanced state-of-the-art, research-based medical care to routine care of uncomplicated illnesses. Clearly, with such a full range of services, your nursing staff needs to be differentiated according to the severity and complexity of the patients for whom they care.

To achieve the appropriate match of nurse skill to patient requirements, you need to address issues of "internal integration": screening for and hiring the right mix of nurses according to experience, competence, and education for the types of patient-care needs of your units; orienting and socializing new nurses consistent with their areas of clinical practice; staffing differentially; rewarding differentially; and varying forms of governance across the units based on personnel capabilities and maturity (Schein, 1991b, 1987, 1985). In some inner city emergency departments, for example, the work context for nurses bears an unfortunate resemblance to an active war zone. The type of nurse who works well under these circumstances is not likely to fit equally well on the postpartum unit.

In cultural terms, the organizational tasks vary sufficiently to lead to the evolution of quite different work cultures on the varying units. While management theories do not generally advocate a heterogeneous approach to administration, it may be that a diversified model would more aptly link form to function in the technically diverse hospital. Many hospitals currently have elements of de facto differentiation among work areas, but it is implicit and evolutionary rather than philosophically designed.

Caresfurst Hospital

Scenario 4.5

A teaching hospital in a dense urban area—let's call it Caresfurst Hospital— provides exceptional nursing care as a competitive strategy. Other teaching hospitals abound in the area, all of which compete on the basis of medical care, research, and affiliation with a prestigious medical school. There's not enough inpatient business to fill all the hospitals in this region, so the business of health care carries imminent survival threats. Caresfurst Hospital is known to provide state-of-the-art medical care, but it is with exceptional nursing care as a strategic niche that the hospital cuts itself apart from the pack.

A hospital vice president, when she first came to town to interview for the position she currently holds, took a taxi from the airport to the hospital. The driver said, "Oh, you're going to Caresfurst Hospital? Everyone in the world knows that [another local medical center] is the best, but everyone goes to Caresfurst."

Indeed, reports about care at Caresfurst sound more like testimonials than stories of hospitalization. One patient who had delivered her baby there related her experience:

> During labor, an older nurse came on who was very calm, clearly in control. Not fazed by anything. She directed the doctors about where I was in my labor. My doctor said I didn't look real good, and gave me Pitocin. Throughout all this, I was reassured about the baby, that the baby was never in distress. The nurse stayed with me the whole time, calming me, watching the fetal monitor . . . . Finally I went into tears. I felt like I was in a tunnel, and losing control. When the surgeon said I'd need a C-section, I completely lost it, sobbing hysterically. The nurse kept focusing me back on the baby. The baby was OK. Pretty soon he'd be here and I could see him. A whole team was with me in surgery. The baby was a very big boy. The nurses were uniformly wonderful—helping with breast engorgement, teaching me and my husband about infant care. . . . They were always available, whenever I needed them, for anything. When I was discharged, the nurses gave me the phone number of the floor and reminded me "We're always here!" Did I

appreciate that! I called them from home maybe 3 or 4 times, usually in the middle of the night when no one else was available. When I needed some advice or support, they were there for me. Now I'm being followed by a nurse practitioner, and she's been great too.

The strategy of Caresfurst Hospital is reflected in its culture. Nurses' clinical practice is emphasized in the philosophy and in the policies and reward system of the hospital. Nursing leadership is strong, and the nursing staff are described by the chief executive as bright people with positive self-images. Experienced nurses participate in the orientation, education, and indoctrination of young physician house staff. The CEO talks about the hospital as being primarily for nursing care. The status system and power structure reflect nursing's primacy. All of these cultural characteristics can be traced back to the hospital's basic strategy in a competitive marketplace: to provide the very best patient care and family support. While most hospitals will say this is what they do, Caresfurst really means it. They've put it in place. The hospital culture and patient-care results provide ample evidence.

Value Culture Map

The value system of an organization's culture provides a map of the territory. When viewed as the topography and main highways of the hospital strategies, the value system can be appreciated as a deep expression of culture. Values are often most explicit and visible in practices for personnel selection, socialization of new members (learning the ropes from peers), rewards and recognition, and purposeful alterations in the organization's strategic direction (McDonald & Gandz, 1992).

It is because of the proximity of the value structure to an organization's survival that values are not easily changed. They are the layer next to the core strategy and tasks, as was seen in Figure 4.1. Values and beliefs held by members of a community cannot meaningfully change unless a fundamental shift in survival strategy has occurred. Thus, culture gurus of the popular press, who advise managers on changing or manipulating the values of their organizations, may propagate a superficial understanding of culture. Values are not a "controllable variable" (c.f. Thomas, Ward, Chorba, & Kumiega, 1991). Typically, organizations needing a change in strategy will institute new leadership and/or empower change agents to act. New leaders introduce value shifts consistent with a change in strategic direction. However, all strategic direction changes may not require a change in values. While executive nurses can directly alter structures, policies, or procedures, significant value change (i.e., a change in the organizational culture) cannot occur without a transformation of mission and task. Transformation may be gradual; it may result from the power of vision. In extreme cases, radical transformation may arise from the threat of extinction. Transformation is currently occurring at varying speeds with the mergers of health care systems.

ONE CULTURE OR MANY?

There are numerous organizational consultants who propose to "diagnose" organizational cultures, yet there is neither a comprehensive typology to do so nor a framework on which theorists would agree. Culture is a pervasive phenomenon not amenable to simple measurement. Although anthropologists use in-depth descriptive methods for studying diverse cultures, the utility of this approach to organizations is limited. Our conceptions of organizational cultures are largely partial and incomplete—we understand *some* of the pieces of a bigger puzzle. Organizational cultures are often portrayed in the literature as idealized types, but they rarely if ever appear in pure form. Organizations evidence mixtures of many cultural types.

The popular work *Corporate Cultures* (Deal & Kennedy, 1982), identified four generic cultures, or "tribes":

1. The tough-guy macho culture (individualistic, risk-taking)
2. The work hard/play hard culture (fun and action, quick feedback on degree of success)
3. The bet-your-company culture (big risks, high stakes)
4. The process culture (little feedback on success, focus on how work is done, tendency to become bureaucratic)

One can identify elements of these cultures within any organization.

According to Jones' conception of cultures (1983), when the nature of work becomes more complex, corporate cultures may move from production cultures (routine work) to bureaucratic (tasks less routine, rules and procedures expand) or professional cultures (task difficulty high, routineness low). Within a hospital setting, these cultures may be present to varying degrees in different departments. Production cultures may, for example, prevail in the laundry function where work is relatively routine and predictable. A bureaucracy culture may fit the billing department, whereas a professional culture is necessary to meet the unpredictable nature of patient care. These cultural types can certainly be found within all kinds of health agencies, but the typology cannot be used fully to characterize an enterprise such as a hospital. To understand health care cultures, one needs insight on cultural pluralism and complexity. Hospitals typically are large, diverse organizations comprised of many types of people, and diverse people have diverse values.

Value diversity is the basis for one model of organizational cultures: the competing values perspective (Fig. 4.2). In the competing values model, characteristics of work cultures fall along four dimensions, according to the degree of:

1. Stability or change, structure or adaptability
2. Competitiveness or cooperativeness, and attention to internal or external environments
3. Risk-taking or conservativeness
4. Focus on tasks or on relationships

This typology characterizes four cultural types. The clan is described as a consensual and cohesive culture that emphasizes relationships and morale. The market

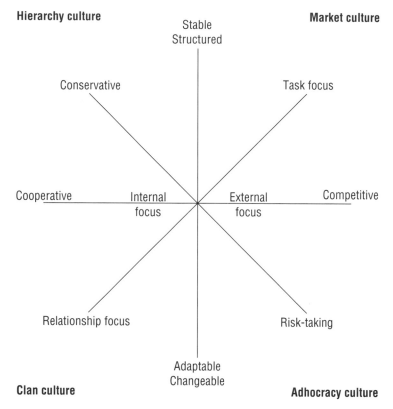

Figure 4.2   *A competing values model of organizational cultures. (Adapted from McDonald &*
Gandz, 1992; Quinn & McGrath, 1985. Used by permission.)

culture differs from the clan. Productivity and efficiency are emphasized in the rational pursuit of objectives. The adhocracy is oriented to change and development, emphasizing transformation and growth. And finally, the hierarchy is oriented to stability and predictability. Regulations and procedures are executed within a structured social hierarchy. These cultures are not easily diagnosed or measured in any precise way. They are generalized types, and a work group is often a mixture of types (Fig. 4.2) (McDonald & Gandz, 1992; Quinn & McGrath, 1985).

Again, elements of all of these cultures can be identified within a typical hospital or agency setting, varying according to task and function. While an operating room might be a structured, stable, and hierarchical setting, the planning department might be most effective as an aggressive, goal-directed market culture. Individual work groups could be clannish or adhocratic. A new ambulatory care team might evidence characteristics of all four cultures. If you were a patient scheduled for surgery, would you prefer an OR team with the culture of the hierarchy or of the adhocracy? Considering the work values of these different types can provide a "culture check": To what extent does your immediate work culture fit the kind of work you do?

Single Cultures

Single, monolithic cultures probably do not exist in reality in pure form, although many successful U.S. corporations of the 1950s through the 1970s were quasi-monolithic cultures. Manufacturing businesses, for example—those making refrigerators, tools, cars, tires—tended to be stable, hierarchical bureaucracies with known values coming from the top management levels. Workers on the assembly lines often developed their own cultures, which could complement or conflict with the dominant culture of executive management. Health care settings, due to the diversity of professional and functional subcultures, have tended to be pluralistic cultures.

A common belief about culture is that organizations that have strong shared values among employees and relatively homogeneous outlooks are more apt to succeed than organizations in which fragmentation of views and goals prevail. Yet both research and practical experience provide convincing evidence that unity and homogeneity are not always positive influences in ensuring organization survival. Organizations that are highly consistent internally are not particularly adaptable, and those lacking a capacity for adaptation may not have a viable future. When an organization has done things in a particular way, its history of success may create a deep but unrecognized threat. Belief in and adherence to the "old ways of succeeding" become the existing cultural value set, greatly inhibiting an organization's capacity for change in the future. Many solid U.S. companies—computer businesses, steel companies, or auto makers—stumbled badly when they continued "business as usual" while the market changed around them. Some hospitals today are tripping over backward-looking attitudes. Increasing facility with forward-anticipation is critical to survival.

Cultural Heterogeneity

Organizational cultures that can use their internal heterogeneity effectively fit best with a complex world. Martin and Meyerson identify three types of organizational cultures: integrated, in which there are shared values across the organization, a culture common to small or new businesses; differentiated, where subgroups are inconsistent or conflicting, typical of many hospitals; or ambiguous (also called fragmented), in which there are uncontrollable complexities, uncertainties, and discontinuities in organizational life. The latter is a state common to many U.S. organizations in the turbulent decade of the nineties (Frost et al., 1991; Martin, 1991; Martin & Meyerson, 1988; Meyerson & Martin, 1987). Health agencies are still more differentiated than integrated, and more ambiguous than they are bureaucratic. Such cultures, while stressful to work in, are adaptive and potentially creative within the current environment.

Subcultures

Subcultures can have varying positive or negative effects on the dominant culture (Aydin & Rice, 1992; Bartunek & Moch, 1991; Gregory, 1983; Perley, 1988; Raelin, 1986; Riley, 1983; Young, 1991). The subcultures' effects may be enhancing—they adhere fervently to and support core values; orthogonal—they accept the core values but also have a separate and nonconflicting set of values particular to themselves; or countercultural—some of their values present a direct challenge to the core values of the dominant culture (Martin & Siehl, 1983; Raelin, 1986; Taft, 1990). On nursing units, the culture of the unit is as significant an influence on staff as is the general culture of the hospital. Use of the Organizational Culture Inventory (OCI), a tool identifying 12 culture types, can provide insight into the variability of the cultures in which nurses work. The types are grouped into four culture styles:

1. Constructive cultures, those valuing achievement and which are humanistic, encouraging, affiliative, and self-actualizing;

2. Aggressive/ defensive cultures, those in which oppositional, power, competitive, or perfectionistic forces may be acting;

3. Passive/ defensive cultures, in which needs for approval, convention, dependency, and avoidance are operating. (Cooke & Lafferty, 1989; Thomas, Ward, Chorba, & Kumiega, 1991)

Yet another way to understand health care cultures is to look at the subcultures of the individual disciplines—nursing, social work, medicine, physical/occupational therapy, hospital administration, dietary—and of the support departments (Aydin & Rice, 1991; Raelin, 1986; Trice & Beyer, 1993). Attributes of gender, race, and social class are correlated with the disciplinary subcultures. Registered nurses, for example, tend to be disproportionately female, white, and middle-class, characteristics that infuse the subculture of nursing. Practical nursing has attracted a greater mix of racial and socioeconomic backgrounds. Although demographic characteristics are changing substantially, physicians have historically been white males from upper-middle or upper-class families, attributes that explain much of the subculture of medicine. The value system of the broader American culture accords status differentially to these clusters of characteristics and to the subcultures. Table 4.1 depicts some of the subcultural characteristics historically associated with three of the health disciplines: nursing, medicine, and health care administration. The typology portrays historical stereotypical differences in cultural orientation across the disciplines, characteristics that are currently in transition (Taft, 1988). The subcultures of the professions consistently fluctuate in the extent to which they:

1. Are congruent with each other

2. Are aligned with the dominant organizational culture

3. Are in tune with the needs and opportunities of society

Relationships among the subcultures are dynamic. Consequently, the culture of the whole may best be characterized as pluralistic. Organizations that experience high degrees of conflict among the subcultures, or disciplines, are also likely to manifest incongruencies as described earlier (Martin, 1991; Martin & Meyerson, 1988; Meyerson & Martin, 1987): differentiation, ambiguity, or fragmentation. **Ethnocentrism** (the tendency to believe in the superiority and importance of one's own cultural view while denigrating the relative importance of others' views) may

Table 4.1 • **Generalized Characteristics of Three Subcultures of Health Professionals**

Characteristics	Nursing	Medicine	Health Care Administration
Major task	Patient care	Diagnosis and treatment of disease	Organizational continuity, managing change and stability
Membership	Historically female, white, middle class; humanistic	Historically male, white, middle and upper class; scientific	Historically male-dominant,* rational
Leading role strength	Comforter, nurturer, health educator	Life-saver and problem-solver; miracle-worker	Keeper of the house, protector
Role centrality	Coordinator of health services	Gatekeeper of health services	Proprietor of health services; holder of the purse strings
Relationships with other professional groups	Collaborative ethic	Autonomy; directing the team Collegiality, equality	Negotiating, seeks cooperation
Model of authority within profession	Hierarchy		Hierarchy
Perspective	Patient-centered, clinical unit/area	Patient- and practice-centered	Hospital's business and market relations
Conflict management	Interpersonal approach	Use leverage available, e.g., resources and authority, to maintain control	Structural and rational approach
Core dilemmas in era of health care reform	Degree of proactivity within context of high uncertainty; traditional vs. new role initiatives	Choice of organizational and network affiliations, and the conditions & extent of affiliations; the future destiny of medical specialists	Where to invest strategic resources in an era of high future uncertainty
Major threats (current)	Decrease in job security; constraints on staffing levels and & other resources; (undesirable) changes in role	Health economics; changes in role; losses in authority, income; malpractice	Organizational survival, job security

*The management of Catholic hospitals, typically run by orders of Catholic sisters, is a notable exception to the generalizations about health care administrators.

further intensify conflicts and misperceptions among subcultures. Each occupational culture may perceive its role as central (Bartunek & Moch, 1991; Gregory, 1983; Taft, 1990).

As noted earlier, subcultural variation in hospitals can be viewed from a nursing unit perspective. Chapter 10 analyzes cultural behavior across types of patient care units. At the unit level, the executive nurse or manager is in a strong position to change the "local" culture. Because unit survival is tied to internal hospital operations, unit work culture is more amenable to direct influence than is that of the organizational culture (Coeling & Wilcox, 1988; Fleeger, 1993).

Executive Nurse Role

The executive, whether a nursing vice president or an operations officer, has a broad view of the organization. The executive participates in the development of strategy and tactics, the allocation of resources, policy-level decision making, and organizational leadership. From these vantage points, the executive understands the plan for continued hospital survival (adaptation) and how future plans may or may not fit with the pre-existing culture. More often than not, the executive is part of the dominant culture of the setting and probably understands how the major cultural subgroups may help or hinder the dominant culture. Considerable attention may need to be focused on the integration of subcultures. As a leader in, and communicator of, organizational survival plans (and therefore as a symbol of the current cultural imperative) the executive provides for hospital personnel and work groups essential leadership for cultural success, translation of strategy into concrete actions. These acts of communication, interpretation, translation, and direction are, under normal circumstances, efforts to bring into alignment the various elements of the health organization. To facilitate congruence among the parts in the pursuit of goals serves both effectiveness and efficiency.

Conversely, under some circumstances, the executive nurse may make a conscious decision to be noncompliant with selected values or norms (del Bueno & Vincent, 1986). The executive may take on a differentiating or a fragmenting role, or may advocate for the subculture of nursing. Such an approach can be deviant, countercultural, or orthogonal. There may be compromises of certain principles that the executive is unwilling to make (e.g., policies or practices that will jeopardize patient safety, or that require dishonest actions) and, under such conditions, it is important to risk a deviant position. The need to make a major organizational change might demand frame-breaking thinking, a questioning of the sacrosanct. The presence of differentiated views within an organizational culture creates the energy essential for change.

There is, of course, risk associated with this, and the executive nurse may test the limits of acceptable deviance. A consistently divergent posture, regardless of the merits of the executive's principles, tends to put the job at risk. There are some organizations that value and thrive on diversity, eccentricity, or perversity. Stories from the computer industry, for example, portray the creative and irascible genius who functions well in a turbulent environment and takes computer technology to a new, unimagined level. Some university faculty are unfailingly outspoken critics of their colleagues or deans. Entrepreneurs, "new paradigm" thinkers, and other "square pegs" rasping against round holes may not always have personalities that blend well with others. The organization that values the creative acts of such individuals, and whose leaders are comfortable with friction and disagreement, supports divergent views as the cultural "way of life" within that setting. Creative conflict has a known, although not guaranteed, association with innovation.

READING THE CULTURE SIGNS

Much has been written in the popular literature about the various manifestations of culture: symbols, rites, rituals, stories, legends, language, humor, and traditions. Cultural manifestations, as described and illustrated in Table 4.2, are the visible expression of a culture and its values. They portray, and continually inform members about, the culture. These definitions have been based on the work of many authors: Trice (1984), Trice & Beyer (1993, 1984), & Schein (1991b, 1987, 1985), del Bueno & Vincent (1986), & Morgan, G. (1986), Hatch (1993), and William Foote Whyte, cited in Jones (1991), Barley (1991) & Martin, Feldman, Hatch, & Sitkin (1983).

Survival Manifested

Typically, the manifestations of culture have a direct or indirect link back to key aspects of survival—either the agency's survival and/or survival strategies for the individuals who work in that setting. Cultural manifestations regularly remind the long-term employee and inform the new employee of "how things are done around here." The training and socialization of new employees, and role modelling of appropriate behavior, are two more explicit means a leader has to influence behavior consistent with cultural realities (Siehl & Martin, 1987).

Stories
Stories provide a rich medium for cultural messages. They implicitly transmit information that is "not talked about." Good stories are simple and memorable. The subjects of stories may be past or current, of negative or positive influence. For example, most employees experience, at one time or another, common human anxieties—feeling insecure, fear of failure, sensing disrespect from others, fear of falling from grace or being "out of favor," feeling subordinate, losing privileges, or being out of control. A common story theme concerns job security: Could I be fired? Laid off? The stories that circulate in a work setting often address these tensions metaphorically. Here is an illustration:

> Employees of a computer software company that has experienced a downturn are worried that the president will be forced to make some radical decisions. Several good alternatives may be available, but employees don't have a good reading on how it might go. There are current stories circulating about The Big Boss: Is the boss "human"? Compassionate? Ruthless? Trustworthy? Experiences employees have had with the boss are widely shared as anecdotes.

Table 4.2 • *The Components and Manifestations of Organizational Cultures*

Culture component	Definitions, descriptions and examples
Culture	A pattern of publicly and collectively accepted meanings operating for a given group of people at the same time. It implicitly interprets a group's own situation to itself. Cultural meanings derive from a group's past experiences with external and internal adaptation
Values	Conceptions of what's desirable. Guides to action and choice. An enduring preference. *Values* may be central (most important, key values) or peripheral, e.g., commitment to patient care; belief in social equality.
Beliefs	Something accepted as true, actual, or real; the mental act, condition, or habit of placing trust or confidence in a tenet or in another person. Convictions, e.g., "I believe in magic."
Norms and taboos, sanctions	Prescriptions and proscriptions of acceptable behavior in a culture. *Norms* = "the shoulds" or "shouldn'ts" of behavior. *Taboos* = "the don'ts." You'll recognize a norm or taboo when you break it! *Sanctions* = the endorsement or countenancing of specified actions by an authority, e.g., shouting at a peer breaks a *norm*, whereas shouting at the Chairperson of the Board breaks a *taboo*. Either, but almost certainly the latter, may result in negative *sanctions*.
Ideology	Relatively coherent sets of beliefs that people share and that explain their cultural realities to them in terms of cause-and-effect relationships. For example, a "traditional viewpoint" or "bureaucratic mentality;" civil rights advocacy; the belief that only men should be leaders.
Metaphors	Images, visual conceptions of the work context. *Metaphors* may vary by gender, ethnicity, and other personal reference groups, or by occupational sub-culture, e.g., the use of sports or gardening metaphors would come from different subcultures. Other common metaphors use military (troops, front line, "the trenches"), sports (captain, team, "go to the mat"), family ("big daddy," sibling rivalry), biological (this place is a zoo), and machine images (well-oiled machine, assembly line).
Symbols and signs	*Symbols* are a medium of cultural interpretation. Anything that represents an association with some wider, more abstract, concept; they make real or more explicit the unconscious or subliminal meanings of cultural values, e.g., the Nightingale lamp. Size and condition of offices; a company logo; hospital locations where heating and cooling are inadequate. A symbol of social equality may be the use of first names among coworkers.
	Signs carry implicit meaning for members of a given group. It is a conventional indicator (e.g., a figure, device, object, emblem, event, word, charecteristic, quality, act, or gesture) which is used to convey an idea; a sign stands for something else, e.g., The disappearance of nursing caps is a *sign* of the times. The sign (the absence of nursing caps) implicitly conveys notions of broad changes in women's and men's social roles.

(continued)

Table 4.2 • The Components and Manifestations of Organizational Cultures (continued)

Culture component	Definitions, descriptions and examples
Ceremonies, rites, and rituals	*Ceremonies and rites* = public events that are planned and dramatic, often conducted before an audience, which in concentrated form recognizes culturally defined accomplishments or acts of social consequence. They heighten and reinforce the shared meanings, the cultural dictates, of what's important. Often involve social roles, and rank and status. May be focused on individuals or on groups. *Rite* = a public and planned event portraying or promoting social acts of positive or negative consequence. *Ceremony* = an occasion connecting two or more rites. *Ritual* = a standardized repetitive set of detailed actions, or scripts, that dictate common processes and practices. Rituals may in some instances be used more to manage anxieties than to produce consequences of practical importance. For example, the charting in patient records may be ritualized (e.g., vital signs q4h); the annual budgeting process is an organizational ritual.
Traditions and customs, conventions	Means of exhibiting and passing down cultural elements from generation to generation. *Tradition* = a time-honored practice or set of practices; modes of thought or behavior followed by a people continuously from generation to generation. *Custom* = a habitual practice followed by people of a particular group. *Convention* = an accepted way of doing something. General agreement on or acceptance of certain practices or attitudes, widely observed in a group; useful to facilitate social interaction, e.g., the tradition of a capping ceremony for student nurses, the custom of wearing a cap, and the convention of putting one's hair up under a cap are all disappearing with changing views of the role of women and men in the American workplace.
Sentiments (e.g., humor, frustration)	*Sentiments* = vague feelings or awareness, sensations. A thought, a view, or an attitude based on feeling or emotion instead of reason, e.g., nurses' reactions to working four weekends in a row; "dark humor" among staff on a children's oncology unit.
Stories, myths, legends, heroes and heroines	*Stories, myths and legends* are narrative tales of fact and fiction. *Stories* give hints on "how to get along here"; "how to succeed, fail, or deal with the boss"; they may also tell members how "special and unique" this place is. *Myth* = a dramatic narrative of actions or events that are imagined or not based on established facts. *Legend* = a narrative, handed down through members, of some extraordinary event that has a basis in history but has been embellished with fictional details. *Heroes and heroines* often concern the founder(s) and significant players in the organization's history who are attributed with bringing life and stature to the enterprise, often overcoming difficult obstacles to do so.
Archetype	An original model or type after which other similar things are patterned; a prototype. An ideal example of a type; quintessence, e.g., Dr. Jekyll was the *archetypal* physician.
Artifacts	Material objects created by people to use in cultural activities. Hospital beds, surgical instruments, patient charts, and IV poles are examples of common *artifacts*.

Stories provide information on events and situations from which employees infer the relative threats to their own jobs.

Negative gossip can move through a workplace like a Texas twister. Is a nursing unit targeted to close? What might happen to my job? What hints do the rumors provide about what I might do, or not do, to enhance my chances of continued employment? In the uncertain world of health care today, stories may circulate about the relative job stability of the chief executive, or other top executives. Change at the top often foreordains changes throughout the organization. What are the current political alignments? How should I behave to avoid an undesirable change in my own position? Stories act like weather vanes.

Needing to feel special, or unique, is a prevalent human need, so stories about the workplace often attribute specialness to one's place of employment. Work stories commonly portray extraordinary feats or acts of brilliance by past or present leaders. Or, they may convey the belief that "there aren't many people who could survive the challenges of working here." Tales may suggest that hiring practices are highly selective, or that "you have to be slightly crazy to work here" (a badge of distinction); or anecdotes may simply remind you that "there's no place like this— this environment is really special." Sometimes the need to feel unique is manifested in "let's pretend" thinking. Stories about specialness are self-enhancing (Martin, Feldman, Hatch, & Sitkin, 1983).

Stories about how an organization deals with obstacles or challenges abound. In large medical centers, a story may start from what employees read about their hospital in the local newspaper. It is circulated through the workplace and, like the child's game of telephone, the insights and speculations of others are added to the original story. In no time an elaborate story has developed (don't you wish official information could be passed so quickly and effortlessly?) The culture processes versions of the "rumor-story" according to the conditions of its own survival situation and the fears and insecurities of its members. A positive story may fuel a burst of confidence and pride in the perceived accomplishments and successes of the organization (Martin, Feldman, Hatch, & Sitkin, 1983). For example, innovation surrounding a medical "first," selection of the medical center as a national site for clinical trials, and reports of an individual patient's "miracle" tale are all stories that create a sense of pride. On the other hand, an unfavorable press report (e.g., the careless handling of radioactive materials) may necessitate a public relations response from the hospital. Individual employees, learning of the hospital's response, will need to make their own peace with the PR statement—specifically, with the perceived truthfulness of the response, the proximity of the events to their own work responsibilities, and the anticipated sanctions that might be brought to bear should their views diverge from the official response.

An Organization's Character
A general indication of an organization's culture is the perceived measure of its "character": the degree of disparity between the espoused values and the values-in-practice (Argyris & Schn, 1974). What is projected outward (to the public) as the image of the institution, or touted as the values and ideals under which it operates, may be perceived by the direct caregivers as disparate from their day-to-day experiences. An incongruence or contradiction exists. Examples of such a disparity in-

clude: a projected image of teamwork on the outside and competition or backbiting in practice; exaggerated claims of professional competencies or skills; characterizations of pure motives when behaviors are in reality based on greed or narrow self-interest; or "prettying up" a situation by misrepresenting the facts or lying (Riley, 1983). The "official" story released of scandal in a government agency, for example, may diverge markedly from the perceptions of the American public. Discrepant portrayals of organizational events lead to inferences about the integrity and trustworthiness of the institution as a whole.

Incongruencies between the espoused values and the values-in-use are not only prevalent in organizations but also inherent to all human collectives (Argyris & Schn, 1974). How often does one hear of the quality services an organization provides (e.g., "excellence in patient care"), knowing that in this setting there are some serious quality problems, or ethical violations, that are not being addressed? There is virtually always a gap between the ideal, (what is espoused) and the real (that which is practiced). And if the real ever catches up to the ideal, the ideal is likely to be elevated still higher. That's the achievement ethic at work.

The critical issue for the culture is not the inconsistency itself but its potency. The impact of the disparity on the culture will be determined by: (1) which organizational values are violated—central or peripheral, and (2) the degree or extent of disparity. Wide discrepancies between values espoused and those in use, and among those values that are most fundamental and important, have a more divisive effect on a workplace culture than will narrow disparities of less significant values. Large misalignments can result, for example, from a change in hospital ownership or governance, a crisis in profitability, or a change in leadership. When an organization is in the process of making major strategic, task, and role changes, it is to be expected that disparities will be great. The turmoil and cultural disruption that come from these circumstances are necessary and expected. But under day-to-day conditions, work proceeds most smoothly when discrepancies between "the company line" and the practices in place are relatively narrow and do not concern the most important or closely held values (McDonald & Gandz, 1992; Nadler & Tushman, 1980; Sackman, 1991).

Missing Signs

Finally, one of the more challenging of cultural manifestations to identify is, paradoxically, what is missing: the absences, gaps, the hidden or invisible, the unspoken (Moore, 1991). When unexpected decisions are made, where did they come from? Who was visibly present, and who behind-the-scenes? Notice who is absent on a key committee. Who is part of a merger steering committee or a community agency and hospital planning group. A health agency culture in one urban area, for example, espouses "one standard of care" for all of its patients. An astute observer might discover, however, that there are separate waiting areas for private and indigent patients; the areas for the former are more lavishly decorated than are those for the latter. Committees organized around merger issues should address issues such as assessing the cultures of all the joining organizations and the activities of each to define the future activities.

In a large medical center, an interdisciplinary quality improvement team, mandated to change admitting procedures to a more user-friendly experience for patients, worked for nine months to develop an innovative and well-integrated admissions process. The team's newly implemented practices were ignored by several private surgeons. Failure to use the new process for admissions to the surgical unit has created some annoying problems: two entirely separate methods are used for admitting patients; there is a likelihood of future mix-ups that will inconvenience patients and families; and costly variances away from efficient resource utilization are occurring. Nonetheless, hospital administration and medical management have failed to take action to correct the surgeons' refusal to use the new process. The failure to ensure compliance has sent negative messages to the hospital culture. For example:

- "Don't try to be innovative or develop patient-friendly processes. Why bother? It won't make any difference anyway."
- "Some [privileged] people can do whatever they want."
- "Obviously, surgeons are more important than the QI Team."
- "Surgeons are more important than patients."
- "Hospital administration doesn't really care about cost efficiencies, or how patients are treated, or what difficulties are created for the rest of us. Favoritism wins out."

Such comments offer telling revelations of the culture.

Culture Created

While there is no one "right" organizational culture, some cultures may provide more positive work environments than others. Certainly those in which individuals feel their work is valued and their impact is meaningful are most rewarding.

All cultures are created by human choices about "how we do things around here." They are our way of creating conditions to ensure survival. Table 4.3 displays eight fictional, simplified hospital types whose cultures have developed based on the pursuit of different strategies.

A close look at the fundamental survival strategies in Table 4.3 provides insight into why a hospital culture develops the way it does. The research-driven medical center, for example, pursues a core strategy of medical innovation, to which medical education is directly linked. Although the medical center's mission places "patient care" as primary, in reality there may be copious cultural evidence that patients don't always come first. This is not to say that patients are jeopardized, or even treated discourteously. One's interpretation of "patient care" can assume a short- or long-term time horizon, or it can be specific to one patient or generalized to future unidentified patients. In a research hospital, priorities in research and education will regularly compete with other pursuits, including direct patient care.

Table 4.3 • Simplified Hospital Culture Types* Deriving from Survival Strategy

Hospital type	Survival strategy and values	Sample characteristics	Examples
Research-driven medical center	• The attraction for patients: Innovation & state-of-the-art diagnostic & treatment methods; cutting edge knowledge in medical science. • Patients referred by: community physicians, self (desire for most advanced treatment), or by national / international network of medical specialists. • Status conferred based on professional reputations & hospital image.	• Medical education usually part of these settings. University affiliation common. • Multiple missions may confuse priorities. • Specialization & subspecialization. • Patients often more complex than in other settings. More tertiary care. • High tech, innovation, fast pace. • Competitive internal environment. • Personnel turnover. • Respect for the authority of persons with advanced knowledge, innovative methods.	• Teaching hospitals or university medical centers. • Examples: –Personnel tend to seek learning & innovation –Physicians, nursing staff, & other disciplines like the thrill of being at the cutting edge of knowledge. For some, striving toward & breaking the knowledge barrier are ends in themselves. The "official line" is that "Patient care always comes first." In reality, however, does it? e.g. –New department heads are selected for their track records in research & grant funding. –It is not unusual for patients to wait in the clinic past appointment times while the residents complete rounds or conferences.

(continued)

*Note: Categories of this table are not mutually exclusive. Hospital cultures are depicted as simplified "pure types" which rarely exist in reality. A mixture of characteristics of two or more of the cultural types is common and expected in any given hospital.

Table 4.3 • Simplified Hospital Culture Types* Deriving from Survival Strategy (continued)

Hospital type	Survival strategy and values	Sample characteristics	Examples
Morally committed institution	• Philanthropic or church-supported organizations. • Ideology driven & defined. • Dependent on volunteer assistance, and an ethic of charity toward "fellow man." • Infusion of fluctuating levels of public funding.	• Resources supplied through philanthropy vary from low to full support levels. • Values strong, explicit; degrees of fervor. • Ideology & beliefs provide energy source, serve to bond members of health team. • Some disparity possible between ideal values & actual practices. • Internal competition not normative.	• Religiously affiliated hospitals. • Free clinics • Community/storefront services provided by indigenous people. • Women's Feminist Health Collective • Examples: –Distribution of free condoms at a family planning clinic. –Catholic hospital: Public anti-abortion notice –Jewish hospital: Mottos of beliefs, creeds, "our ways" framed on walls. Names of big philanthropic givers mounted in brass. –Photos of community volunteers on walls.

(continued)

Table 4.3 • *Simplified Hospital Culture Types* Deriving from Survival Strategy (continued)*

Hospital type	Survival strategy and values	Sample characteristics	Examples

Physician-dominant hospital	• Basic assumption: Physicians are the lifeblood of the hospital, bringing patients in the door. Except through the ER, patients don't walk in by themselves. If not happy, MD's can move their patients to other hospitals.
	
	• Future survival depends upon a continuing cadre of active & loyal medical practitioners.
	
	• Although the future may be different, surgery has been the most lucrative business.
	
	• The community is an important customer.
	
	• Future: Links with physician networks; high level of loyalty desirable.
		• Most U.S. hospitals share these characteristics to some extent.
		
		• Administration views physicians as primary customers.
		
		• There is administrative resistance to alterations in policies, processes, or procedures which require physicians to change and might inconvenience or annoy them.
		
		• Community involvement & activities—with families, groups, & local government. Employees may live in community.
		
		• Conservative regarding change. Little momentum to change, until forced.
		
		• Warm, friendly family feeling.
			• Community hospitals.
			
			• Nurses working in these hospitals may seek a more calm working environment, preferring relatively "high touch, low tech" settings.
			
			• Examples:
			
			  –A community hospital conducted an experiment of keeping patient records outside of patient rooms, rather than at the nursing station. Advantages: Nurses did much less running, & charting completeness & accuracy increased markedly. Attending MD's complained, however, because they didn't want to walk down the halls to review charts. Result: Charts were returned to the nursing station.
			
			  –QA/CQI coordinator, "I love this size of hospital. Coming from a university hospital, I find that my work here can really make a difference."

(continued)

Table 4.3 • Simplified Hospital Culture Types* Deriving from Survival Strategy (continued)

Hospital type	Survival strategy and values	Sample characteristics	Examples
Public hospital	• Public funding, wholly or in part. Health & safety net for citizens.	• Severe financial constraints, resource limitations common.	• Veterans Administration hospitals • Public municipal/county/state hospitals.
	• Dependent on continued good will of public.	• Agency image fluctuates with level of resources.	• City health department; community mental health center.
	• Board members often political appointees from the community.	• Budgeting decisions are far-removed from caregivers.	• Examples:
	• Some hospital appointments may be politically connected.	• Bureaucratic; stolid, limited innovation.	–Board members of a municipal hospital may have little in-depth understanding of health care.
	• Attract under-insured patients or specific populations as part of public mission.	• Scandal-prone. Periodic bursts of public inquiries, pressure, accusations. Little changes below the surface.	–Employees of a county hospital system: Pride in the hospital's ideology; public mission, and its commitment to the poor.
	• High visibility, subject to media attention.	• Job security a priority with many long-term employees.	–Hired to upgrade the level of nursing care, a new nurse exec at a VA hospital left in frustration 18 months later. Her repeated attempts to upgrade care were met with sabotage, sandbagging, and civil service grievances by the "old guard." With civil service protection, individual caregivers could not effectively be held accountable.
		• Civil service system protects some employees with minimal performance levels.	

(continued)

Table 4.3 • *Simplified Hospital Culture Types* Deriving from Survival Strategy (continued)*

Hospital type	Survival strategy and values	Sample characteristics	Examples
Specialty health agency	• Specialty organization, and/or one-of-a-kind in a given geographic area. • Clear, focused mission & expertise; niche. • Development of stable continuing referral sources. • Maintenance of positive reputation critical. • Surveillance of health policy developments in the public sector consistent with or contrary to agency's interests.	• Ongoing nurturing of referral relationships. • Ideological commitment among caregivers. • Ongoing concern with limited service mix, fear of obsolescence; drive to maintain advanced methods of care. • Adaptability necessary as survival insurance. • Strong sense of organization as "special place." • Strict norms of confidentiality with high-profile clients. • Tight culture, tendency toward isolation from professional colleagues outside of agency; an island in the sea.	• Center for psychiatric and substance abuse services for the rich & famous. • Children's rehabilitation hospital. • Single publicly supported general hospital in a dense urban setting, no competition. • Single psychiatric hospital in an urban area, offering comprehensive range of therapies. • Examples: –A Visiting Nurse Service is challenged by the readiness of hospitals to open their own home-based care programs. To hold a competitive edge, they maintain a staff that performs state-of-the-art procedures, and is frequently inserviced. The agency also has on staff a political liaison whose responsibilities are to provide surveillance on health policy, and be actively in contact with key legislators. –Counseling for families of children with birth defects, or those recovering from abuse/neglect. –A suspect in the murder of a prominent socialite "disappears" from public view. He has withdrawn to the protection of an exclusive psychiatric hospital.

(continued)

Table 4.3 • *Simplified Hospital Culture Types* * *Deriving from Survival Strategy* (*continued*)

Hospital type	Survival strategy and values	Sample characteristics	Examples
Networked hospitals & agencies	Linkages among institutions for economies of: Administration; purchasing; consolidation & integration of services; and/or capturing of patient populations and referral relationships. • Vertical and horizontal integration.	• Some agencies in network apt to be large, complex, diverse. • Frequent changes in interorganizational relationships as needs change. Time drain on managers. • Inter-institutional ambivalence re network linkages. • Sibling rivalry & competition among institutions. Occasional strident turf conflicts. • Resistance to imposition of practices from other institutions. • Power sensitivity & resource guarding between hospitals. • Tending toward formal agreements. • Caregivers have difficulty staying "current" with interorganizational arrangements.	• Teaching hospital linked to group of geographically dispersed community hospitals. • Vertical linking across continuum of care: outpatient facilities, inpatient hospital, long-term care facility, home health services, physical therapy practice, physician group practices. • Examples: –A consortium of all hospitals in a low-population rural state, organized to address common needs and to share resources. –Multihospital systems formed for national, regional, or local linkages. Between-hospital referrals within the network capture patient populations.

(*continued*)

Table 4.3 • Simplified Hospital Culture Types* Deriving from Survival Strategy (continued)

Hospital type	Survival strategy and values	Sample characteristics	Examples
Competitive & opportunistic organization	• Aggressive; explicit acknowledgement of pursuit of own self-interests. • Continuous environmental scanning for new opportunities. • Effective links with governmental and social power structures. • Makes friends with VIP's.	• Continuous bold forays to expand services or add to existing services; plays "hardball." • Macho or "cowboy" culture which rewards strategic and technical success. • Competitive internal climate. • Criticism from external community & other agencies common. • Ethic of "charging ahead," not intimidated by criticism.	• Private national hospital chain. • Large, prestigious medical center with a service area beyond local region. • Multi-hospital system. • Examples: –For an elite medical center, a Certificate of Need (CON) is approved to expand bed capacity—even though there are sufficient numbers of pre-existing beds in that community. The local newspaper launches an investigation into the channels of "social pull" & "favoritism," hoping to uncover irregularities. A listing of the members of the Board of Trustees of this institution reveals that they are individuals with numerous business & political connections throughout the state. –When seeking to purchase a hospital in a given area, a national hospital chain sends an "advance person" to assess the local political climate and to determine if sufficient backing can be generated to support the chain's strategy. –A large urban teaching hospital opens satellite clinics within selected affluent communities.

(continued)

Table 4.3 • Simplified Hospital Culture Types* Deriving from Survival Strategy (continued)

Hospital type	Survival strategy and values	Sample characteristics	Examples
Patient-centered institution	• The competitive strategy is to excel at providing a patient-focused and user-friendly environment. • Belief that consumer satisfaction and a strong institutional reputation will compete well in the community and ensure continued survival.	• Organizational processes, inter-departmental relationships, and service delivery are designed with the patient's viewpoint as the central organizing principle. • Friendly, humanistic internal environment. • Some interdisciplinary conflict, but functional. • Often an ethic of moral commitment. May be female-dominant. • "What is good for the patient and family" is primary concern with any organizational change. At times, this belief may be a barrier to innovation.	• Hospice. • Children's hospital. • Community hospital with philanthropic roots. • Home-based care. • Examples: –A community hospital & medical center creates a new oncology unit designed to reflect their patient-centered philosophy. They hold a series of focus groups with oncology patients and with patients' families to determine what architectural designs to incorporate into the unit. –An interdisciplinary service team cares for hospice patients. Caregivers voluntarily attend funeral services when the patient dies. –A children's hospital integrates treatments and therapies into developmentally appropriate activities. –Committed pediatric practitioners take their advocacy for children to the statehouse. –A major urban medical center interviews all AIDS patients at their first post-hospital appointment to determine how care could be improved.

INTEGRATIVE PRINCIPLES

The model of the clan, market, adhocracy, and hierarchy depicted earlier (see Figure 4.2) is based on four dimensions that can provide the infrastructure of workplace culture to achieve integration of culture and effectiveness:

- The extent of focus on the internal and/or external environment
- The degree of hospital stability, direction, and control versus orientation toward change, flexibility and variety. (Denison, 1990)

An examination of the focus on the internal or external environment addresses such questions as: "Is the hospital responsive to society's needs, or is it consumed with the tasks of its own internal functioning?" "Can this culture change to meet new challenges, or will it join the resting place of the dinosaurs?" "Where are the pockets of innovation, and where is the resistance located?" Change within health care organizations during the decades of the 1980s and 1990s has picked up momentum to the degree that many believe there is too much focus on the external environment, and insufficient support for stability and the internal workings of patient care delivery. The magnitude of change that came about with the institution in 1983 of DRG-based reimbursement resulted in part from a relative lack of concern with the external environment and resistance to change prior to that period—specifically, the failure of providers to control steadily rising costs that greatly outpaced inflation. Most health care agencies today are functioning as market and/or adhocracy cultures, as could be seen on the right side of Figure 4.2. However, because the market in most regions is also volatile, a result of restructuring of the entire health industry, there is little stability even within the market culture.

Subgroup cultures in the health disciplines may be at varying points of understanding the overall need for adaptation. Nurses, for example, tend to have a good understanding of the internal environment of organizations but little command of industry economics or external market relationships. Physicians have resisted adaptation, in large part because of impending loss of control and declines in income. All disciplines, and all organizations, need continuity and adaptation simultaneously to survive, but the balance between these two forces, necessary for optimal functioning, cannot be prescribed. The abilities of organizational leaders, including the executive nurse, to orchestrate forward progress successfully with attention to all points on the internal-external and stability-change dimensions separate an innovative organization from a plodder.

Based on the dimensions of stability-change and internal-external focus, four integrative principles of culture are identified in Denison's recent work (1990). Effective organizational cultures tend to embrace certain principles, including:

- Those organizations assuming an Internal Point of Reference tend to follow principles of: Involvement and Consistency
- Those organizations assuming an External Point of Reference tend to follow principles of: Adaptability and Mission

Levels of involvement, consistency, adaptability, and mission are sufficiently important to organizational culture to warrant detailed description.

Involvement

A central tenet of organizational behavior is that effectiveness in organizations is greatly enhanced by the involvement and participation of employees in decisions affecting their work life. With involvement, the individual and work group tend to exercise higher levels of ownership and responsibility which, if applied widely throughout the organization, will contribute to effective organizational functioning. In nursing, there is a prolific literature about nurse empowerment, shared governance, and participative decision making. Research supports the positive influence of involvement on organizational effectiveness. Both formal and informal involvement contribute to effectiveness, but over time the more formal mechanisms appear to be the most critical for success. Involvement of nurses on key hospital-level committees and task forces, for example, is a critical structural and formal medium for a nursing voice. If one assumes that health agencies today evidence a high degree of concern with the external environment, a focus that negatively impacts employees' sense of ownership, then involvement of staff in decision making expands in import as a cultural norm.

Adaptability

The capacity of an organization to read, interpret, and respond successfully to signals from its external business environment bodes well for its effectiveness. Both present and future survival depend on external adaptation, accompanied by internal reorganization (Schein, 1991b, 1987, 1985). With health industry reform, for example, primary care assumes a greater role in the health care delivery system—a manifestation of an external adaptation. In order to achieve internal integration, health agencies must expand the contingent of primary care providers. In addition to rendering primary care services, these providers will serve as gatekeepers for additional utilization of health services. Ambulatory care will continue to expand while inpatient care shrinks. A reliable rule is that external adaptation cannot occur without concomitant internal integration.

Similarly, the ability to respond to internal customers is essential. How would hospitals and health agencies change if every department treated its relationships with the other departments with the customer-mindedness of L. L. Bean? Departments and divisions need flexibility and "customer-mindedness" to work well together. In hospitals, this has been most strikingly demonstrated in the past by the orientation to physicians as key customers. The perceived "customer" base of health care organizations today is expanding to include patients' families, insurance groups, large corporations, other members of health networks, contracting businesses or cooperative purchasing groups, and even the U.S. government (the largest purchaser of health services). In some cases, as in the development of health networks, who is "internal" and who is "external" is changing. Adaptability to both internal and external environments positively influences organizational effectiveness and, ultimately, survival (Denison, 1990).

Consistency

The consistency principle predominates in some of the popular press on organizational culture. The essence of the notion is that a set of values, beliefs, and practices shared widely and relatively consistently by organizational members will guide behavior and result in effective performance. Internalized values guide behavior and synchronize functioning within a setting, creating "normative integration." We know, for example, that personnel systems that reward the high performance of employees are more likely to produce desired outcomes than practices that reward behaviors not connected to performance, such as employee longevity or loyalty (Kerr, 1975). Consistency between desired behaviors and resulting rewards will encourage members to deploy their energies toward what they believe is important for the organization.

The consistency principle, however, does have the potential to conflict with the principle of adaptability. A strong, cohesive culture that does not change to meet the needs of society is not likely to produce an effective organization. Research suggests that high consistency is, in fact, associated with high performance in the short term; over the long term, however, extreme consistency may be a neutral or negative influence on organizational effectiveness. Detroit's automobile industry provides the example of companies who remained consistent with past practices while their customers were asking for something different. Japanese-made cars had cut heavily into the domestic market before auto makers responded with radical changes in the design and quality of American cars.

Mission

Commitment to a shared mission has been identified as a critical cultural attribute for success. The informed participation of members in the vision and goals of their institution strengthens long-term organizational performance. Vision, according to Denison, "allows an organization to shape current behavior by envisioning a desired future state" (1990, p. 14). While any enterprise will undergo virtually constant change, superficial turbulence can be navigated by holding a clear and steady course. A strong mission provides employees with purpose and meaning. In some settings, meaning from work can assume spiritual intensity. Staff members working in the early months of the Clinton White House, for example, were imbued with a religious fervor.

In assessing the extent to which an organization promotes involvement of employees, consistency of values and norms, commitment to a vision and clear mission, and flexibility and adaptation to the external environment, the reader will find that adherence to these principles varies considerably. Inconsistency in application may be an accident of history or a construction of management. In highly turbulent environments, such as the health industry, consistency of values may become either impractical or potentially fatal. Executive management might intentionally create, or encourage, a state of heated disagreement among key players; dissonance can be an essential precursor to "unfreezing" a system and allowing for the consideration of new possibilities (Lewin, 1951). During times of external threat, involvement of employees in major decisions may be suspended until the crisis passes. Trust between managers and employees may be challenged when leaders must act rapidly with minimal employee participation. However, trust need not be destroyed if (a) a trusting relationship pre-exists, (b) employees understand the nature of the crisis, and (c) employees are regularly kept apprised of the situation and given opportunities to discuss it with their leaders. The principles of consistency, involvement, mission, and adaptability, while desirable cultural attributes, must therefore be assessed relative to the environment, the organization's current success in the marketplace, and its future survival prospects.

RELEVANCE OF ORGANIZATIONAL CULTURE

Knowledge of organizational culture is important to the executive for one overarching purpose: understanding the workplace will aid you in accomplishing what you believe to be important. With increasing awareness of cultural meanings, you can select approaches to issues that are congruent with "how things work around here." Greater effectiveness is the desired result.

In addition to aiding effectiveness, understanding the local culture has secondary benefits. Pain and frustration are reduced. One can more strategically pick the battles worth fighting in that culture. An increasingly realistic anticipation of culture shifts, such as when a new CEO comes aboard, may reduce the attendant shock level of radical change. Interdepartmental conflicts, or conflicts due to agency mergers, are more readily diagnosed, and perhaps resolved, when cultural values and survival assumptions are surfaced. Ways to focus and maximize one's influence on nursing practice and the nursing culture become evident when the survival issues are understood.

In settings suffering from extreme scarcity of resources—a state common to many hospitals today—survival choices become more urgent, strategic, hard-nosed, and unsympathetic to practices that might be "nice" to do but won't contribute directly to the immediate fortunes of the hospital. When your values and the values of your workplace do not fit well together, you can better understand the sources of tensions, and you can make an informed choice about staying, altering your aspirations, looking elsewhere for work.

Finally, and most significantly, an executive nurse who has a deep comprehension of culture can influence an organization at its core. Opportunities for advancing patient care practices, expanding nursing roles, or developing new patient services become easier to identify. Of particular importance to the advancement of nursing is the development of resource links with the practice of nursing. Nurses are central to the societal goal of health and the patient care mission of health agencies. A direct connection of nurses to economic flows would enable the profession to develop comprehensive practice more consistent with national health needs and priorities. If nurses are able to command resources directly, both patient care and nursing practice stand to benefit. Reimbursement for advanced practice is one clear link to resource generation—but more need to be developed. Nurses should be leaders in the development and monitoring of clinical quality indicators, not only in nursing but also in cross-disciplinary teams. The health promotion expertise of nursing must be used strategically within health agencies. There is an urgent need for solid research on the clinical impact and effectiveness of nursing interventions. And we must ask ourselves: Are our visions for patient care and the profession of nursing a good fit with societal needs? With the current economic realities of the industry?

The decade of the 1990s is witnessing a dramatic reorganization of health care delivery systems. Many of the changes are good for patients and families, good for the national economy, and good for nurses. Some are frightening to medical specialists, threatening to the utilization of hospital facilities, worrisome to the public, and chaotic and upsetting to hospital employees. Fewer hospitals will be around in the year 2000 than now, but more community- and home-based methods of caring for society's health needs will be in place. It is hoped that long-term care and psychiatric services will become more accessible.

In forcing new strategies for survival, the magnitude of changes that have occurred and will occur in health care are dramatically altering organization cultures. Shifts in financial and technological emphases—from cost-based reimbursement to DRGs, from inpatient to outpatient treatments, from illness intervention to health promotion—are seismic. This is a period of unparalleled opportunity for nurses.

From an individual survival perspective, many of the challenges of leadership call for substantial personal strengths:

- Thinking big, taking risks
- Living with constant and often disorderly change
- Working comfortably with complex information and conflicting factors while staying in touch with what's important
- Experiencing an ongoing state of employment insecurity
- Contributing to others' states of ongoing employment insecurity
- Living with high internalized levels of responsibility for the fate of our organizations—and the dependents of those organizations
- Maintaining clinical and management values concurrently
- Thinking on your feet in a variety of politically charged settings
- Playing hardball, every day
- Developing an ability to reframe and entertain bold new creations

We cannot allow the past to constrain our future.

Summary

It is believed that wisdom is gained with the confluence of age, experience, and common sense. Wisdom is a recognized capability of judgement that springs from deep insight and sound, mature knowledge. It is the ability to see beyond the obvious, through the fog of ambiguity, into enduring truths that are present in the subtleties and tacit meanings of life. A wise person can find the simple patterns within the seemingly complex.

The capability to understand human cultures, with all their murky imprecision and layers of meanings, provides considerable guidance on the road to wisdom—a direction of particular consequence when one is leading others.

Acknowledgments

The author acknowledges with gratitude the careful review, good ideas, and support of several colleagues in the preparation of this chapter: Pamela Tscherne, Denise Emmitt, Gail Bromley, and Shelia Pittman. Having thoughtfully read early rough drafts of the manuscript, they provided me with critical comments and insightful suggestions. Feedback and encouragement from Carolyn Vacanti, Diana Biordi, and Harriet Coeling were also valuable during the formative stages of the writing. My husband, Rick Taft, is acknowledged with special appreciation—foremost for his "care and feeding" of the author, but also for task support. From skillful editing to gofer runs, he added value at critical junctures. My thanks to all of you.

Discussion Questions

1. Describe your work culture and identify strengths and weaknesses that have an impact on quality patient care.

2. What business-as-usual practices or behaviors might be changed to produce greater efficiency, and how would you implement the change in your work setting?

3. In community health nursing, the notion of patient- and family-centered care and health promotion are not new ideas. Nurses' awareness of the need for more health promotion and less costly invasive interventions has been far ahead of that of society. Now, the "great discovery" of patient-centered care and health promotion in our society is making news. Nurses knew this decades ago! Why didn't you listen? But, who is the "you"?

References

Argyris, C., Schn, D. A. (1974). *Theory in practice: Increasing professional effectiveness.* San Francisco: Jossey-Bass.

Aydin C. E., Rice, C. E. (1992). Bringing social worlds together: Computers as catalysts for new interactions in health care organizations. *Journal of Health and Social Behavior, 33* (June), 168–85.

Aydin, C. E., Rice, R. E. (1991). Social worlds, individual differences, and implementation: Predicting attitudes toward a medical information system. *Information and Management, 20,* 119–136.

Barley, S. R. (1991). Semiotics and the study of occupational and organizational culture. In P. J. Frost, et al., eds. *Reframing organizational culture.* Newbury Park, CA: Sage, 36–54.

Bartunek, J. M., Moch, M. K. (1991). Multiple constituencies and the quality of working life: Intervention at FoodCom. In P. J. Frost, et al., eds. *Reframing organizational culture.* Newbury Park, CA: Sage, 104–114.

Blau, P. M. (1986). *Exchange and power in social life.* New Brunswick, NJ: Transaction.

Coeling, H. V., Wilcox, J. R. (1988). Understanding organizational culture: A key to management decision-making. *Journal of Nursing Administration, 18* (11), 16–24.

Cooke, R. A., Lafferty, J. L. (1989). Level V: Organizational culture inventory. Plymouth, MI: Human Synergistics.

Czarniawska-Joerges, B. (1991). Culture is the medium of life. In P. J. Frost, et al., eds. *Reframing organizational culture.* Newbury Park, CA: Sage 285–297.

Deal, T. E., Kennedy, A. A. (1982). *Corporate cultures: The rites and rituals of corporate life.* Reading, MA: Addison-Wesley.

del Bueno, D. J., Vincent, P. M. (1986). Organizational culture: How important is it? *Journal of Nursing Administration, 16* (10), 15–20.

Denison, D. R. (1990). *Corporate culture and organizational effectiveness.* New York: Wiley.

Fleeger, M. E. (1993). Assessing organizational culture: A planning strategy. *Nursing Management, 24* (2), 39–41.

Frost, P. J., Moore, L. F., Louis, M. R., Lundberg, C. C., Martin, J. (1991). *Reframing organizational culture.* Newbury Park, CA: Sage.

Gregory, K. L. (1983). Native-view paradigms: Multiple cultures and culture conflicts in organizations. *Administrative Science Quarterly, 28* (3), 359–376.

Hatch, M. J. (1993). The dynamics of organizational culture. *Academy of Management Review, 18* (4), 657–693.

Jones, G. R. (1983). Transaction costs, property rights, and organizational culture: An exchange perspective. *Administrative Science Quarterly, 28* (3), 454–467.

Jones, M. O. (1991). On fieldwork, symbols, and folklore in the writings of William Foote Whyte. In P. J. Frost, et al., eds. *Reframing organizational culture* . Newbury Park, CA: Sage.

Kerr, S. (1975). On the folly of rewarding A while hoping for B. *Academy of Management Journal, 18* (4), 769–783.

Lewin, K. (1951). *Field theory in social science.* New York: Harper & Brothers.

Martin, J. (1991). A personal journey: From integration to differentiation to fragmentation to feminism. In P. J. Frost, et al., eds. *Reframing organizational culture.* Newbury Park, CA: Sage, 352–355.

Martin, J., Feldman, M. S., Hatch, M. J., Sitkin, S. B. (1983). The uniqueness paradox in organizational stories. *Administrative Science Quarterly, 28* (3), 438–453.

Martin, J., Meyerson, D. (1988). Organizational culture and the denial, channeling, and acknowledgement of ambiguity. In L.R. Pondy, et al., eds. *Managing ambiguity and change.* New York: Wiley.

Martin, J., Siehl, C. (1983). Organizational culture and counterculture: An uneasy symbiosis. *Organizational Dynamics, 12* (2), 52–64.

McDonald, P., Gandz, J. (1992). Getting value from shared values. *Organizational Dynamics, 20* (3), 64–77.

Meyerson, D. E. (1991). Acknowledging and uncovering ambiguities in cultures. In P. J. Frost, et al., eds. *Reframing organizational culture.* Newbury Park, CA: Sage, 254–270.

Meyerson, D., Martin, J. (1987). Cultural change: An integration of three different views. *Journal of Management Studies, 24,* 623–647.

Moore, D. L. (1991). Inside Aunt Virginia's kitchen. In P. J. Frost, et al., eds. *Reframing organizational culture.* Newbury Park, CA: Sage, 366–372.

Morey, N. C., Luthans, F. (1985). Refining the displacement of culture and the use of scenes and themes in organizational studies. *Academy of Management Review, 10* (2), 219–229.

Morgan, G. (1986). *Images of organization.* Newbury Park, CA: Sage.

Nadler, D. A., Tushman, M. L. (1980). A model for diagnosing organizational behavior. *Organizational Dynamics, 9* (2), Autumn, 35–51.

Perley, M. J. (1988). Understanding the culture of health care. *Aspen's Advisor for Nurse Executives, 4* (1), 1, 4–5.

Quinn, R. E., McGrath, M. R. (1985). The transformation of organizational cultures:A competing values perspective. In P. J. Frost, et al., eds. *Organizational culture.* Newbury Park, CA: Sage, 315–334.

Raelin, J. A. (1986). *The clash of cultures: Managers and professionals.* Boston: Harvard Business School Press.

Riley, P. (1983). A structurationist account of political culture. *Administrative Science Quarterly, 28* (3), 414–437.

Sackman, S. A. (1991). *Cultural knowledge in organizations: Exploring the collective mind.* Newbury Park, CA: Sage.

Schein, E. H. (1991a). The role of the founder in the creation of organizational culture. In P. J. Frost, et al., eds. *Reframing organizational culture.* Newbury Park, CA: Sage, 14–25.

Schein, E. H. (1991b). What is culture? In P. J. Frost, et al., eds. *Reframing organizational culture*. Newbury Park, CA: Sage, 243–253.

Schein, E. H. (1987). Coming to a new awareness of organizational culture. In L. E. Boone, D. D. Bowen, eds. *The great writings in management and organizational behavior.* New York: Random House.

Schein, E. H. (1985). *Organizational culture and leadership.* San Francisco: Jossey-Bass.

Shafritz, J. M., Ott, J. S. (1987). *Classics of organization theory. 2nd ed..* Chicago: Dorsey.

Siehl, C., Martin, J. (1987). The role of symbolic management: How can managers effectively transmit organizational culture? In J. M. Shafritz and J. S. Ott, eds. *Classics of organization theory. 2nd ed.* Chicago: Dorsey, 433–445.

Taft, S. H. (1990). Consulting for professional organizations: Issues and challenges. In C. N. Jackson, M. R. Manning, eds. *The organization development annual. Vol. 3. Diagnosing client organizations.* Alexandria, VA: American Society for Training and Development, 76–85.

Taft, S. H. (1988). Professional cultures of medicine, nursing, and health care administration: A study in internal integration in a changing organization. Unpublished doctoral dissertation. Cleveland: Case Western Reserve University, Department of Organizational Behavior.

Thomas, C., Ward, M., Chorba, C., Kumiega, A. (1991). Measuring and interpreting organizational culture. In M. J. Ward, S. A. Price, eds. *Issues in nursing administration: Selected readings.* St. Louis: Mosby, 11–119.

Trice, H. M. (1984). Rites and ceremonials in organizational culture. In S. B. Bacharach, S. M. Mitchell, eds. *Perspectives on organizational sociology: Theory and research.* Vol. 4. Greenwich CN: JAI Press.

Trice, H. M., Beyer, J. M. (1993). *The cultures of work organizations.* Englewood Cliffs, NJ: Prentice-Hall.

Trice, H. M., Beyer, J. M. (1984). Studying organizational cultures through rites and ceremonials. *Academy of Management Review, 9* (4), 653–669.

Wiener, Y. (1988). Forms of value systems: A focus on organizational effectiveness and cultural change and maintenance. *Academy of Management Review, 13* (4), 534–545.

Young, E. (1991). On the naming of the rose: Interests and multiple meanings as elements of organizational culture. In P. J. Frost, et al., eds. *Reframing organizational culture.* Newbury Park, CA: Sage, 90–103.

INNOVATOR AND EVALUATOR OF NEW ORGANIZATIONAL MODELS

PART II

Maryalice Jordan-Marsh
Susan R. Goldsmith
Paula V. Siler
Elisa Sanchez
Peggy Nazarey

CHAPTER 5

The Community Design Model

Introduction

In a reform climate, national trends offer new opportunities for innovative approaches to organizational change. As current strategies for improving health care delivery become increasingly ineffective, it is clear that new competencies and new partnerships are required. Traditionally, health care providers have interacted with each other in a parallel play, "hand off" (to the next person) style. Schools of medicine and nursing have emphasized individual expertise and independent decision making (Farrell & Robbins, 1993). This style of interaction is becoming increasingly dysfunctional in an era of cooperation and teamwork. In the twenty-first century, successful leaders will construct and participate in meaningful partnerships with multiple stakeholders across the health care continuum (Farrell & Robbins, 1993).

This chapter focuses on strategies for managing transitions at the organizational, team, and individual levels. Specific attention is given to structural innovations that can be initiated by the executive nurse in concert with an interdisciplinary team. These strategies and innovations are described in the context of the Community Design Model. The Community Design Model is an organizational design developed at Harbor–UCLA Medical Center that serves as a framework for broad organizational change.

NATIONAL TRENDS AND PARADIGM SHIFTS

Recent major trends have changed the context of health care delivery. These include changing social norms, cost constraints, burgeoning technology, increasing regulation, and the evolution of a radically different work force (Seitz, Donaho, & Kohles, 1992). These external forces will precipitate changes at many levels. The effect of these issues on health care policy at all levels is similar to what might happen to players in a game where the rules (and even the players) have changed. Those left in the game recognize the need for new strategies, and for approaches to both resolving old problems and responding to emerging obstacles. Proactive strategies can be as extensive as systemic reform and broad organizational change, or as focused as creating self-directed work teams within a unit. At all levels, there have been paradigm shifts in responses to change. These paradigm shifts include the following.

- At the national level, widespread public sentiment for change led to the establishment of President Clinton's Health Care Reform Task Force. The task force looked at basic reconfigurations of payer and service arrangements under the umbrella of managed collaboration (Dauner, 1993). These changes, although beyond the scope of this paper, provided the backdrop for subsequent shifts occurring at the institutional (or organizational), group (or team) and individual levels.

- At the institutional level, the trend is toward broad organizational change that is comprehensive and systemic in nature. The focus is on reengineering basic business philosophy and decision-making practices. "Why do we do what we do?" is as important as "How can we improve on what exists already?" (Hammer & Champy, 1993). Reengineering is driven by the need to become more customer focused and cost effective. Transformation of this type requires new configurations of players, from different disciplines and levels, collaborating on change efforts.

- At the group level, teams have been reactivated as the basic work unit (Howe, 1993). Work is redesigned and roles reconceptualized to accommodate the specialized needs of the team, and to facilitate customer-centered decision making. Continuous quality improvement, with its emphasis on stakeholder representation in process improvement, has been instrumental in crystallizing this shift.

- At the individual level, new expectations (philosophical and behavioral) are evolving for the person as a team player. Interdependence, consensus decision making, mutual accountability, open communication, and cultural sensitivity with shared vision and values are essential tools for the effective team player. Shared accountability through formal and informal leadership roles is expected from individual team members.

The reform climate invites meaningful change at all levels. The executive nurse and other leaders in the health care field can wait for changes to be dictated by external groups (through government mandates and payer requirements) or they can take the initiative at the local level through broad organizational change. Development of a shared vision and values, an organizational design model, and behavioral change at the individual level assist leaders in initiating this level of change.

VISION, MODEL, AND BEHAVIOR INTERPLAY

Executive nurse leadership roles have evolved dramatically from the decades when nursing practice was dictated by physicians. One trend realized in the 1980s was a move away from the subordinate director of a service unit to the accountable "leader" of a professional clinical department (Aydelotte, 1988). With increasing visibility and input into organizational decision making, executive nurses no longer simply follow instructions. In many organizations, the executive nurse has become a key member of the organizational executive team, and is accountable for a major component of patient care delivery. In the 1990s, the executive nurse often assumes a leadership role in the initiation of broad change and creation of the strategic focus for the organization.

The contemporary executive nurse has new opportunities and supports for being involved in creating and articulating the organizational vision and values, selecting and/or designing the model for change, overseeing implementation, and documenting outcomes. Today's executive nurse is a transformational leader who "commits people to action, who converts followers into leaders, and who converts leaders into agents of change" (Bennis & Nanus, 1985, 3). This twenty-first-century leader acts as a facilitator of change, has experience in process improvement, is statistically minded, and works through teams.

Three ingredients of successful change efforts are primary tools for today's executive nurse: (a) a guiding vision and values, (b) an organizational design that supports the vision, and (c) the ability to design and inspire behavioral change at the individual level (Fig. 5.1). Vision and values are the basis for change at the organizational level. Vision and values are unique to the organization and encompass short- and long-range projections. Organizational design reflects the way the organization operates and sets in motion the way change will be planned and maintained. Organizational designs can be applied in many settings. Behavioral change refers to shifts that individuals make to adapt to the vision and embody the values.

The remainder of this chapter describes strategies of the executive nurse at Harbor–UCLA Medical Center, working in concert with an interdisciplinary team (referred to here as the "Executive Leadership Team") in creating a shared vision

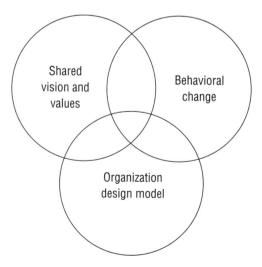

Figure 5.1   *Three ingredients of broad-scale organizational change. (Copyright © 1993, Harbor–UCLA Medical Center.)*

and values and an organizational design model, and inspiring and supporting behavioral change at the individual level. This work is characterized by major structural innovations and transitions at the organizational, team, and individual levels.

ORGANIZATIONAL LEVEL
Structural Innovations and Transitions

Structural innovations and transitions at the organizational level are based on the development of a program for broad organizational change. Strategies to initiate this change include developing a shared vision and values and an organizational design model. The vision and values of a community of patient care leaders, and the Community Design Model (CDM), were initiated by the executive leadership team at Harbor–UCLA Medical Center. This work was advanced by participation in an innovative nursing program. Strengthening Hospital Nursing: A Program to Improve Patient Care (SHNP) is a jointly sponsored initiative by The Robert Wood Johnson Foundation and The Pew Charitable Trusts. Direction and technical assistance are provided by St. Anthony's Health Care Foundation, Inc., under the leadership of Barbara A. Donaho, RN, MN, FAAN. Strengthening Hospital Nursing Program includes 68 large and small, teaching and nonteaching hospitals in 19 states and the District of Columbia. Participating organizations are developing innovative models for improving patient care services through institutionwide restructuring.

Development of shared vision and values is the first stage of facilitating broad organizational change. Vision is the catalyst for broad organizational change. It is a statement of a preferred future that represents the organization's values and reflects what has meaning and importance. A clear vision is essential to successful organizational restructuring. The interactive "backwards" planning approach, identification of an "ideal present" (Flower, 1992), replaces the traditional crisis-intervention model predominant in health care. Ackoff's interactive management model (Flower, 1992, p. 65) starts by asking where you want to be right now and then planning backwards from where you want to be to where you are. The executive nurse facilitates the transition to this new orientation through planning and stakeholder involvement. A primary role of the executive nurse is to engage stakeholders in the vision, provide support for new values, and offer guidance for broad-scale organizational change.

At Harbor–UCLA Medical Center, the vision is to become a community of patient care leaders. In this vision, everyone is a leader and everyone is a member of the campus community (as a stakeholder). The executive leadership team at Harbor–UCLA was responsible for initiating and facilitating the envisioning process. The process began with formation of a values statement entitled "We Care," and expanded to incorporate development of a shared vision. This process included the collaboration of over 35 campus representatives and the coordination of over 200 responses from stakeholders across the campus.

The Community Design Model

The next step in broad organizational change is the selection or development of an organizational design that drives the strategic management of change.

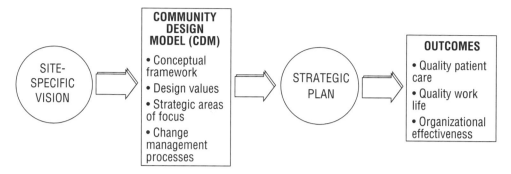

Figure 5.2 *Reengineering process using the community design model. (Copyright © 1993, Harbor–UCLA Medical Center.)*

Organizational design is a way of operating tailored to an organization's unique vision, philosophies, and strategies. Organizational design addresses how the work is accomplished on a day-to-day basis while simultaneously supporting the vision. It also serves as a framework for guiding organizational change. If the organizational design does not support the vision, it negatively impacts both the short- and long-term goals. An organizational design identifies how people relate to each other, the organization, and the environment in accomplishing common goals. As resources become increasingly limited, mental models of relationships become more important (Senge, 1990). The framework provides direction for a strategic plan shaped by the vision and values that characterize these relationships and for an evaluation plan of the outcomes of the organizational design.

The CDM is an example of a framework for broad organizational change that is vision-centered and has a conceptual base. The purpose of the model is to assist organizations in the process of achieving their vision. The CDM has potential for application in diverse settings with distinct visions. The CDM is a framework for organizations whose goals are to achieve: vision-based, quality, customer-centered service; a quality work life for staff; and organizational effectiveness. The model has four key components: A conceptual base, strategic directions, outcome indicators, and strategic management processes (Fig. 5.2).

Conceptual Base
The conceptual base of the CDM is built on the assumption that success requires creating an internal sense of community, in combination with the expectation that every stakeholder (patients, faculty, staff, students) is a leader. The conceptual base is built on six major constructs (Fig. 5.3), with a coordinating focus on strategic management. The complementary constructs are community, transformational leadership, harmony, transitions, and the learning organization.

Strategic Directions
Strategic directions are a means of transforming the vision from "vapor to paper and paper to practice" (Miura, 1992 personal communication). The assumption in the CDM is that attention to these four strategic directions will create an organiza-

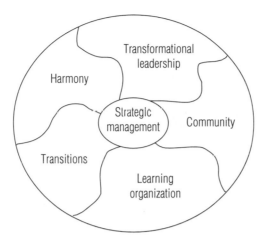

Figure 5.3 *Community design model conceptual framework. (Copyright © 1993, Harbor–UCLA Medical Center.)*

tion that is long-lasting and responsive to changes that support quality customer-centered service, quality work life, and organizational effectiveness. The areas of strategic focus in the CDM are: creation of a community initiative; establishment of a leadership culture of continuous improvement; development of a user-friendly environment that empowers stakeholders; and development of systems to facilitate transitions.

Outcome Indicators
The development of outcome indicators is an important part of applying the CDM. Outcome indicators reflect the organizational vision and are the focus of measuring and evaluating strategic plan elements. Our outcome indicators are culture, structures, systems, and learning/competencies.

Strategic Management Processes
The CDM outlines various processes that support restructuring through reengineering. The critical attributes of the model include a focus on teamwork, empowerment, a sense of belonging, decentralized decision making, and the development of human potential. The structures required to support the change efforts address developing interdependence through teams, shared decision making at the service level, communication, and governance across the institution.

Processes for facilitating change are critical to successful implementation of the model. These are the use of interactive planning in strategic management, attention to transition management, shared vision and values, flattened hierarchies, recognition and rewards, information flow, and development of a learning organization. The methods to accomplish this are work redesign, role reconceptualization, systems development, leadership development, team building, and diversity management.

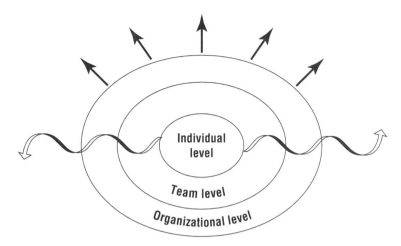

Figure 5.4   *Expansion of organizational change. (Copyright © 1993, Harbor–UCLA Medical Center.)*

TEAM LEVEL

Change agents can be most influential if they view themselves, not as a force upon an inert object, but as an initiator of motion that sets off other motions, creating a ripple effect. Senge refers to this cause-and-effect phenomenon as *systems thinking* (Senge, 1990). The executive nurse in a change agent role facilitates systems thinking by creating a core team that will precipitate formation of subsequent teams/rings. The advantage of this approach is that each previous team is a member of a larger team, to the point where all organizational members are part of one large team with each ring having an effect on all others (Fig. 5.4).

Structural Innovations

In applying broad organizational change, it is beneficial to identify what works already, capitalize on it, and expand it to become part of change efforts. At Harbor–UCLA, many preexisting factors set a firm foundation for broad change efforts. These included: successful internal partnerships between nursing, medicine and administration; successful external partnerships between the medical center and UCLA schools of medicine and nursing; and implementation of a team model at the executive level (as well as within the department of nursing).

Organizational innovation called for an executive leadership or design team that would cross traditional boundaries. This new team would act as a catalyst and prototype for the creation of other teams. At the onset, the team configuration included the top executives: the hospital administrator, the director of nursing, and the medical director, whose influence was balanced by adding senior and mid-level executives with specialized responsibilities that spanned administrative and clinical departments; the associate hospital administrator for operations; the director of nursing research; and the director of professional practice affairs for nursing. An additional element was the inclusion of staff members responsible for facilitating the change effort: a project coordinator, an organizational development specialist, and a project administrative assistant. Staff backgrounds and educational experiences are diverse, ranging from business to education, with only one from health care. These diverse perspectives continually challenge the executive team to question basic assumptions and communicate understandably to non–health care stakeholders.

The configuration of the design team at Harbor–UCLA is one example of a microcosm team. A *microcosm team* is one in which all disciplines and interests in the organization are included (Senge, 1990). The team does not literally include every organizational stakeholder group, but creates a balance among members, so that diverse stakeholder interests are considered. Through a deliberate understanding of group process and strategic management, each member of the team makes it a point to consider all known opinions and needs. For example, recognizing that one team cannot be aware of all interests, the design team gathered information through planning teams, focus groups, and surveys.

Transition

At the time this executive-level design team was developed, there was little precedent or guidance. Lawler observed that "a great deal is known about how to structure and manage production teams in an organization, but virtually no research discusses work teams at the senior management level" (Lawler, 1992, p. 274). Driving the inception of the design team was an intuitive need to make the team reflective of the medical-center community. Community values were symbolized at the design-team level with respect to (a) the tension between development of internal expertise versus dependency on external consultants, (b) diversity of the group with respect to background, and (c) a clinical versus administrative orientation. Deliberate strategies were used in the design team's development to create a sense of belonging, facilitate accountability and ownership, provide opportunities for team learning, and build from a base of shared vision and values.

Using the team-as-microcosm approach allows for pilot testing of change strategies. For example, a team that can adopt "reflection-in-action" (Schön, 1990), that is, can extrapolate from its own responses to anticipate the effect of changes throughout the organization. Buy-in and resistance can be understood, predicted, and planned. An objective facilitator can assist a microcosm group in its self-reflection and action.

Using microcosm teams as the core planning and implementation unit can also accelerate change. Team members experience behavioral change through previously described pilot testing of change efforts. Individual change creates a ripple effect throughout the organization as members communicate and engage in new behaviors among other stakeholders. At the design-team level, team configuration is critical, because members perceive themselves as directly accountable for "walking the talk." It is imperative that microcosm team members represent the leadership ranks (formal and informal) of the organization, touching into many departments and organizational levels. In creating the microcosm team, some members should be selected for their content or process expertise. Team members who recognize and accept their role as change agents can use learned strategies to spread change efforts to their respective stakeholder groups.

INDIVIDUAL LEVEL

Integrated delivery systems are altering the way health care providers interact within the health care community. Health care provider roles, behaviors, and skills are undergoing significant reevaluation and adjustment. New competencies are required for all health care executives (Farrell & Robbins, 1993). These core competencies are the basic skills required to bring about the organizational vision and design model.

Internal Community Structure

In the CDM, groups relate to each other in the context of an internal community. Individuals create and maintain this community across groups through transformational leadership. Community building and transformational leadership are core competencies.

As health care groups undertake reform in the 1990s and struggle to become patient centered and worker sensitive, the concept of community has broad appeal (Department of Nursing, 1990; Friedman, 1993). The community approach offers to bring people together to achieve a common goal without compromising diversity or individual identity (Thomas, 1991).

In building community, people (and their relationships) are recognized as the organization's greatest resource (Hammer & Champy, 1993; Lawler, 1992). Development of stakeholders as potential leaders, in the context of the community, is a cornerstone of the Community Design Model.

Core Competencies

Transformational leadership is an interpersonal orientation to bringing about change in groups and/or organizations. The mission of the transformational leader is to engage individuals and groups in shifting to new relationship paradigms to accomplish common goals. Transformational leadership competencies include (Healthcare Forum, 1992):

- Mastering change to help organizations view change as an opportunity for new alternatives and calculated risk taking.

- Systems thinking to understand interrelationships and patterns in solving complex problems.

- Shared vision to craft a collective organizational vision of the future.

- Continuous quality improvement to engender a never-satisfied attitude, which supports an ongoing process to improve clinical and service outcomes.

- Redefining health care to focus on healing, changing lifestyles, and the holistic interplay of mind, body, and spirit.

- Serving the public to weld social mission to organizational objectives and actions (Block, 1993).

Transformational leaders are instrumental in building community as they help inspire vision and translate that vision into reality (Bennis & Nanus, 1985).

Transitions

At Harbor–UCLA, the executive nurse has initiated and supported many strategies and innovations at the organizational, team, and individual level to assist in community building and transformational leadership. These innovations are standardized across the team model and encouraged at the individual level (Table 5.1).

*Table 5.1 • **Building Community Through Transformational Leadership***

	Strategies/Innovations

Organizational Level Interventions	• *Community Design Model/Organization Design*
	• *Outcome Dimensions*
	• *Strategic Plan*
	• *A Constellation of Empowerment Strategies*
	  –Decision-making model
	  –Third-party facilitation
	  –Ground rules and guidelines
	  –Win/win agreements
	  –Decentralized decision-making
	  –Visible agenda and group memory
	  –Oversight (versus implementation)
	  –Feedback loop plan: no surprises, no "dumping," delegation
	• *Changes in the New Roster of Players*
	  –New co-leader partners
	  –Principle of inclusion versus exclusion
	  –Non–health care stakeholders
	  –Interdisciplinary teams which mix administrative, clinical people
	  –Votes for support staff who attend meetings
	  –Continuity through a consistent staff member attending a broad range of meetings

Team Level Interventions	• Ground rules • Centering exercises (warm-ups and other structured experiences) • Check-in time at beginning of team meeting (setting the expectation that members share issues from the workplace and links to their personal lives) • Humor and metaphors • Formal and informal structures • Accountability for outcomes at the team level • Strategic management tool kit
Individual Level Interventions	• Deliberate modeling of behaviors that reflect new values and expectations • Creative tension: experimentation and failure are learning strategies • Internalizing and sharing the CPCL vision • Hands-on leadership • Visualizing, diagramming, use of visual metaphors • Active participation versus attendance • Ownership • Lateral thinking: constellations • Systems thinking

(Copyright © 1993, Harbor–UCLA Medical Center.)

Summary

At no other time in history has there been a greater need for leadership (Farrell & Robbins, 1993). Executive nurses can help fill this void through transformational leadership and broad organizational change. This change is facilitated through development of a shared vision, adoption of an organizational design model, and creation of new expectations and support for behavioral change at the individual level. The Community Design Model is one option for broad organizational change that is consistent with national trends toward building a sense of community and individual leadership. The Community Design Model offers the executive nurse the opportunity to create true change at the organizational level, which will enhance reform at state and national levels.

Discussion Questions

Interactive planning is critical to the implementation of the Community Design Model.

1. Describe the planning steps you would use to initiate and implement this model in your own health care setting.

2. How would you use the organizational, team, and individual interventions?

References

Aydelotte, M. K. (1980). Myrtle K. Aydelotte. In T. M. Schorr, A. Zimmerman (Eds.), *Making choices, taking chances: Nurse leaders tell their stories* (pp.7–14). St. Louis: C. V. Mosby.

Bennis, W. G., & Nanus, B. (1985) *Leaders: The strategies for taking charge.* New York: Harper & Row, 1985.

Block, P. (1993). *Stewardship: Choosing service over self-interest.* San Francisco: Berrett-Koehler.

Dauner, C. D. (1993). California health reform decisions. *California Hospitals*, May/June, 13–16.

Department of Nursing. (1990/May). Harbor-UCLA Medical Center: A community of patient care leaders transitioning to a culture of empowerment. Grant proposal. Torrance, CA: Harbor-UCLA Research and Education Institute, Inc.

Farrell, J. P., & Morley M. R. (1993). Leadership competencies for physicians. *Healthcare Forum Journal*, July/August, 39–42.

Flower, M. New tools, new thinking. *Healthcare Forum Journal*, March/April, 62–67.

Friedman, E. (1993). Concepts of community. *Healthcare Forum Journal*, May/June, 11–17.

Hammer, M., & Champy, J. (1993). *Reengineering the corporation: A manifesto for business revolution.* New York: HarperCollins.

Healthcare Forum. (1992). *Bridging the leadership gap in health care.* Executive summary. San Francisco: Author.

Howe, G. S. (1993). Team spirit. *Executive Excellence*, July, 19.

Lawler, E. E. (1992). Identify work design alternatives. In *The ultimate advantage: Creating the high-involvement organization*(pp. 77–121). San Francisco: Jossey-Bass.

Schöen, D. A. (1990). *Educating the reflective practitioner.* San Francisco: Jossey-Bass.

Seitz, P. M., Donaho, B. A., & Kohles, M.K. (1992). Initiatives to restructure hospital nursing services. In L. H. Aiken, C. M. Fagin (Eds.), *Charting nursing's future: Agenda for the 1990s* (pp. 98–107). Philadelphia: J. B. Lippincott.

Senge, P. M. (1990). *The fifth discipline: The art and practice of the learning organization.* New York: Doubleday Currency.

Thomas, R. R. (1991). *Beyond race and gender: Unleashing the power of your total work force by managing diversity.* New York: American Management Association.

Sharon Aadalen
Annette McBeth
Lynette Froehlich
Mary Kay Hohenstein
Shirley Raetz
Kathryn Schweer

CHAPTER 6

Transforming Health Care Systems

Introduction

The executive nurse for the twenty-first century is the shaper, as well as the product of, twentieth-century technological and social change (Murphy & DeBack, 1991). In the face of appalling access inequities in a system dominated by medical care, nursing leadership has called for a national health policy (Milio, 1981) and health care reform (ANA, 1991). As this reform is taking shape locally and nationally, executive nurses role-model leadership by collaboration and partnership, thus redefining leadership and power for health care in terms of relationships (Burns, 1978; Wheatley, 1992).

Leadership can be transactional (exchange of valued things) or transformational. Leadership for the twenty-first century will be transformational, engaging people so that leaders and followers raise one another to higher levels of motivation and morality. The touchstone for measuring quality of leadership (for the individual executive nurse, nursing profession, and systems of health care) is its degree of actual accomplishment. Executive nurses for the twenty-first century know that power is a byproduct of moral leadership. The empowerment of all contributors to health care and the celebration of the dignity of both leaders and followers are inherent in moral leadership. Nursing as a profession has earned the public trust, and executive nurses preserve this trust through leadership integrity.

Speaking in this chapter are the voices of executive nurses in service and education organizations within Health Bond, the project funded by the Robert Wood Johnson Foundation/Pew Charitable Trusts in south central Minnesota to strengthen hospital nursing and improve patient care. Executive nurses from the three member hospitals and two partner schools within this consortium shared their perspectives through individual interviews conducted in July 1993.

EMERGENT STRUCTURES

New health care structures and models are being tested throughout the country. Decentralized, innovative care delivery systems within hospitals and beyond-the-walls models of health care are forming. A call has been issued by the American Hospital Association for the formation of community care networks. Bipartisan legislation in Minnesota is calling for the formation of integrated service networks. Over the past four years, Health Bond has been demonstrating the development of service-education partnerships. Consortium-shared governance and collaborative relationships evolving through Health Bond activities have formed essential building blocks for an emerging community-care network within south central Minnesota.

TRADITIONAL POWER

During much of the twentieth century, executive-nurse power and authority, in the majority of health care settings, was maintained through:

- Position
- Management focus (centralized planning, direction, problem solving, control, and discipline)
- Autocratic (top-down), rigid processes
- Fiscal focus
- Rewards, punishment

Positional Power

Ascribed positional power was a preeminent value in bureaucratic, hierarchical health care organizations; leadership was not. James McGregor Burns (1978, 18) notes, "To control things . . . is an act of power, not leadership, for things have no motives. Power wielders may treat people as things. Leaders may not." Annette McBeth, vice president at Immanuel St. Joseph's Hospital (ISJ), points out that the traditional view of leaders was deeply rooted in an individualistic, competitive, and nonsystemic world view. The world was seen as technical, mechanical, and rational, reducible to discrete parts through analysis, and put together again through fairly simple summation. Hierarchical, bureaucratic organizational structures were unquestioned.

Among administrative positions, in many settings, there was a hierarchy of power. The executive nurse in a hospital may not have been on equal footing with nonnursing administrators, and as such was more a reactor to internal and external environmental changes.

In the academic setting, the dean of a school of nursing was in a different position from other deans who did not have to prepare graduates for licensure. Given nursing's later arrival in academia, the nursing dean (and nursing faculty) had a continuing challenge being accepted as peers scholars and administrators.

Management Focus

The health care position at the top of an organization, department, or corporation was the seat of power. Centralization of decision making in the hospital's chief-executive position in small rural primary-care facilities like Health Bond's Arlington Municipal Hospital (AMH) or Waseca Area Memorial Hospital (WAMH) resulted in ineffective utilization of scarce human resources.

A large percentage of the executive nurse's time predictably focused on short-term issues rather than on trends and collective learning. The executive nurse was micromanagement-oriented; this person, not the immediate supervisor of a service or unit, handled operational issues.

Autocratic Top-Down Process

Shirley Raetz, executive nurse at WAMH, one of Health Bond's rural primary-care hospitals, described the executive nurse as "The Boss. What she said, everybody did."

An autocratic, hierarchically organized, inflexible system of rules and regulations resulted in an "unnurturing" environment in some organizations, noted Mary Kay Hohenstein, instructional dean for the health and safety division, South Central Technical College (SCTC).

Fiscal Focus

If the nursing department had control of its own budget, the executive nurse had total budgetary control. McBeth (ISJ) recalls that in acute care the focus was on the dollars. The executive nurse may have kept an eye on clinical outcomes, but without question the bottom line was the driving force.

Rewards and Punishments

Kathryn Schweer, dean of the school of nursing, Mankato State University (MSU), recalls that if events didn't go the way the executive wished (even if successful), the executive nurse (or his or her boss) could punish. Sometimes innovators were punished for not being successful in the traditional way. The executive had power to reward or punish people, behaviors, projects. If things went well (in the direction the executive desired), the person may have been promoted.

EMERGENT SOURCES OF POWER

Executive nurses in the 1990s retain positional power, the ultimate "buck stops here" authority, according to Schweer (MSU). They continue to be expected to set the direction, be enthusiastic and energetic, and make necessary decisions appropriate to their responsibility, authority, and accountability. The executive nurse continues to have to react to change and system redesign (highly likely when a new president comes to campus or a new chief executive comes to a health care system). Hohenstein (SCTC) notes that the executive nurse facing the 1990s is more likely to be an equal partner at the planning table.

Health Bond executive nurses agree. For the future, the authority of their leadership lies in their ability to work with and through people and be transformers of current reality to a new shared vision of a desired future. These executives clearly describe executive nurse leadership for health care into the next century using these kinds of terms:

- Visionary
- Ethical
- Empowering
- Reflective
- Health-outcome oriented
- Generalist
- Collaborative
- Community-oriented
- Team player

The adoption of systems theory (von Bertalanffy & Rapoport, 1956 and seq.) across disciplines during the second half of the twentieth century has had a profound effect on the world view of health care executives. Executive nurses have been "early adopters" of this innovative way of thinking (Havelock, 1969; Rogers, 1983). Further developments, such as chaos theory (Gleick, J., 1987) have challenged the way we think about everything . . . and resulted in the evolution of a new focus on leadership for the future (Wheatley, 1992).

Visionary

The effective executive nurse for the future has "commitment to a vision and articulated goals, and the ability to help people work together to build 'shared vision,' 'our vision,'" according to the executive nurses in Health Bond. Contrasting the traditional view of leadership with the new view of transformational leadership, McBeth states that, "All the analysis in the world will never generate a vision."

Peter Senge (1990, p. 205) speaks of the discipline of "shared visioning" as one of the disciplines of the learning organization. In the Health Bond Consortium, executive nurses have role-modeled shared visioning at the organizational, interorganizational, intercommunity, and interregional levels. These executives know how important it is to be responsive (versus reactive) to other change makers and stakeholders in their spheres of influence. McBeth (ISJ) states:

> It's critical there be a high-level working relationship with any of the individuals who are leading health care in the community. Region 9 Development Commission is a key player bringing people together from a nine-county region (county commissioners, laypeople, business community representatives, education and service health care providers) who have traditionally been in competition with each other to a focus on a common goal. I choose to become involved with Region 9 Development Commission because it gets me into the community in a different way (from my position in the hospital).

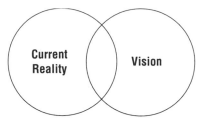

Figure 6.1   *Overlapping image: Vision and current reality. (From P. Senge, 1990.* The Fifth Discipline: The Art and Practice of the Learning Organization. *New York: Doubleday. Used by permission.)*

Raetz (WAMH) recognizes that the executive nurse's focus can no longer be on one's own organization, patients, and staff. "We have to look at the whole of the health care system and how patients and families move through it, from regional primary care to tertiary care centers (as needed) and home again. Good communication is essential."

Froehlich (AMH) describes the executive-nurse role as helping staff to identify shared values that can lead to shared visioning. "Always question traditions and examine paradigms to help create new ways to continually test and challenge current theory. Simultaneously, the executive nurse provides leadership for truth telling about where we are . . . [about] current reality." This leader helps colleagues to hold within their mind's eye an overlapping image of the vision of the future and current reality (Fig. 6.1).

The executive nurse plays, like a harp, the creative tension resulting from the gap between the vision and current reality to move the collective energy of group, organization, and community systems toward the vision (Fig. 6.2).

Peter Senge (1990, 357) points out that the principle of creating tension in organization is not new: "It is the creative tension of personal mastery, one of the disciplines of learning organizations" (Senge, 1990, 139–173). Martin Luther King Jr. said, "Just as Socrates felt that it was necessary to create a tension in the mind, so individuals could rise from the bondage of myths and half trusts . . . so must we . . . create the kind of tension in society that helps men rise from the dark depths of prejudice and racism" (King, 1986, 52–59).

In his book *The Future Executive*, Harland Cleveland (1972, 22) wrote:

> The wise executive will take as his major task . . . inducing . . .
> a degree of tension within the organization, enough loud and
> cheerful argument among its members so that all possible out-
> comes are analyzed, the short-term benefits are compared with
> the long run costs, the moral dilemmas are illuminated, and the
> public relations effects are analytically examined.

McBeth (ISJ) sees creative tension as an integrating principle: This principle. . . "teaches us that an accurate picture of current reality is just as important as a compelling picture (vision) of our desired future." She cautions, "Vision without an understanding of current reality will more likely foster cynicism than creativity." Leading through creative tension is different from solving problems. In problem-solving, "the energy for change comes from attempting to get away from an aspect

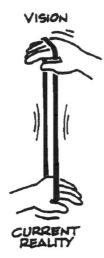

VISION

CURRENT
REALITY

Figure 6.2 *Creative tension between vision and current reality. (From P. Senge, 1990.* The Fifth Discipline: The Art and Practice of the Learning Organization. *New York: Doubleday. Used by permission.)*

of current reality that is undesirable." Executive nurses who lead through creative tension draw on "the energy for change that comes from the vision—from what we want to create put together with current reality."

What do Health Bond executive nurses vision as a preferred future? Froehlich (AMH) has a vision of a transformed rural primary care hospital whose staff works with physicians, health care consumers, patients and families, and other health and human services professionals and organizations as educators for health care reform. Froelich knows that it isn't enough for the executive nurse to have a vision; the executive must engage all types of people and community groups in shaping the vision and sharing commitment to it. She expects herself and other executive nurses to be involved in health care reform and to keep respective local communities current, involved, and educated.

McBeth (ISJ) advocates the community health model (i.e., health promotion and protection, disease prevention) as the template for shared envisioning about future health care reform, systems redesign, and innovation regardless of consumer/patient population. Hospitals are transforming into community or regional health centers. Health care system redesign goes beyond the walls of any hospital or provider. Executive nurses are uniquely prepared to provide the leadership for this paradigm shift, according to McBeth. "We are the only ones who can do this; we are in a pivotal position. The focus is on patient care, care coordination, and patient care outcomes, and the executive nurse is the clinical person on the team to provide this leadership."

Ethical

Strong ethical character, principled actions, and the courage of one's convictions, are all descriptors Health Bond executive nurses use to describe nursing leadership for the future. Jean Watson, Director of the Center of Human Caring,

University of Colorado, provides a nursing focus for the ethical issues. She asserts that "caring in nursing is a philosophy or moral commitment toward protecting human dignity and preserving humanity" (Bevis & Watson, 1989). The ethical components of nursing leadership are made visible by the act of caring in nursing. Health Bond executive nurses demonstrate and strengthen their own commitment to ethical leadership through participation in their respective state and national professional organizations as well as by the relationship of trust they have built among themselves.

Empowering

"Open communication and decentralization of decision-making, . . . spreading power through empowerment of others" is an emergent source of executive nurse power and authority according to Schweer (MSU). A participatory style, and involving stakeholders in change processes early and often, are mentoring strategies for decentralizing decision making, according to Hohenstein (SCTC). The executive nurse guides staff to make decisions and is a facilitator and coach. Raetz (WAMH) believes that encouraging greater staff involvement in decision making and inspiring staff to be leaders results in organizational effectiveness. Staff nurses "are closest to the patient, and work with the physicians every day; their ideas must be respected because they know what works." Staff empowerment is a function of risk-taking abilities, skill at sorting out what works and what doesn't work, and self-confident courage of the executive nurse.

Peter Senge (1990, 233–269) describes team learning as a different process from team building. Executive nurses must be very effective at creating environments for team learning about dialogue and discussion if true empowerment of people in the health care work force is to happen. Senge argues that team learning is the discipline that must be practiced if continual improvements in quality of care and services are to be realized (Senge, March 1992).

A learning from the Health Bond consortium experience has been the significant role the executive nurse plays in creating new structures or groupings of people (novel mix of talents). When executive nurses identify the parameters of expectations for resource use, and monitor change progress and outcomes for such groups, they can enhance individual and group decision making and design skills, whether in the area of curriculum or care delivery system innovations. Educational programs have stressed this executive-level responsibility and the importance of work groups' being sure they are clear on their responsibility, authority, and accountability before they start their work (Cox & Miller, 1991).

Empowering leadership is caring leadership. Morath and Manthey (1993, 77) state that "whether it is in the board room, in medical staff meetings, or in the hallways, the nurse administrator uses every interaction to teach about nursing and the value of caring." These leaders describe caring as "a very powerful act that provides the courage for people to change, heal, and grow." From caring flows quality. Caring is humanistic and freeing. It liberates.

Reflection

Donald Schon (1983, 1984) asserts that the leader of the future must be a "reflective practitioner." Constructive, critical reflection is evident as McBeth (ISJ) describes her views on the knowledge, competence, and skills required of an executive nurse in the future. She poses such questions as: "What are the skills I need to advocate for health care along the patient, family, health-care consumer's continuum?" "What is my background in community health?" "What do I need to learn?"

McBeth reflects on the key responsibility executive nurses have for learning, building organizations, and forging community groups who are continually expanding their capabilities to shape the future. Executive nurses for the 1990s and beyond must be designers, teachers, and stewards. They must be able to create a learning environment, a learning organization, and an approach to learning between organizations, other providers, planners, and laypeople in community.

Raetz (WAMH) takes responsibility for providing an atmosphere that fosters an understanding of why change is happening in health care, and for being proactive to change how we're providing patient care. Raetz is concerned about providing her staff with the tools and education to assist people in making change.

As Health Bond executive nurses work with others, they try to get inside the experience of the other, to understand diverse and at times divergent perspectives. The processes of letting go (of the past) and of letting in (new ideas, new approaches, new possibilities) are apparent in their interactions. Peter Senge speaks of the discipline of critiquing mental models (1990, 174–204). McBeth describes this skill as "bringing to the surface and challenging prevailing mental models (paradigms)."

Schweer (MSU) describes this process as listening: "Being sensitive to broad areas; sensitive to people; listening perceptively; listening to broaden one's own view; listening for possibilities to create." Executive nurses who take seriously being a reflective practitioner have made the paradigm leap from the "technical rational" ways of knowing (theory is separate from practice) to the emergent reflection-in-action process (Smyth, 1986), in which theory emerges out of practice and practice informs theory (praxis). Kemmis (1985, 140) provides insights into the nature of critical reflection:

1. Reflection is not a purely internal, psychological process; it is action-oriented and historically embedded.
2. Reflection is not a purely individual process; like language, it is a social process.
3. Reflection serves human interests; it is a political process.
4. Reflection is shaped by ideology; in turn it shapes ideology.
5. Reflection is a practice which expresses our power to reconstitute social life by the way we participate in communication, decision-making and social action."

Reflection-in-action is what allows the transformational leader to be, as Schweer describes it, "a knowledgeable guider of change processes."

Health Outcome Oriented
A focus on patient outcomes is an emergent source of executive-nurse leadership, according to McBeth (ISJ). "Have we improved the health status (physical, spiritual, emotional function) of the populations we serve?" "What are the perceptions (level of satisfaction) of the population being served?" "Have we achieved cost containment while assuring continuing improvement in quality?" These are the measures the executive nurse of the future must use.

The executive nurse who role-models responsible self-health practices (spiritual and behavioral as well as physical), is a credible role model for the twenty-first century. Morath and Manthey (1993, 76) assert that the executive nurse provides leadership through being, knowledge, and actions.

> . . . Nurse administrators who clearly articulate and organize their lives around what is meaningful have a personal power to instill commitment and help others work together and bring forth their best contributions. This includes being a model for the personal characteristics required for optimal collaborative performance: caring for the self, self-respect, self-knowledge, and self-confidence.

This leader has a sense of humor, and celebrates with others their accomplishments—often. This leader holds personnel accountable for domains of delegated responsibility and authority, yet the executive nurse "does not expect perfection of anyone involved in change processes," states Raetz (WAMH). The executive nurse "educates," which means "to lead forth." When problems occur, the emphasis is on asking what we learned from this situation.

Transformational leaders expect to succeed. They trust the people they work with to want to learn and to create outcomes that exceed the vision any of them could create alone. They are systems thinkers: The whole is greater than the sum of its parts (von Bertalanffy & Rapoport, 1956 and seq.). It is natural for them to think about the care of patients and families and of health services in communities for consumers, because they think in wholes and interdependent, inter-related parts. They promote the discipline of systems thinking among colleagues (Senge, 1990, 6–7).

Generalist Working with Specialists

The executive nurse for the twenty-first century must be an integrator who can assure whole-brain perspectives (right-brain creative, inductive, intuitive and left-brain analytical, synthetic, and deductive) operating in organizations. Work groups and teams must be put together that provide whole-brain functioning. The executive nurse must be skillful at integrating specialists as well as health care consumers into effective interdisciplinary teams by drawing on knowledge of human and organizational dynamics, systems and change theory, and interpersonal communication.

This leader reads widely, both from general literature and from other health, medical, and human services disciplines, and learns continually. The executive nurse of the future thinks broadly and then is able to simplify and communicate effectively with individuals of all ages, from all walks of life.

Morath and Manthey (1993, 77) identify tools the executive nurse will use: ". . . Strategic visioning, interactive planning, financial management, change management, methods and processes of continual quality improvement, and methods of reengineering, while making clear the reasons behind their actions to colleagues, fellow administrators, and physicians." Translating these strategies into practice is the executive nurse's challenge. Russell Ackoff's Interactive Planning Process is presented in Figure 6.3 as a model to assist in the translation. Interactive planning begins with the examination of current reality and identifying the ideal vision

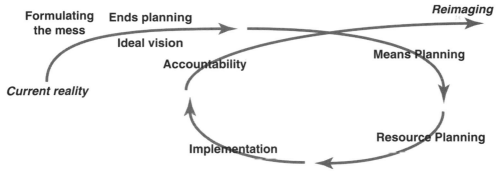

Figure 6.3 *Russell Ackoff's interactive planning process. (From Ackoff, R. L., 1981.* Creating the Corporate Culture. *New York, NY: Wiley.)*

(ends planning), and is followed by means and resource planning, implementation, accountability, and reimaging.

NEW ROLE EXPECTATIONS

Health Bond executive nurses described their roles during the past five years and what they anticipate to be role expectations into the twenty-first century. Table 6.1 summarizes these contrasts.

Changing health care structures require executive nurses to have high-level skills in systems thinking, communication and relationship management; and, more important, they must be able to nurture the development of direct communication, relationship management, and creativity in work groups, organizations, and community coalitions.

Using External Consultants

Health Bond executive nurses have used external consultants to assist in this process. Hospital and nursing-education program executives have found that external consultants can help them to realize shared visions and goals. These executive nurses are committed to the development of leadership within the region, and are positioning nurses in advanced roles to be internal consultants in their own organizations and external consultants for other organizations within the region. In applying for the RWJF/Pew Charitable Trusts grant, the in-service and academic executive nurses envisioned the position of director for the consortium to be that of role modeling an integrated service/education partnership position. Thus they designed the position of consortium director to be a combination internal and external consultant to the respective organizations in the project.

Health Bond executive nurses view one another as external consultants within their own community. Table 6.2 presents Health Bond's executive nurse perspectives on the relative strengths of internal and external consultants.

Schweer (MSU) values a retreat setting for reflection and sharing, processing change, and visioning, whether an internal facilitator or a consultant is used.

Table 6.1 • **Expectations of Executive Nurse Functioning, 1987–1993 and 2000–2005**

1987–1993	2000–2005
1. Manage education and service for illness care within own organization, institution	1. Lead interdisciplinary "beyond the walls" teams to provide health promotion, accident and disease-preventive "wellness care"
Germ theory of disease	Understanding that over 90% of health care is necessitated by dys-functional behaviors
Incentives: Get people into acute care	Incentives: Keep people out of acute care
Vision the future, believe in it; create the enthusiasm to move toward it	Create public policy based on future shared visioning that integrates public and private interests; teach and role model shared visioning
2. Emphasis on innovation in health care delivery redesign, reform; tests and technology	2. Beyond delivery system innovation to answer the question "What makes for health in populations, community?"
3. Expectation of broader knowledge base in education and health careers	3. Keeping on top of information explosion: executive-nurse expertise in communication technology
4. Discipline, department, organizational focus to interdisciplinary teams (including health care consumers and community providers); partnerships; collaboration; mentorship	4. Transformational leadership for interregional, interstate, and inter-national integrated systems
Advertising to marketing perspective (listening mode) and consumer-led health care	Accountability for population, community, state, national, interna-tional health
Expert-led architectural changes to program de-sign; staff, consumers, lead architectural change	Ecological, environmental global resources, conservation commit-ment
5. Shame, blame, and punishment for risk taking, mistakes help us learn, enhance ability to revise our theories	5. Rewards for "outrageous ideas and experiments"; visioning positive futures; inquiry approach is the norm
6. Increased functioning in external environment in ways supportive of changing leadership role	6. Global perspective: expertise in diverse cultures
Shift from being internal expert to use of inter-organizational collaboration and external consultants to acquire broad base of knowledge executive nurse needs to do job	Executive leadership identifies what needs to be done; is knowl-edgeable about who, in local or external environment, has needed skills; identifies leverage points for change in systems.

Table 6.2 • **Strengths: Internal and External Consultants**

Internal Consultants	External Consultants
1. Allows staff to become aware of "gems" of expertise and knowledge within own organizations; value and use inner strength of organization, human resources	1. Bring new ideas; are accepted as "expert" more readily For certain organization and inter-organizational issues, an external consultant is essential
2. When paired with an external consultant, is a powerful partnership for change, staff development	2. Peer consultants outside of own organization or system, to discuss problems, concerns and possible strategies and ideas
3. In academia, deans or academic VPs on same campus can function as internal consultants; limits relate to unique position of nursing dean preparing students for national licensure	3. Can validate direction of leader wanting to be both in academia and service
4. Executive nurse as internal consultant can assist colleagues and staff to sort through traditions and encourage everyone to challenge them	4. Crystallize faculty, staff action

"Getting away is important in coming to consensus about where we are going, what we are expecting, what students (our customers) expect of us, and what is changing in the health care setting." Health Bond's member-hospital executive nurses have also used the retreat format extensively for leadership development among staff.

The executive-nurse role is to work with people in the health care setting to identify external or internal consultation sources who can assist the work group in developing a shared vision and identifying the resources necessary to make that happen. The ultimate purpose of external consultants has been strengthening human resources within the region. Health Bond organizations have used external consultants in the following ways.

One-Shot Consultation
One-shot consultations consist of brief meetings by one or more external consultants, from the same source, with internal groups (e.g., medical staff, board of directors, department heads, nursing-service personnel) around a common topic (e.g., quality improvement):

- Arlington Municipal Hospital used consultants from an urban-based health care system to provide two-hour programs to their medical staff, board of directors, and department heads on quality-improvement roles and responsibilities.

- Arlington Municipal Hospital involved a consultant/facilitator from the state hospital association for a day-long board of directors and medical staff retreat focused on long-range strategic planning.

Two Days to One Week Consultation

This time allows for educational programming with a particular consultant related to two or more topics (e.g., nursing diagnosis and collaborative problems):

- Mankato State University involved a curriculum consultant for a two-day educational program to which other nursing program faculty and students were invited, and a single day of consultation for the school-of-nursing faculty that was focused on the educationist approach (i.e., it was learner-focused, in contrast to the Tylerian behavioral-objectives approach) (Bevis & Watson, 1989).

- Health Bond sponsored a consultant on nursing diagnosis and documentation to provide a week-long consultation and educational experience for nurses from both education and service within southern Minnesota. Consortium member-hospitals staff (multidisciplinary) and education-partner faculty and students had the opportunity to participate in two half-day sessions on documentation issues. On three succeeding days, the same program, on nursing diagnosis and collaborative problems, was presented to nurses from education and service; 665 nurses attended. School-of-nursing faculty also had a half-day consultation on further integration of nursing diagnosis and collaborative problems into the curriculum.

One-Shot Consultation with Two or More Consultants

This setup brings in people with a range of expertise to inform new developments and design new systems and strategies (e.g., documentation-and-information system development for patients' continuum of care).

- Immanuel St. Joseph's Hospital brought together consultants from public health/community health care, information systems, and patient classification systems to work with acute care personnel in envisioning documentation flow and information management across the continuum of care (physician office, primary and secondary care hospital, emergency services, tertiary care, home care).

Long-Term Consultant Relationship

When considering a major reevaluation or addressing complex internal issues, a long-term relationship with a single consultant or a consulting firm may be desirable:

- Waseca Area Memorial Hospital has established a relationship with a futurist from the University of Minnesota to work with staff and patients in its four outpatient chemical-dependency clinics in researching a clinical intervention called "One Day Plus" for post-acute stages of recovery (Harkins & Gordon, 1993).

- The Minnesota Technical College System engaged an external consulting firm to assist them with an enrollment management project across all campuses.

- Health Bond has a contract with an international consulting firm related to leadership development and care delivery system innovations. All consortium members and partner schools have available consultation and educational programming.

Consultant Roles Within a Consortium

There are times when it is necessary to monitor internal and external consultants to ensure well-integrated results that are in accord with the original vision.

- The consortium-director position has the responsibility and the authority to oversee this mix of internal and external roles within Health Bond. The position was designed to provide a model for joint service and educational positions. The goal of the search was to identify a team player who valued the role that nursing would play in the evolving consortium, had experience in education and service, had expertise in evaluation and research, and would assume full consortium-level executive responsibility for the five-year implementation grant. The executive nurses demonstrated upstream thinking in seeking a doctorally prepared nurse for this position, an idea they had to sell to their respective executive officers.

The Joint Appointment Model

In the joint appointment model, a full-time position exists in service or education. If the position is filled in service, then time is subcontracted to a nursing-education program for clinical or course instruction. If the position is based in an academic setting, then time is subcontracted to the service-provider organization.

The Health Bond consortium director is in the state university system, where the director is an associate professor. During the first two years of the RWJF/Pew Charitable Trusts grant, the consortium director role was defined as a full-time position. The director divided time among all five Health Bond member hospitals and partner schools and worked continually with representatives of all five organizations; the Health Bond staff and the consortium shared governance structure.

The consortium director has been part of strategic-planning activities for patient services and the institution as a whole at the grantee hospital. The director attends periodic board meetings, medical staff meetings, and departmental patient-services meetings in all consortium hospitals.

At the school of nursing at the state university, the consortium director attends faculty meetings, serves on the strategic planning committee, and fulfills a faculty role (related to the director's areas of education, research, and practice expertise). Having the director as a faculty member is what has made the model work. The director's "presence, guidance, communication effort, persistence, and teaching activities have established the director as a faculty member and simultaneously kept the consortium focus prominent."

The consortium director's role with the technical college has taken a different direction. The director works closely with the dean of the health and safety division and the director of the practical nursing program; communicates with the executive administration; and interacts continually with faculty members within the practical nursing program and the health-and-safety division to assure their increasing involvement in Health Bond Consortium committees and activities. The consortium director has provided leadership, along with faculty from both schools, for collaborative planning on an LPN–BSN program.

Beginning with year 3, the director's focus shifted to 90% administrative and 10% faculty time at the school of nursing. The director has continued to attend faculty meetings, co-chair the strategic planning committee, and facilitate five seminar groups in the undergraduate research course. The director has also been a member of the steering committee for an innovative, collaborative MSN program in the school of nursing, a participant in grant writing, and a facilitator of the LPN–BSN initiative.

During year 4, the position will be 80% director and 20% faculty; in year 5, 65% director and 35% faculty. When the five-year RWJF/Pew Charitable Trusts grant ends, the position becomes a fully integrated joint appointment with a 50% commitment from the service setting and 50% from the state university system.

Health Bond is currently working on other joint appointments (e.g., with the school of business) in addition to joint appointments with the school of nursing (clinical experts from the grantee hospital will have time subcontracted from the service setting to the state university school of nursing). A critical issue being resolved through this model is that any individual in a joint appointment will have a defined full-time position within a given system (service or education) for benefit purposes.

Project Directors

Project directors within each of the Health Bond hospitals are working as internal consultants within their own organizations regarding care delivery system innovations. In this capacity, they work directly with the external consultant and with executive nurse, management, and staff inpatient services related to care delivery redesign and staff empowerment. These internal consultants are being positioned regionally for care delivery system redesign. As a first step, they are getting experience by being consultants to one another across Health Bond member hospitals.

Other Disciplines

Other health and human services disciplines are having the opportunity to function not only as internal consultants within their own organization but also as external consultants to other Health Bond member hospitals and regional nonmember hospitals. Examples include respiratory therapy, physical therapy, occupational therapy, nutrition, hospice, and cardiac rehabilitation.

Nursing Faculty

Faculty from the school of nursing are increasingly called on to serve as consultants and educational facilitators to hospitals within Health Bond. Arlington Municipal Hospital sought consultation from the school of nursing as follow-up to a JCAHO visit. Nurses from Arlington Municipal Hospital then shared what they learned about nursing process with colleagues at Waseca Area Memorial Hospital. Waseca nurses consulted with colleagues at ISJ when they were developing their own Medicare-certified hospice program, and again when they planned an annual education program on oncology. A project director at Immanuel St. Joseph's Hospital invited faculty members from nursing programs at the state university and the technical college to be part of the design team for a care delivery system innovation related to Partners-In-Practice. Faculty are being called on to consult with nurses at Immanuel St. Joseph Hospital as nurses apply what they continue to learn about nursing diagnosis and collaborative problems to their clinical practice with specific patient populations.

The line between an internal and an external consultant begins to blur within a health consortium. This happens as the walls between "us" and "them" crumble as a result of shared vision, shared governance structure, and innovative interdisciplinary service and educational efforts.

Summary

Health care systems for the year 2000 and beyond will be interlinking networks of providers and services, payors and health care consumers. The "business" will be the health of communities, regions, populations—and the global village. Responsible stewardship of limited resources will provide all people access to wellness care.

Health Bond executive-nurse perspectives suggest a new descriptor for twenty-first century executive nurse leadership: *interpreneurship.* This represents an advance over the existing definitions of an entrepreneur as "one who organizes, manages, and assumes the risks of a business or venture" (*Webster's Ninth,* 1990) and the 1980s reference to an entrepreneur as an individual innovator within an organization.

The executive nurse will be an integrator of leadership and followership; novice zeal and expert grace; courage and playfulness; generalist and specialist; commitment and celebration; energy and ease; creativity and conservation; dignity and humor; truth telling and envisioning. This transformational leadership will influence others to see the promise of both individual health and health for a global village.

Discussion Questions

1. What role expectations for 2005 will be unique to your health care setting?

2. Is the executive nurse in your organization a transformational leader? Why or why not?

3. What needs to change in your environment to implement transformational leadership?

References

Ackoff, R. (1981). *Creating the corporate future.* New York: Wiley.

Ackoff, R. L. (1989). The circular organization: An update. *The Academy of Management Executive. 111*(1), 11–16.

American Nurses Association (1991). Nursing's agenda for health care reform. Kansas City: Author.

Bevis, E. O., & Watson, J. (1989). *Toward a caring curriculum*. New York: National League for Nursing, Publication #15–2278.

Burns, J. M. (1978). *Leadership*. New York: Harper Torchbooks.

Cleveland, H. (1972). *The future executive*. New York: Harper & Row.

Cox, S., & Miller, D. (Eds.). (1991). *Leaders empower staff*. Minneapolis: Creative Nursing Management.

Gleick, J. (1987). *Chaos: Making a new science*. New York: Penguin.

Harkins, A., & Gordon, S. (1993). Futures in substance abuse damage control: Development of personal recovery alternatives through guided story-telling. *Futurics: A Quarterly Journal of Futures Research 17*(1,2), 1–4.

Havelock, R. G., et al. (1969). *Planning for innovation through dissemination and utilization of knowledge*. Ann Arbor: Center for Research on Utilization of Scientific Knowledge, Institute for Social Research.

Kemmis, S. (1985). Action research and the politics of reflection. In D. Bond, R. Keogh, R. D. Walker (eds.), *Reflection, Turning experience into learning*. London: Kogan Page.

King, M. L., Jr. (1986). Letter from a Birmingham jail. *American Visions*, January/February, 52–59.

Morath, J., & Manthey, J. (1993). An environment for care and service leadership: The nurse administrator's impact. *Nursing Administration Quarterly, 17*(2), 75–80.

Milio, N. (1981). *Promoting health through public policy*. Philadelphia: F. A. Davis.

Mish, F. C. (ed.). (1990). *Webster's ninth new collegiate dictionary*. Springfield: Merriam-Webster.

Murphy, M. M., DeBack, V. (1991). Today's nursing leaders: Creating the vision. *Nursing Administration Quarterly, 16*(1), 71–80.

Rogers, E. (1983). *The diffusion of innovations*. New York: Free Press.

Schon, D. A. (1983). *The reflective practitioner: How professionals think in action*. New York: Basic Books.

Schon, D. A. (1984). Leadership as reflection-in-action. In T. J. Sergiovanni & J. E. Corbeilly, (eds.) *Leadership and organizational culture: New perspectives as administrative theory and practice*. Urbana, IL: University of Illinois Press.

Senge, P. M. (1990). *The fifth discipline: The art and practice of the learning organization*. New York: Doubleday Currency.

Senge, P. M. (1992). Building learning organizations. *Journal for Quality and Participation, 15*(2), 30–38.

Smyth, W. (1986). *Reflection-in-action*. Victoria, Australia: Deahin University Press.

von Bertalanffy, L. & Repoport, Anatof. (eds.) (1956 and seq.). *General systems*. Ann Arbor: Society for General Systems Research.

Wheatley, M. J. (1992). *Leadership and the new science: Learning about organization from an orderly universe*. San Francisco: Berrett-Koehler.

Linda D. Schaffner

Total Quality Management
Impact on the Executive Nurse

Introduction

A wave of excitement about **total quality management (TQM)** began in health care in the late 1980s and early 1990s. Hospital chief executive officers(CEOs) viewed it as a means to improve operations and reduce costs of services. Leaders and educators went to seminars and began to read the experts. Sophisticated models for implementation of TQM were presented by growing numbers of consultants. To most executive nurses these new models did not look all that different from the nursing process. Quality care has been included in nursing's mission and goal statements for years. Executive nurses have spent their careers focusing on how to improve quality of care.

A tremendous amount of energy, money, and time has been spent in recent years to bring TQM to health care. Many organizations have thrived in a TQM environment but, on the other hand, many models have failed to produce the intended results. The key to success appears to be the extent of leadership commitment and direct involvement throughout the entire process. For the executive nurse, it is therefore important to have a complete understanding of TQM and to be assertive about remaining involved at both the planning and implementation levels of a TQM program.

HISTORY

Total Quality Management found its early roots in the work of Joseph Juran, W. Edwards Deming, and Philip Crosby. Each of these experts began their careers in manufacturing industries and focused on statistical quality-control techniques to achieve improvements in products and service.

Juran and Deming introduced TQM to the Japanese after World War II and assisted them to become manufacturers of high-quality products. Crosby developed a successful quality management program at International Telephone & Telegraph (ITT).

Juran (1989) describes a trilogy of separate yet parallel managerial processes to manage quality: quality planning, quality control, and quality improvement. **Quality planning** focuses on identifying and creating products and services that meet customer needs. **Quality control** involves reducing variability in order to increase consistency in quality. **Quality improvement** involves process changes in the system in order to correct problems. Juran believes that top management must direct all organizational activity and set priorities in order to achieve optimal organizationwide quality. He urges top management to increase its pace of quality improvement through concentrating efforts on "the vital few" rather than on "the useful many" (Dienemann, 1992).

Deming (1986) uses fourteen points as guidelines for quality improvement:

1. Create constancy of purpose for improvement of product and service.

2. Adopt the new philosophy.

3. Cease dependence on inspection to achieve quality.

4. End the practice of awarding business on the basis of price tag alone.

5. Improve constantly and forever the system of production and service to quality and productivity, and thus constantly decrease costs.

6. Institute training on the job.

7. Institute leadership.

8. Drive out fear.

9. Break down barriers between departments.

10. Eliminate slogans, exhortations, and targets for the work force.

11. Eliminate work standards (quotas) . . . Eliminate management by objective (MBO).

12. Remove barriers that rob the hourly worker of his right to pride of workmanship.

13. Institute a vigorous program of education and self-improvement.

14. Put everyone in the company to work to accomplish the transformation.

In general, Deming emphasizes changing the philosophy and the management style of the organization by empowering the worker and focusing on leadership and team building. Deming offers a system of knowledge that complements the knowledge that health care workers already have in subject matter and values. His principles help establish a policy for developing a clear mission and a clear idea of what quality means.

Philip Crosby's school of thought includes four "Absolutes of Quality Management" (Burrus, 1992):

• Quality is defined as conformance to requirements, not "goodness."

• The system for causing quality is prevention, not appraisal.

- The performance standard must be zero defects.
- The measurement of quality is the price of nonconformance, not indexes.

Crosby (1979) developed a quality maturity grid as a guide for helping firms implement and assess their quality management programs. He placed emphasis on the costing out of the price of poor quality, on doing things right the first time, and on changing the organizational culture to expect quality.

These three quality gurus agree on the key elements of TQM, and each has developed large consulting organizations with training-and-implementation programs. They differ on issues concerning program emphasis and methodology. Health care organizations need to examine carefully what best fits their own philosophy and culture before embarking on a consultant-designed program.

The term **continuous quality improvement (CQI)** has evolved out of quality assurance/quality assessment and performance-improvement efforts over the years in health care. In particular, the Joint Commission on the Accreditation of Healthcare Organizations (JCAHO) has influenced quality management and methodology in hospitals through its development of standards and a prescriptive review process. Regardless of whether a hospital has adopted a formal TQM program, JCAHO has moved organizations into a direction of continual improvement, outcomes-oriented monitoring, and comprehensive evaluation activities.

The terms TQM and CQI have been used interchangeably when discussing quality management in health care. Basically, there are four core concepts of TQM that are consistent in all models:

1. Focus on the customer.
2. Reduce variation.
3. Continuously improve.
4. Work as a team.

Based on these four core concepts, TQM is a management approach that seeks to identify and then reduce the gap that may be present between customers' and health care providers' perceptions of the quality of care received. Therefore, the skills and ideas of everyone are needed to bring about improvements and enhance services through TQM.

TQM AND NURSING

Nursing is not new to the measurement and management of quality. Since Florence Nightingale we have been collecting and analyzing data. Tools developed in the 1960s and 1970s illustrate the profession's advances in quality assurance/quality improvement efforts:

- Slater Scale: was designed to evaluate the competencies of a direct care provider.
- QualPACs: focused on the patient as a basis for evaluating nursing care.
- Rush-Medicus: related processes of care to outcomes of care through an extensive criteria list of patient-specific and nursing-unit items.

- Norma Lang: implemented standards in a nursing quality assurance (QA) model. Initially, nursing QA tended to focus retrospectively on specific events and settings, but by the late 1980s nursing systems began to focus more on the entire patient care episode and in the design of QA programs that focused on both process and outcome measures.

The TQM Movement

Nursing greeted TQM with a degree of skepticism. It was difficult to evaluate whether it was the latest fad (following customer service programs and quality circles), or a new terminology for the scientific process, or the nursing process. The first challenge for the executive nurse became evident: it is essential that the executive nurse be involved in the organization's decision to implement a TQM program. Models and methods differ greatly, and the executive nurse must engage in research to understand the relationship of TQM to what is already known about quality management.

TQM and quality improvement (QI) are not the same thing, yet they are not isolated from one another. TQM is a total process that involves changing the very fabric of an organization. It requires the commitment of everyone and results in a cultural transformation for all parts of the organization. TQM is a journey. It does not mean that you will implement a new program next month and then be finished. Organizations with experience will testify that it takes five to ten years for the transformation to be considered successful.

For the executive nurse who is new to TQM—or perhaps struggling with an implementation model—it is recommended that time be spent talking with a peer who has experienced it firsthand. The ideas and model offered here are based upon the experience at Bethesda, Inc., of Cincinnati, Ohio. Other models exist in the literature, but it is beyond the scope of this chapter to present them.

Ongoing challenges that the executive nurse will face in implementing TQM include:

- Obtaining buy-in
- Differentiating TQM from nursing QI
- Applying TQM in the clinical environment
- Educating the entire staff
- Sustaining momentum

Discussion of each of these challenges follows.

OBTAINING BUY–IN

The first issue related to buy-in is the commitment of the executive nurse. The executive nurse must be personally committed to the idea that TQM is valuable and that it is the right thing to do. Involvement in the decision to implement TQM is key, and active participation by the executive nurse as a member of the steering committee for implementation will help to assure program success across the entire organization.

Bethesda, Inc., is a private, not-for-profit, diversified health care organization in Cincinnati that is made up of two acute-care hospitals of approximately 700 beds with over 1300 members of the medical staff. The corporation also includes a tri-state home health agency with offices in thirteen cities and a durable medical equipment company; a senior services division operating two skilled-care nursing facilities and two adult day care centers; and a diversified division that operates two work capacity centers, five occupational health centers, and numerous contractual corporate-health services provided to businesses.

Bethesda's commitment to TQM was initiated by the chief executive officer, L. Thomas Wilburn, Jr., an industrial engineer by training, who has served for over twenty years as a thoughtful and innovative leader in our organization. In the summer of 1988, Wilburn attended the National Demonstration Project Conference, where he heard reports from twenty-one hospitals involved in TQM activities of various types. Also in 1988, members of Bethesda's senior management attended the four-day seminar presented by W. Edwards Deming, where we became convinced that there was much about TQM that made sense. We had researched the teachings of Juran and Crosby, but selected Deming as the foundation for our TQM initiatives.

Fortunately, some members of our board of trustees who were from industry were knowledgeable and experienced in TQM, so obtaining support for the investment in time and resources came easily. In January 1989, a steering committee was established that included members of senior management and selected medical staff. GOAL/QPC was selected as a consultant to get us started, and staff appointments (a vice president and a medical staff consultant) were made in order to ensure ongoing program direction and follow through.

Early on, acceptance was a problem. Exposure to TQM had occurred primarily at the senior management level and implementation of the program took a strong academic approach. Although the executive nurse had been included in Deming's seminar and in the early process of decision making about TQM, she was not made a member of the initial steering committee and became more of an observer than an active participant during the first stages of implementation. The director of corporate education was promoted to VP of TQM, and our corporate education department (along with the consultant) embarked on extensive training sessions as the essential first step of our program. Our initial project teams were composed primarily of line staff, and for the most part middle management had little or no involvement in team activity. The process seemed lengthy as we methodically followed each step at the direction of our TQM facilitators, educators, and consultant.

The results were mixed. We had process successes and failures. But we learned a great deal and several things happened along the way that enabled us to move forward more easily.

Purpose and Goals

We adopted a clear statement of purpose and goals that helped to translate and communicate to all of our employees and medical staff what TQM was all about. Our purpose statement is:

To adopt a leadership philosophy that supports, encourages, and expects all employees to participate in the continuous improvement of services to meet the health care needs of the community and to support and encourage physicians, customers and suppliers to be involved in these continuous improvement activities.

Our goals are:

1. To empower all employees to investigate work situations and improve systems to enhance delivery of service and quality of care.
2. To support and recognize departmental and crossfunctional teamwork.
3. To establish an environment that leads to efficiency and productivity and promotes creativity.
4. To identify and meet the needs of internal and external customers.

The steering committee added the executive nurse to its membership after medical staff and administrators began to struggle with applying TQM to patient care. Also, we modified our educational approach to become one of "just-in-time" education that was tailored to the needs of active project teams.

A major issue that surfaced was middle-management commitment. This issue took a substantial amount of time to address. It was clear that more direct involvement was needed by managers. We began to educate and train them as facilitators and actively appointed managers as leaders or sponsors of project teams. Until TQM became a part of the way we did our work, we were constantly struggling to balance old ways with new ways.

Perhaps the greatest challenge has been obtaining medical staff commitment. While the philosophy and goals are not a problem for physicians, the *process* of implementation can be a really difficult issue. Physicians are comfortable with their traditional quality activities of monitoring and looking for "bad apples." They are not able to dedicate the time that project teams need. They want results quickly. We solved some of the issues by using sophisticated data tools to illustrate the need for improvements in patient care on the front end; utilizing physicians as consultants to teams rather than as members of teams; using specifically trained nurse analysts to assist physician clinical-department chairs/committee chairs with the use of TQM tools in medical staff meetings and QA activities; and focusing specific TQM educational segments into continuing medical education (CME) programs.

DIFFERENTIATING TQM FROM NURSING QA/QI

Historically, the responsibility for nursing QA/QI has been delegated from the governing body down through the organizational structure to the executive nurse. It is a responsibility that all executive nurses accept seriously, and virtually all hospital nursing executives have established comprehensive programs to manage the quality of nursing care within their organizations.

With the advent of TQM as an organizationwide strategy, executive nurses have had to examine their traditional QI programs and carefully determine how the processes differ, or can be integrated with, TQM. At the earliest opportunity, the executive nurse must articulate the complementary and enhancement attributes of TQM in a way that has meaning for nursing staff (who are committed to the value of their current nursing systems).

Key points for consideration include:

QI	TQM
Externally driven	Internally driven
Reactive	Proactive
Follows organizational structure	Follows patient care
Department focused	Crossfunctional
Inspection oriented	Planning oriented
Responsibility of few	Responsibility of all
Uses audits and indicator monitoring	Uses TQM tools (flow charting, Pareto charts, cause-effect, run/control chart, QFD, Hoshin)
Follow-up of special causes	Follow-up of special or common cause deviations

It is important that executive nurses recognize the opportunities for improving QI programs through the use of a TQM approach. The nursing process is a strong foundation for TQM. However, TQM represents a different thinking process and, for professional nurses who are grounded in the nursing process, education and support throughout is necessary.

Looking at the nursing process in terms of the TQM "PDCA" cycle helps in the translation.

QI	TQM
Assess	Plan
Plan	Do
Implement	Check
Evaluate	Act

It is also important to articulate process thinking as it relates to core processes and critical processes in TQM. Process thinking involves knowing and understanding the core processes and the critical processes of patient care within the total system. Bethesda's Process Improvement Model is depicted in Figures 7.1 and 7.2.

Core processes are the vital, few, macro processes that if executed well will result in the achievement of the organization's mission and vision and customer satisfaction. Core processes describe the key functions of an organizational unit. Core processes are typically stable over time. An example of a high-level core process is the process of treatment.

Critical processes are the small group of subprocesses that are elements of the core processes and which, if improved, will have the greatest impact on desired outcomes. For example, subprocesses of the process of medication might be: (a) prescribing/ordering, (b) preparation/dispensing, (c) administration, and (d) monitoring effects on patients.

BETHESDA PROCESS IMPROVEMENT MODEL

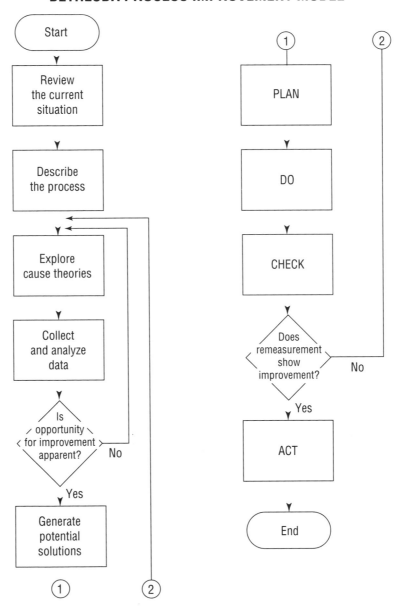

Figure 7.1   *Bethesda Process Improvement Model. (From Bethesda, Inc., Cincinnati, Ohio. Used by permission.)*

At Bethesda, a key factor in the successful nursing QI integration with TQM was a decision to train our "nursing quality improvement coordinators" as TQM facilitators and to involve them as project team leaders. These nurses were already highly skilled and respected for their expertise in quality management. They had developed a sophisticated program of nursing QI that had evolved to an extensive

PROCESS IMPROVEMENT MODEL

1. Review the current situation
- Identify the problem
- Identify customer/supplier perceptions
- Determine quality characteristics
- Gather available information

2. Describe the process
- Identify purpose of the process
- Construct a flow chart
- Determine operational definitions
- Gather baseline data

3. Explore cause theories
- Construct cause & effect diagrams
- Look for root causes
- Ask "why" five times

4. Collect and analyze data
- Collect new data or review existing data to validate cause theories
- Use the seven QC tools to display and analyze data

5. Generate potential solutions
- Evaluate and select best solutions

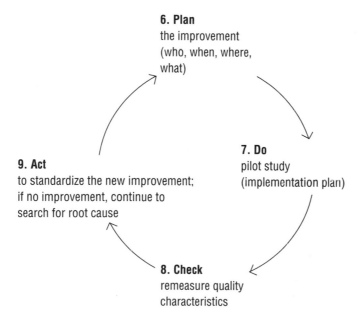

6. Plan
the improvement
(who, when, where,
what)

7. Do
pilot study
(implementation plan)

9. Act
to standardize the new improvement;
if no improvement, continue to
search for root cause

8. Check
remeasure quality
characteristics

Figure 7.2 *Bethesda Process Improvement Model. (From Bethesda, Inc., Cincinnati, Ohio. Used by permission.)*

model of unit-based staff involvement. They were quick to adapt to changes of terminology and to identify problems and opportunities for application of TQM out of our traditional nursing QI monitoring activities. Activities such as statistical methods, and data presentation and processes, were coming together.

TQM CLINICAL APPLICATION

Where TQM really has meaning for nursing is in its clinical application. Once we were able to be clear about the enhancements offered to traditional QI, and the nursing quality improvement coordinators became knowledgeable in TQM, we made significant strides in our implementation and integration efforts. We focused the application of TQM techniques on areas that we had found difficult to solve through our existing nursing QA/QI program.

For example, within the division of nursing, problems with timely administration of preoperative prophylactic antibiotics continued to occur despite continuing "individual counseling" and "in-servicing." The housewide nosocomial infection rate was below the national statistical rate published by the Centers for Disease Control (CDC), but we were interested in lowering the rate further. Also, our hospital standard (which was supported in the literature) called for the prophylactic antibiotic to be administered within 1 hour of the incision time, and we knew through our monitoring activities that our compliance with the standard was inconsistent. A multidisciplinary TQM team was formed that included physician consultants, and the group embarked on its work through the Bethesda Process Improvement Model (see Fig. 7.1).

A variety of TQM tools and techniques were used throughout the process of improving preoperative antibiotic administration, and bottom-line results were impressive. By following through with the recommendations of the TQM team, we were able to improve our compliance with the standard from 51% of antibiotics administered within the 1-hour time frame to 91% administered according to the standard. The antibiotic administration process that was designed and successfully piloted has continued and is consistently remeasured to ascertain whether we are maintaining the improvement (Dressman, 1993).

We did learn a great deal from this team experience. While the topic may not have been unique, it was one that had meaning in our system and had not been solved through traditional QI activities. The project pointed out the value of statistical data in a way that made sense to clinicians in all disciplines. The medical staff got involved and took responsibility for helping to improve quality. And, most important, it enabled us to see the merits of integrating TQM tools and techniques with a basically sound QI program in order to achieve better and lasting results in improved patient care.

EMPLOYEE EDUCATION

There is no way to avoid universal employee education. Implementing TQM requires a massive educational effort. It is important to recognize at the beginning that it is an expensive undertaking. Every employee needs to receive at least a basic TQM orientation and overview. Content should include the organization's vision, mission, philosophy, goals, and the basics about TQM tools. This information needs to be a part of new employee orientation, without exception.

Following basic orientation, every employee needs at least an annual update. At Bethesda we added it to our mandatory education day. Out of the 8-hour schedule for JCAHO and clinical requirements, we allocated 45 minutes for TQM core concepts, process analysis, and employee participation.

Information and Education

The more difficult task is to reach every *current* employee with adequate information during a TQM program implementation. Executive nurses must involve staff on all shifts and manage both scheduling and assignments. In addition, there is a need to balance mandatory clinical and regulatory educational needs with a limited budget for in-service and continuing education. TQM must become a priority, and it is necessary to do whatever works best to schedule all staff for the programs. Depending on the amount of depth your organization chooses for the first program, a 2- to 4-hour block of time will be needed for each employee.

For project teams, we started doing approximately 16 hours of education before the team started its work. With experience, we found that this was tedious and people did not retain it. Conducting a brief start-up program served us better, and then we moved to teaching the TQM tools in a just-in-time fashion that proved to be more effective.

Topics that were better offered in a just-in-time fashion included the following:

- Flow charts
- Cause-and-effect diagrams
- Pareto charts
- Histograms
- Run charts
- Scatter diagrams
- Control charts
- Quality management and planning tools

For advanced education, we developed a set of modules that managers and key support staff (such as clinical nurse specialists) could take on an elective basis.

For all new managers, a 3-hour introduction to TQM is mandatory. The content includes purpose and goals, Deming philosophy and methods, core concepts, the TQM model, daily management of critical processes, Hoshin planning, and cross-functional management.

For current managers and selected support staff, we recommend a series of TQM classes that are 2 to 3 hours each:

- Introduction to the process improvement model, quality tools, and variation
- Management's role in implementation of TQM team solutions
- Managing in a team environment
- Introduction to daily management

- Introduction to Hoshin planning
- In-depth course on Hoshin planning
- TQM project team education
- TQM sponsor education
- TQM team leader education

Facilitator Training

In addition, a facilitator training program has served us well. We started our program with an extensive training of a select group of core facilitators. This core group was multidisciplinary in makeup, and they served full-time as facilitators. Subsequently, we have trained current managers and selected staff to serve as part-time facilitators, so that they could use the skills in their home departments or work with multidisciplinary project teams in other parts of the organization. For facilitators, training involves five 8-hour days. The curriculum covers in-depth training about TQM tools/techniques and group process expertise. Part-time participants must be willing and able to commit 8 hours per week to facilitate TQM teams and activities. At present, we have over 90 part-time facilitators, prepared and active in our organization.

Having trained a small group of core facilitators proved helpful. Because they received advanced training and are experts in TQM, these facilitators are able to take on the really difficult projects and to serve as coaches for managers who want to use TQM in their departments. The further you get into TQM as a clear culture of the organization, the more you value the experts and the more you begin to seek out advanced knowledge. From an educational standpoint, we've added programs for leadership staff in quality function deployment (QFD), breakthrough thinking, Hoshin planning, and paradigm prism. The additional tools and techniques proved invaluable as we addressed the arena of health care reform.

Educating the medical staff was another issue. We had hired a physician with an MBA to work with our doctors. Most of what we tried in the beginning did not work (e.g., the typical retreats and CME programs). The physicians on early TQM teams had very low tolerance for the tedious all-day educational programs, and they soon dropped out if the process involved too many meetings. One of our best successes with the medical staff was to involve a group of nurses whom they trusted in "translating" the value of TQM to patient care and medical staff activities. We trained our utilization-review nurses and nurse analysts as TQM facilitators. This group of nurses worked directly and regularly with medical-staff department, section, and committee chairs. They were experienced and respected clinicians who took their new knowledge of TQM and applied it to familiar medical-staff activities in a subtle but effective way. Though much that was accomplished resulted from one-on-one education in a just-in-time mode, it worked. Even though we have a large medical staff (over 1300 physicians) and the effort focused only on the leadership group, it had an amazing spin-off effect. As leaders used TQM in meetings and QA activities, other members of the medical staff absorbed it. Gradually, TQM has become a part of the medical-staff culture for physicians who work in our institution. The attending staff are now more willing to help out as consultants to TQM teams, and they are very receptive to data when quality patient care improvements are suggested.

Education never stops in a TQM environment, and it is a constant challenge. Each advancement in our understanding of the process and each new element we want to introduce has educational/communication implications that cannot be treated lightly. We've found that it is impossible to educate or communicate too much.

SUSTAINING MOMENTUM

The most difficult aspect of TQM implementation is maintaining excitement and pace. What needs to happen requires rigor, discipline, and time. Employees and physicians want to see results, and they want those results to be evident quickly. But TQM does not happen that way.

What really matters is that TQM becomes a part of the everyday way that work is done. Gradually, the organizational culture becomes so ingrained in TQM that doing anything without it is impossible.

This is not an easy road. It is easier to sustain momentum if the continual educational efforts, structured process-improvement activities, and ongoing strategic planning of the organization does not deviate from basic TQM philosophy and principles. But when you have a large group of employees and physicians that are all at different levels of TQM buy-in and educational knowledge, it is a challenge to be on top of all the gaps and issues. This is the responsibility of the leaders.

Tips for Success

A few suggestions that might help to sustain the momentum follow.

Prioritize
Select what you work on very carefully and aim for high-profile projects that can truly make a difference. If you can do a few things right, and they are things that matter, you can achieve an impact that people will remember.

Alignment
To undertake multiple activities that involve a lot of people can be useful, but a more powerful effect results if the organization is able to translate seemingly divergent efforts into a project that has significant quality-improvement impact for a broad group of internal and external customers at the same time.

Speed
There is a real need to do things quickly, but there is also a need for discipline to achieve best results. The balance is difficult, but if the foundation is firm it is possible to move ahead rapidly with continual improvement while simultaneously addressing priority redesign/restructuring in a changing health care environment.

Totality
The "T" in TQM must be meaningful. *Total* quality involves more than process improvement. The philosophy becomes the way strategic planning is done in the organization. It involves long-term thinking about the future, and it allows for

creative breakthroughs. You simply cannot treat TQM as a separate program that you pull out for resolving problems or simply as a replacement for your current QI activities.

Involvement

It sounds trite, but people must stay actively involved if momentum is to be sustained. TQM is not a process where you can sit back and watch to see what happens. For nursing, TQM offers a wonderful opportunity to lead, and to be visible champions. The skills needed in a TQM environment come naturally to nurses, and for those who choose to do so there are many chances for role enhancement outside of traditional boundaries.

Successes

What truly sustains momentum in the final analysis is the ability to see results and hold the gains. It's important to share the success stories widely and repeatedly. The successes don't have to be monumental, but they do have to be real. Even the small wins can have broad organizational impact when shared by a team of employees who made it happen.

STRATEGIC PLANNING

TQM changes the strategic planning process of the organization. Rather than depending on current performance data and the external environment as a basis for planning, the TQM approach is customer driven. This means that the needs and expectations of both internal and external customers are used to drive the planning process. TQM-based planning views the organization as a system, and it fosters widespread involvement in the development of proactive goals. Some specific tools that are helpful in strategic planning include the quality function deployment (QFD) system and Hoshin planning.

Quality Function Deployment (QFD)

Quality function deployment is a system for designing products or services based on customer demands. It is the outgrowth of the Japanese system called company-wide quality control, which involves all employees in the organization in the continual improvement effort. A first step in the use of this advanced TQM tool is to define who the primary customers are. For example, the primary customers of a health care organization might be patients and their families, physicians, employers, employees, and third-party payers. Three basic classes of customer wants can be defined. The first class consists of what the customers tell you they want, which you then give them (specifications). In this part of the process, customers and suppliers continually throw information back and forth until there is a common understanding. The second class of customer wants are called "expected quality." This class consists of what the customers do not tell you they want, but assume they will get. For example, people assume that a product will be safe. The third group of customer expectations is called "exciting quality." These consist of new ideas generated by the supplier. The customers do not expect the quality characteristics in this category, but they are delighted when they experience them. QFD methodology statistically analyzes and prioritizes customer needs in a way that enables the organization to identify breakthrough objectives as the basis for planning (King, 1989).

Hoshin Planning

Hoshin Planning is a management system that allows you to organize and orchestrate the efforts of all functions within the organization so that the organization moves toward a desired future state. It is an American version of a fully integrated top-down/bottom-up management system originally developed as part of Japan's TQM. In its simplest terms, Hoshin planning is a ball game of "catch" between management and staff. Management begins by identifying a vision and breakthrough objectives that will allow the organization to achieve the vision. Top management then passes these priorities down through the organization to determine the feasibility and practicality of the objectives. Department managers in turn share their views on how they can achieve the breakthrough objectives in their specific areas. The point of Hoshin is to build consensus and vertical alignment among staff. Integral to this process is the use of seven TQM management and planning tools: affinity diagrams, interrelationship diagrams, tree diagrams, matrix diagrams, prioritization matrices, process decision program charts (PDPC), and activity network diagrams (King, 1989; JCAHO, 1992).

Strategic Planning

Strategic planning involves both long-term plans (typically 3 to 5 years) and short-term plans (usually written for 1 year). The emphasis must be on developing strategic plans rooted in the customer and specifying continual improvement and breakthrough goals. In the current environment, external factors can play a key role in the formation or modification of strategic plans—and the response must be rapid. It is therefore important to have some flexibility in the plan and an effective system of plan deployment.

   The executive nurse must know how to use the sophisticated planning systems and the advanced management tools. Again, it is essential that the nursing leader be involved in the entire process of TQM and strategic planning.

TQM Implementation

To cite an example of the power of TQM in strategic planning, Bethesda, Inc., used its solid foundation in TQM and the strength of the TQM philosophy to restructure the organization. In 1993, we had a corporate breakthrough objective "to determine the way to structurally organize a health care provider so that it is customer driven and to implement that organization form at Bethesda. . . ." The organizational requirements for restructuring in an evolving market included the following:

1. Integration across the continuum of care and the associated providers.
2. Increased interdependence between departments and divisions across the system.

3. Improved communication and decision making within governance and management.

4. Consistent management of cost and quality to enhance health status at the lowest possible cost.

5. Rapid customer-oriented responses to market developments.

6. A high degree of operational flexibility and innovation.

Using these requirements, we embarked on a restructuring process that had "the needs of the customer, patient, and market" as the "guiding force in the design of our system." Our goal was to become a fully integrated system. We recognized and involved physicians as integral partners in the design of the overall organization and the delivery of services.

This has not been an easy transition, but at each phase of the process we've been consistent in our use of TQM. We are now a very different organization than we were when we began. Traditional "smokestacks" in a hierarchy are gone, and we now think of core processes. We've streamlined management and eliminated the vice presidents and directors in our organization. Job titles include core area leaders, transformation coordinators, and core process owners. Process management teams have been established and are busy mapping/redesigning the core processes of the organization.

New Structure

The old Table of Organization looks radically different (Fig. 7.3). In fact, it doesn't look like a chart of lines and boxes at all. Organizational services are aligned into five core areas, which are designed to make Bethesda flexible and amenable to change as our customers' needs change:

1. **Member acquisition services** are designed to enroll and retain members (customers) in our health care system. To do that, we need to understand and anticipate customer expectations and translate those to drive organization response.

2. **Health status management** is designed to optimize the health status of the people we serve as measured by the effectiveness of intervention strategies.

3. **Health services/physician services** are designed to provide appropriate clinical services to customers and to continually enhance the value of these services. The bulk of traditional services are in this area, but reorganized across the continuum of care rather than by specialty lines.

4. **Internal services** are designed to supply the direct providers of care with the information and materials needed to deliver appropriate health services and to provide the appropriate environment and physical necessities.

5. **Integrating services** are designed to enable the organization to act as a seamless system for serving its customers.

Once the five core areas were defined, the leadership team worked to identify core processes within each area. We ended up with 22 core processes as a starting point. These allowed us to move forward in our transformation to a customer-driven organization that can meet the challenges of both the current and future health care environment.

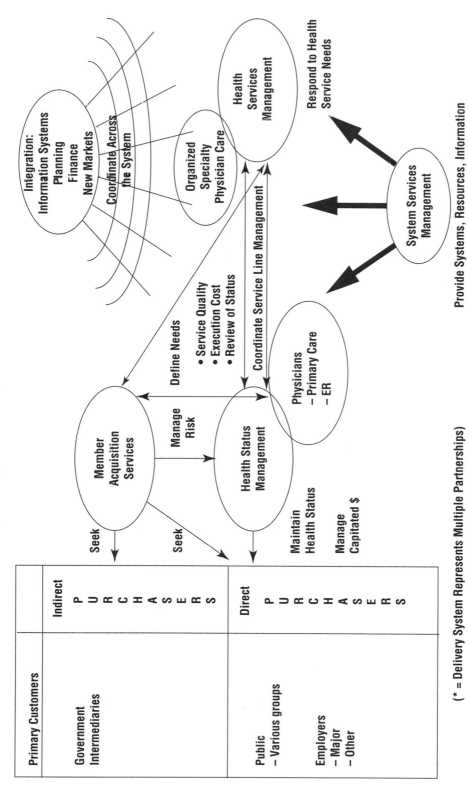

Figure 7.3 *Integrated System Concept Chart. (From Bethesda, Inc., Cincinnati, Ohio. Used by permission.)*

129

Nursing Implications

What did all of this mean for nursing? The former corporate nursing officer became a core area leader for health services/physician services, sharing this responsibility with another administrator and a physician executive. The executive nurse from one of our hospitals became a transformation coordinator and assumed the corporate nursing officer duties in a staff rather than line position. Directors of nursing and department managers became core process owners, and in the process of selecting the best candidates for these positions, it was readily apparent that the nursing directors/managers were often the best prepared people to assume these broader roles. The TQM position descriptions are:

- **Leadership Team (Core Area Leaders)**. This is the core team responsible for development of the customer-driven organization and for driving the integration of the core areas. The leadership team defines "what needs to be done"; others, such as core process teams, define "how it will be done."

- **Transformation Coordinator**. This is the person who coordinates the process of transforming work processes from a traditional functional operation to a customer-driven operation. They use process management and work to facilitate the culture changes and reengineering necessary to transform traditional roles to self-managed teams, coaches, and leaders.

- **Core Process Owner**. This is the person who is ultimately accountable for overall performance and outcomes of a customer-driven core process from beginning to end. The core process owner is expected to lead the process management team and to initiate changes in the core process, as recommended by the team, to ensure optimal process performance.

PRODUCTIVITY AND COST IMPLICATIONS

Mission, not financial crisis, should be the driving force behind productivity gains. As the TQM learning process evolves, it is evident that the approach to productivity improvement needs to change. Typically, productivity measurement activities will lack a mechanism to incorporate customer needs or process improvement ideas, and they do not offer a way to adjust staffing to short-term workload changes. It is possible, however, to implement a productivity improvement program that has its roots in TQM. At Bethesda, we called our new system of productivity "continuous operational assessment and response," or COAR.

COAR

There are five integrated modules in COAR: department business planning, reporting of biweekly weighted workload and person hours, systemwide variable staffing, cross-functional employee training and job redesign, and global outcome measures and forecasting. The central idea of COAR is measuring and responding to the environment at the appropriate level as quickly as possible. With the help of our management engineering department, managers now have a timely and more useful workload monitoring system readily available for decision making. Even though variable staffing was not a new concept for nursing, it was new for most other departments, and the idea of cross-training became a broadly accepted concept in the organization rather rapidly when fiscal pressures became a priority (Reifenberger, 1992).

Productivity, Quality, and Cost

Productivity and quality are related, and that relationship can best be illustrated by looking at waste. Doing the wrong things and doing things wrong are the simplest examples of opportunities for improvement when viewed from a TQM perspective. Often, the way we do things is self-serving rather than a consideration of what is important from the customer's set of expectations. To achieve both quality and productivity, it is necessary to have good data and to set improvement targets. If customer expectations are clear, then doing the right things, the right way, with the right number of people, will lead to optimal productivity and quality.

Quality and cost are related as well. The new world of managed care is painfully forcing health care providers to reduce the costs of care while continuing to demand quality. Measurement of quality has taken some rather unexpected turns, depending on who is doing it and how it is being done. But the measurement of costs is fairly clear to the outside world; they simply look at billed charges or discount prices, depending on who is doing the looking. The principles of TQM may be applied to achieve the highest possible quality at the lowest possible cost when goals are defined in measurable terms. The aim is to avoid waste and change the process so that quality failures do not occur. Quality and cost control depend on effective management systems with reliable data and a shared understanding of how to interpret it.

Nursing is often seriously affected in productivity improvement and cost-reduction initiatives for obvious reasons. Nursing makes up the largest percentage of the workforce, in numbers and in salary dollars. In a TQM environment, however, we need to look at patient care as a continuum, with multidisciplinary caregivers in addition to nurses. Many models of patient care redesign are being implemented these days, and each organization has to take an approach that seems to fit their situation best. The bottom line is that we can no longer afford any waste. All clinical disciplines must work together in the interest of efficient and effective patient care systems that result in quality at reduced cost. The tools and techniques associated with TQM can help caregivers in the presentation of data and in decision making related to redesign efforts.

POSITIONING OF THE EXECUTIVE NURSE

The executive nurse's role can change dramatically in a TQM environment. It is a positive change, and it is exciting.

In any TQM implementation, the executive nurse is a knowledgeable and essential partner on the team. Specifically, areas of involvement should include:

- Strategic planning
- Patient care as a cross-functional process
- Teamwork

- Leadership
- Medical staff collaboration
- Customer-driven horizontal operations

The executive nurse needs to be actively involved at the highest level of any planning related to TQM. Because the work of a health care organization is patient/client centered, it is the executive nurse who can best provide the expertise and talent needed to implement a TQM program.

Patient care involves many clinical disciplines and support services, but it has traditionally been the nurse at the bedside who is responsible for coordinating all activities into a plan of care that is in alignment with the physicians' medical plan for the patient. In a TQM environment, collaboration and teamwork are at the heart of what works best for the patient and have been proven to lead to the best-quality outcomes when functioning effectively. The executive nurse must therefore find ways to create and foster multidisciplinary teamwork. TQM should not be a nursing-driven initiative. It is essential that the executive nurse utilize and influence a broad implementation approach involving as many clinical disciplines as possible.

Another key issue is that most executive nurses find it difficult to hire new nurse managers into a mature TQM organization if they have not attained some basic knowledge and experience in the philosophy, tools, and techniques of TQM. The managers' role must include the broader and larger organizational goals and the manager in a TQM organization must readily adapt to priority functions as a teacher, coach, and facilitator. It is essential that leadership in a TQM organization actively listen to the customer and to the staff with the purposes of learning and action in mind. Also, these leaders must be able to truly empower their employees in a way that sets an example of TQM commitment and behaviors. Employees must be given ownership in order to build their own commitment, and a vision of success must be created by those who manage and guide the organization. Executive nurses and nurse managers who are accustomed to traditional roles of directing and control will not be comfortable in a TQM world. These individuals may need to face the harsh reality of leaving if they cannot or will not transform.

Summary

The ultimate goal of the highest possible quality patient care delivered at the lowest necessary cost equals value in a TQM organization. That goal cannot be achieved without nursing, and it is the responsibility of the executive nurse to serve as the champion of the effort. Nurses have an opportunity to use their education and skills in a TQM environment as never before. The real reasons that nurses became nurses in the first place can be enhanced, and their sense of professional and personal fulfillment can be achieved, if they honestly commit to TQM.

Discussion Questions

1. How would you implement TQM in your health care setting?

2. Do you think it would enhance your work environment? Why or why not?

References

Burrus, W. M. (1992). Differences: Between the CQI gurus. *Quality Matters, 1*(1). Landmark Communications, December, 1–6.

Deming, W. E. (1986). *Out of the crisis.* Cambridge, MA: Center for Advanced Engineering Study, Massachusetts Institute of Technology.

Dienemann, J. (1992). *Continuous quality improvement in nursing.* Washington: American Nurses Publishing.

Dressman, K. L. (1993). Lessons learned from an early TQM effort: Surgical prophylaxis. *Journal of Nursing Care Quality.* Aspen, 73–80.

Gaucher, E. J. & Coffey, R. J. (1993). *Total quality in healthcare.* San Francisco: Jossey-Bass.

Joint Commission on Accreditation of Healthcare Organizations. (1992). *JCAHO: Striving toward improvement, building a house of quality* (pp. 131–164). Oakbrook Terrace, IL: Author.

King, B. (1989). *Better designs in half the time: Implementing quality function deployment (QFD).* Methuen, MA: GOAL/QPC.

King, B. (1989). *Hoshin planning. The developmental approach.* Methuen, MA: GOAL/QPC.

Reifenberger, J. (1992). Hospital emphasizes its mission to guide productivity improvement. *Modern Healthcare,* August 3.

CHAPTER 8

Lauren Jones

Developing a Learning Organization

Introduction

In most health care settings, employees are encouraged to arrive at multiple solutions when problem solving. We have a tendency to come up with *the* definitive solution—and, if that doesn't work, it's back to the old way. Yet there are many solutions to specific problems, and executive nurses can challenge employees to devise several solutions, each of which can be tried, even if they are not the solutions of choice for the executive nurse. Trying several solutions sends the message that nothing is permanent and that systems are dynamic. Dynamic organizations are in constant flux, and a thinking staff can anticipate change and adopt strategies that will meet the changing needs of health care.

This chapter will discuss the behavioral consequences of pyramidal structures and strategies to create a **learning organization**, an organization that encourages thinking throughout its structure, and not just at the top.

If you have a minute, and your organizational chart is handy, try connecting the boxes denoting positions on the chart. Do you notice the pyramid created by connecting the dots? Does it look similar to Figure 8.1?

CURRENT ORGANIZATIONAL STRUCTURES

When hospitals, as we know them, began, they were functionally based (i.e., primarily focused on medicine and nursing). As medical care became more complex, we added functional areas such as radiology, pharmacy, dietetics, accounts receivable, housekeeping, and so on. As you can see (and may have experienced firsthand), those functional areas became entities unto themselves. These kinds of areas are called "silos," because that's the shape created by the functional approach. In silos, budgets are considered independent, and accompanying territo-

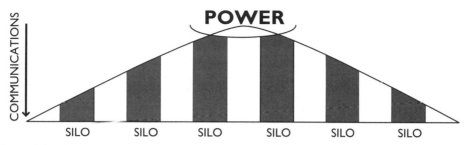

Figure 8.1 *Power. (From Jones, L. 1993. We need to re-expand our organizational brains.* Journal for Quality and Participation, 16, *3: 28–31.)*

ries are emphasized and defined. Rewards and recognition systems directly encourage silo loyalty. As staff are promoted within their silo, it gives them a defined span of control that results in vertical communication within the silo. Often, the silos are so encapsulated that employees within a particular silo look either up or down, with little opportunity or incentive to communicate horizontally across other silos. Now, consider how patients and their families move through the health care organization—horizontally. It is hard to think of an example that illustrates a patient who would come in contact with only one silo. Yet, the pyramidal structure of many organizations neither promotes horizontal communication nor fosters understanding of the big picture.

Think back to your last executive meeting. My hunch is that each vice president or director gave a report almost parallel to that of colleagues. Usually the CEO is paying attention, but the other attendees are probably focused on their own reports. There's almost an unwritten law that says, "You don't mess with my silo, and I won't mess with yours." Often, executives focus on their own silo, maybe to the exclusion of other silos. There is also an another unwritten law created by the silo structure. *Thinking* only occurs at the top of the pyramid or, in some instances, at the top of the silo. Employees aren't expected to think, just *do*.

BEHAVIORS IN A PYRAMIDAL ORGANIZATION

What are the behavioral illustrations of a pyramidal organization? You can probably identify many of them throughout the day. The employees who ask permission to do anything different, even though something is obviously required to change: "I knew it was wrong, but I thought that's the way you wanted it" or "I didn't think we could change this without asking you." These are classic examples of comments made by employees who are used to "bumping" decisions up the silo and assuming that decision making and thinking are done on the next rung up the organizational ladder.

Most of this thinking is based on the vertical nature of communication in a pyramidal organization. Information usually flows down, and generally the silo doesn't promote circular communication (top-down-top). As a result, communication is often indirect and passive. Employees who do not receive timely, direct information tend to make it up: "Well, you know why they are meeting, don't you?" or "I'll bet I know what's going on."

Sometimes, the nature of the pyramidal structure forces executives to hold information or communicate it in a formal manner. Unfortunately, the formality can cause the perception that information is a secret, known to only a chosen few. Again, the secretive nature of any information can lead to distortions and passive-aggressiveness on the part of those who feel left out of the communication—in short, dysfunctional communication patterns.

The dysfunctional behaviors practiced in many health care organizations have been well documented (Schaef & Fassel, 1990). Most people who seek a nursing career tend to be nice people who want to help. Couple this with the fact that most nurses are women, and you may have a large population of caregivers who are rescuers, enablers, and martyrs.

Most women have been socialized to be individually competitive. They were encouraged to be the brightest, the cutest, the funniest, the "whatever-est." Now, however, we are expected to be team players, helping each other and working together.

Now, most of you who are reading this are saying,"Wait a minute. We help each other in our department." Granted, but do we do this to the exclusion of other silos? Does it become us against them? Interestingly, the *us* and *them* can be A.D.N. versus B.S.N.; nurses versus everyone else; nights versus days; staff versus management; nurses versus administrators; unit versus unit; or nurses versus physicians.

In that kind of environment, what gets valued is politeness and compliance. Those values can also translate into a passive-aggressive environment where direct communication is not valued and a nonconfrontive atmosphere results. You often hear nurses comment that they disagree with a decision, or someone who made the decision, but wouldn't think of telling that person: "I don't want to hurt their feelings." Unfortunately, they would rather share their opinion with several dozen close colleagues. The lack of confrontation has produced myriad policies and procedures. In many organizations, if you track the origin of a particular personnel policy, you will find that it was written to deal with one individual but went on to become a policy insulting everyone.

The best scenario is an attendance policy. The employee who was chronically late was not coached individually; it was easier and less confrontive to issue a policy that mandated timeliness. The usual result was that the offender ignored the policy and the majority of employees who were appearing on time were affronted because they were already showing up on time.

It would be an interesting exercise for executive nurses to examine their current policy and procedure manuals. In most instances, the number of policies and procedures is inversely proportional to the amount of thinking expected. Most staff nurses (however, not all) are thrilled to be included in a decision-making process, but often that is not valued in our current organizational structure.

LEARNING CYCLE

If our organization is pyramidal, how do we develop a learning organization? We start first by breaking a learning organization into components of a learning cycle (Fig. 8.2).

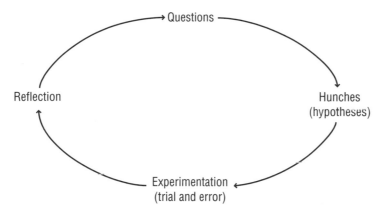

Figure 8.2   *The Learning Cycle. (From Handy, C., 1990,* The age of unreason. *Boston: Harvard Business School Press.)*

Overall, this cycle emphasizes the importance of *questions* as they lead to *hypotheses*. The hypotheses get tested through arriving at several *solutions* and testing them out. Evaluating the various solutions or experiments requires a time of reflection, not only to look at the solutions themselves but also at the process used in arriving at the solutions. The *reflection* also provides an opportunity to see if any of the content or process could be standardized to other silos or throughout the organization. We will look at each phase of this cycle in depth to allow for better understanding and to provide an assessment tool for use in your organization. A learning survey was developed (by the author) for the purpose of assessing an organization's readiness to create a learning organization. Sample questions have been included with each phase of the cycle.

Questions

In most organizations or departments, questions are not viewed positively. On the contrary, they are viewed as problems to be fixed as quickly as possible. You can see where that leads to the popular term *crisis management* (or "firefighting"). Unfortunately, many managers are promoted to leadership positions based on their firefighting ability. True leadership has very little to do with firefighting and everything to do with long-term planning and systems development. When questions are viewed as problems in an organization, silence and status quo are often valued. The focus is on doing rather than thinking. Many managers don't encourage questions in their silo because they view questioning as a challenge to their authority. They much prefer a silo that is composed of compliant workers who just *do*.

Most leaders will quickly tell you that it is important for staff not only to do, but also to understand the system in which they do. Understanding the system allows staff continually to evaluate and improve the system that ultimately affects patient care.

Not understanding a system results in a focus on detail and complexity. An example of this is the concept of shared governance. That term can also apply to continuous quality improvement (CQI), or participative management.

Departments or organizations that do not understand the concepts will immediately jump to by-laws and rules and regulations before employees have had an opportunity to embrace the ideas and assume some ownership and investment in the ideas. Many health care executives become very frustrated when they find out that there aren't (nor should there be) specific handbooks on CQI or shared governance. The struggle is necessary in adapting the concepts to your own organization or silo. Yet, the struggle cannot begin without asking many questions.

It is important for the executive nurse to look at how questions are viewed. Many nurses were educated in nursing schools that eschewed questions. Instead of answering a student's question, the response often was: "Why don't you know the answer?", which quickly led to not asking questions. That same behavior has carried over to our silos and organizations. Many nurses who question are labeled troublemakers.

Establishing Ground Rules

To engage this first stage of the learning cycle, it is important to establish ground rules for conduct within units, departments, or meetings, so that a safe atmosphere is created for risk-taking and subsequent learning. Since each group of employees has different organizational issues, ground rules will vary with each group. Some groups not comfortable challenging a manager might have a ground rule that says "All voices are equal" and "There are no repercussions for anything said in here."

One specific ground rule that should be contained within the diverse sets is "No voting." We have a tendency to base decisions on a show of hands, only to pay for the dissenting votes later. Voting members are often heard defending or maligning decisions to their colleagues: "Well, I didn't vote for that and I won't support it." Consensus is more time-consuming initially, but it pays off in the long run.

Consensus

Reaching consensus means going to each member and asking what it would take to support a particular decision. Some might need more time or more data; others may support the decision if they are assured that it will be evaluated in a short period of time. Consensus produces much more ownership (buy-in) than the ostensibly easy voting process.

Whatever the ground rules developed, they need to be *visible* and *signed*. They may sound rather benign, but they act as a facilitator and allow groups and teams to accomplish work using adult behaviors. The concept of ground rules will be referred to again throughout this chapter.

Sample Questions

It might be helpful to use the following questions in your own organization to assess the use of questions as a learning tool.

"Questions in my organization mean. . . ":

1. You're attacking your immediate supervisor.

2. You're rocking the boat.

3. You should know the answer.

4. You are not loyal.

5. You are not a team player.

6. We are all trying to improve.

7. We are all part of the solution instead of the problem.

8. We don't have questions; we go right to solutions.

9. I'm on automatic pilot when I get here and don't question many things.

Hypotheses

Many middle managers have trouble with hypotheses. Many believe that they should have the definitive answer—that there is no room for hypothesizing at all. Their use of questions can be crucial to the success of a team in getting them to stretch and think. It is most difficult for managers to lead a team in developing and testing several hypotheses when they either know the right direction or think they know the right direction.

The hypothesis stage of the learning cycle is often overlooked as teams or several employees jump into solutions. The hypothesizing stage takes time and involves a great deal of data collection before arriving at solutions. And even though we were all educated in the scientific method (i.e., the nursing process), many nurses are not accustomed to methodically collecting and displaying data.

Late-Day Admissions   *Scenario 8.1*

Recently, a group of nurses was complaining that they were getting "a lot" of admissions at 3 P.M. Understandably, this practice was affecting scheduling, change of shift, and reports. Pursuing their comment, I asked how many was "a lot," only to be told "pretty many." The nurses were asked to take a pencil and paper and jot down every time they admitted someone after 3 P.M. Within five days, they had data to support flex scheduling.

The nurses in the scenario were not ignorant or stupid. They had the skills— they just needed to resurrect them. Often, employees who don't feel empowered in an organization revert to global, vague terms. Their powerlessness is exhibited by a sense of hopelessness and frustration because the person on the rung above them in the silo is not "fixing" things.

During the hypothesizing phase, the gathering of data is crucial in determining the solutions that employees propose. Data not only strengthen proposed solutions but they also decrease the likelihood of blaming another silo and jumping to the wrong solution. Later, we will discuss the role of the executive nurse in providing educational opportunities so that employees can be successful in problem solving.

Sample Questions

The following questions may represent where your organization/department/unit is in using hypothesizing.

1. We are encouraged to think about hunches.

2. When a question arises, we are encouraged to think about "why."

3. When a question arises, we are expected to "fix it" fast.

4. We do not spend much time on hunches, or on reasons that some things may be happening.

5. We are encouraged to think through questions and come up with possible causes or solutions.

6. We all know "why" something is happening in our organization.

Trial and Error/Experimentation

The trial and error/experimentation phase is usually the one that gets the most attention. As previously mentioned, we all "know" what the cause of a problem is (usually an individual or silo) and we eagerly leap to *one* solution. However, the process of data collection can often lead to the real cause of a problem or issue instead of the overt symptom.

Scenario 8.2 **Picking Up the Meds**

An example of this is a unit that was complaining about pharmacy not delivering stat medications. In order to ensure timely administration of the medication, nurses would have to go to pharmacy for the medication. Of course, if the unit was busy, there could be quite a time-lag before a nurse was able to get off the unit and pick up the medication. Staff's constant complaints to their nurse manager were greeted with " I know, but pharmacy is short-staffed and if we want the meds we have to get it." Finally, after many months of frustration, and numerous complaints, the chief executive nurse went to the CEO.

Interestingly enough, the head of pharmacy also went to the CEO to complain about the treatment his employees were taking from nurses. He cited numerous examples of verbal abuse and ended his comments with "I know there's nothing you can do about it. I just wanted you to know. Nurses have been like that in every hospital I've worked in."

Fortunately, the CEO was bright enough to know that she didn't have the answer. So, she asked the executive nurse to assemble several interested staff nurses who would join interested pharmacists and technicians to look at the problem and come up with solutions. It wasn't until the medication process was flow-charted that people truly understood the process and were able to propose objective solutions. Briefly, the solutions included fax machines on the units and increasing the number of pharmacy technicians.

The meds scenario illustrates several points:

1. Data collection and flow charting made those involved more objective.

2. The people who were part of the process became part of the solution.

3. Assumptions were debunked about rival silos.

4. There was an improvement in collegial relations through erosion of silos.

Risk-Taking

If the consequences are not serious, it is often a useful learning experience for teams to test a hypothesis that is doomed. The key factors are the severity of the consequences and the opportunity to process the experience and determine what could be done differently next time. Teams quickly learn that mistakes can be valuable when risk taking is encouraged.

Sample Questions

Try the following sample questions to evaluate your organization, department, or unit's level of learning in the trial and error stage of the learning cycle.

1. We are encouraged to come up with several solutions to an identified problem.

2. In our organization, it's either this one new way or back to the old way.

3. Our team gets frustrated when our solution is not implemented.

4. There usually is only one way to solve a problem.

5. There's no need to waste time problem solving; most of the time we all know the best way to solve the problem.

6. We don't "try out" solutions, we implement them and they become policy.

Reflection

The last phase of the learning cycle—reflection—is perhaps the most difficult because it requires time and it is often not valued in organizations. This phase allows us to step back and take a critical look at what we're doing, where we're going, what's working, and what might be improved.

Most executive nurses are accustomed to executive retreats where they can engage in strategic planning. However, this practice need not be limited to a yearly occurrence nor to the executive group. Employees need an opportunity to step out of their business-as-usual routine and critically evaluate solutions, team/unit/department relations, patient care processes, and their own roles as learners and caregivers.

The reflection phase provides the opportunity for employees at all levels in the organization to evaluate and standardize, if possible. If, however, we only value the doing in the organization and not the thinking, we will not be inclined to value the reflection phase.

Reflection need not involve going off-site and spending money on expensive accommodations. It may, however, involve providing floats to allow staff to attend a meeting without feeling that they have shirked their patient-care duties and increased the workload of their colleagues. We will discuss more specific strategies when we focus on creating a learning organization.

Standardization

You can see that the reflection phase is another opportunity to standardize processes, when appropriate. Some strategies that are effective within one unit or department or shift may be useful in other areas. It also helps to further erode silos and moves the organization toward a systems orientation. The reflection phase usually leads to more questions, which further perpetuate the learning cycle.

Sample Questions

The following samples can be used to assess the value of the reflection stage in your organization.

1. We value doing in our organization, not thinking.

2. We value thinking in our organization, not doing.

3. We are supposed to solve problems, but we have no time for it.

4. Management should solve problems.

5. We don't look at solutions once they've been implemented.

6. Only upper management has retreats.

7. We evaluate solutions shortly after we implement, and adjust accordingly.

From Pyramid to System

Engaging this learning cycle throughout an organization creates a structural change from a hierarchical, pyramidal configuration to a system like that in Fig. 8.3.

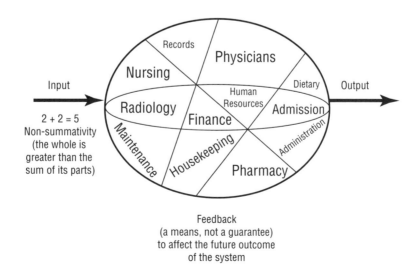

Figure 8.3 *Interrelatedness/Interdependency.*

Upon review, there are several components of a system that may be antithetical to the traditional, pyramidal structure. The focus on the interrelatedness and interdependency of a system underscores the need to obviate the silos and emphasizes the horizontal communication among services.

Non-Summativity

A system allows everyone to be involved in some aspect in the delivery of health care; hence the concept of non-summativity. If we all count in an organization and are all valued for our skills and gifts, it is easy to support the concept that the whole of any organization is greater than the sum of its parts. That same concept also translates into "all of us are smarter than one of us." Again, this may be a difficult concept to embrace if the power resides at the top of the organization or at the top of a silo. It is also difficult if those at the top want to keep the power at the top.

As organizations continue to face downsizing and doing more with less, it becomes imperative for all health care executives to create a work environment that promotes and rewards thinking. Complex organizations must rely on their empowered and accountable employees to continually evaluate, improve, and design processes that will move the organization into the twenty-first century. Where do executives begin to create this kind of environment? How can they look to the future and convince their employees to move in that direction? These are important questions to ask, particularly in light of the many external regulations that continue to plague health care and force many health care executives to react to changes on a short-term basis. The remainder of this chapter will discuss how to create a learning organization that will weather many economic storms and positively affect the future of health care. This content is applicable to all types of health care settings.

HOW TO CREATE A LEARNING ORGANIZATION

The first step in creating a learning organization is to question your own beliefs about yourself and about people in general (the first phase of the learning cycle). What is your purpose in life? Why are you on this earth? What are you here to accomplish? These are sometimes uncomfortable topics. And, as mentioned previously, reflection requires time.

Personal Reflection

The reflection on your personal beliefs is vital in determining the course of your department or organization. Your leadership role and the course you steer will be based on your belief system. If you react to structural change with, as one CEO shared with me, "you're not suggesting the inmates run the asylum are you?", you will create an organization or department based on hierarchy, rules, and compliance to rules. Of course, the consequences of such an organization are that you are responsible for any new ideas and must police the adherence to the rules. That might work if everything remained static and you didn't mind paying salaries for skills you don't intend to use. Your employees will show up, put in their time, and leave. Unfortunately, I'm not sure how many patients or family members would want someone caring for them who's on automatic pilot.

A focus on belief systems really forces people to question their assumptions (paradigms) about themselves and others. If the paradigm "Physicians are always right" exists in your organization, collaboration will be a difficult (if not impossible) value to market.

Organizational Theme

Following is a discussion about the steps that will allow you to develop a collective belief system within your organization or department. This collective belief system will facilitate the creation of the learning organization we have been discussing. The term for this integrated, collective belief system is an **organizational theme** and can be applied within a unit, department, or organization. The specific components of this theme are the mission, vision, values, and behavior, and each component will now be discussed in depth.

Mission

Most organizations have a mission (i.e., some reason for being in business). A **mission statement** describes what business you're in and why, and the statement is readily shared with new board members, the community, and new employees. A brief mission statement succinctly explains the purpose of the organization but does not indicate its future direction. For that, you need a vision.

Vision

The next component of an organizational theme, vision, is a bit more complicated. An **organizational vision** describes and defines where the organization is going and ideally what it will look like. In keeping with the reflection phase of the learning cycle, it is important to create an environment that promotes a relaxed atmosphere for imagining and which steers away from business as usual. The following suggestions may help you conduct this vital exercise.

- Play soft instrumental music in the background with the lights dimmed.

- Within the context of your ground rules (described in the Question section of this chapter), ask your team members to think about the following questions:

    — "What will this medical center look like, ideally, 5 years from today?

    — What services will be offered?

    — What will the employees be saying?

    — What will the physicians be saying?

    — What will the patients be saying?

    — What will their families be saying?

These are but a few of the questions to ask yourself and your staff. You can add to the list as you are conducting the exercise.

Recently, a nurse manager tried this in a long-suffering unit composed of nurses who were depressed and powerless. She dropped me a note to describe the change in morale and productivity that was obvious soon after the session discussing the vision. Several staff nurses commented that they didn't think they had any control over their work environment and were surprised and energized about the things they could control. Without a vision, organizations or departments are doomed to a short-term focus that moves from day to day with no look toward the future. As a frequently referenced idea from *Alice in Wonderland* indicates: If you don't know where you're headed, any direction will lead you there.

Determining our direction allows us to design, implement, and evaluate systems that will continually improve patient care. Communicating that direction fosters employees who are growing professionally and who do not defend their behaviors with attitudes expressed by "We've always done it that way and it's always worked in the past."

There are some executives who may be saying "I've already created a vision and handed it out to everyone." First, congratulations on having a vision; you're already one step ahead. Second, if someone handed you such a paper, what might your first reaction be? "Who do they think they are?" "Who came up with this?" The bottom line is, it might be best to communicate your *draft* vision among your employees for their input and feedback. Some will get involved and dissect the draft, while others will think it's a trick or an exercise in futility because it's already a *fait accompli*.

Beginning this practice accomplishes three things:

1. It begins to build ownership and investment.

2. It begins to promote and enhance accountability.

3. It allows you to keep your vision dynamic and to change it as you near your goal.

Most of us know about how NASA achieved in 1969 Kennedy's vision of putting an astronaut on the moon, and the subsequent languishing of NASA. Many analysts will tell you that NASA never changed its vision; it had no new vision to replace the lofty one already accomplished.

You want employees to buy in to the vision—to embrace the direction you have projected. But how can you ensure some standardization and commonality in the approaches to achieving the vision? This can be accomplished by establishing organizational values, which is the next component of an organizational theme.

Values

Values are part of the soul searching we discussed previously; they provide the guiding principles to achieve your vision. They bring to the foreground beliefs about human beings, work, patients, and their families. These may be thoughts that people have individually, but they are not usually shared publicly.

Values describe how an organization or department or unit will reach its vision. They are the collective tenets held by members of an organization. As such, you can see how important it is to elicit feedback and input from all employees using a process similar to the one described in the vision section. Ask the question "If this is where we say we are going, what values or guiding principles will take us there?"

It also helps to identify the current **organizational values**. They be quite different from the values needed to aspire to the new organizational vision. Many traditional health care organizations valued compliance and conformity to policies, procedures, and physicians. An organization that sees itself on the cutting edge of health care in its new vision will have to adopt new values. Sample values for such a vision might include collaboration and creativity.

There should be general agreement on the values throughout the organization. Employees who do not share similar values will be square pegs in round holes, and you may be able to identify some of those folks as you are reading this. Specific values serve as an excellent recruitment tool and readily differentiate you from your competitor. But how can you measure these values? How can you describe what these values imply? This can be accomplished by developing and identifying the last component of an organizational theme—behaviors.

Behaviors

This component is probably the most difficult for executives and yet easiest for staff. The mission, vision, and values can be a bit obscure for those staff who are relatively concrete and sensory in their approach to work. Sensory employees tend to ignore things they cannot see, hear, feel, taste, or touch.

The **behavioral component**, however, provides the specificity and detail that most employees enjoy. While the vision describes where the organization is heading and the values describe how it will get there, the behaviors define what will be done. In other words, behaviors are expressions of the values.

For example, if one of the values of an organization is collaboration, a specific behavior might involve active participation on a team. Other behaviors that express the value of collaboration might include direct communication and confrontation with dignity and negotiation. These specific actions not only communicate the organization's expectations to all employees so that they may be successful, but they also provide the concrete benchmarks for coaching and performance improvement.

These behavioral expressions of values provide the performance expectations that integrate the mission, vision, and values of the organization (or the organizational theme). In short, the organizational theme is a reliable and powerful strategy that encourages all employees to "sing off the same sheet of music."

Organizational Theme Summary

In summary, an organizational theme is composed of an established mission (what/why an organization is in business), a vision (where an organization is ideally headed), values (how the organization will achieve its vision), and behaviors (what actions will express the values). The purposes of an organizational theme are to:

- Create an integrated approach to organizational effectiveness.
- Promote a systems orientation by viewing the organization as a whole, as opposed to individual turfs.
- Foster horizontal communication throughout the organization.
- Support professional growth as a learning organization.

The executive nurse has a key role in coaching staff as they move from the pyramidal structure to a systems orientation, where they are accountable for continually improving the system of health care delivery. The remainder of this chapter will be devoted to the coaching role.

EXECUTIVE NURSE AS COACH

What is a coach? For many people, several images may come to mind: Vince Lombardi, Woody Hayes, Mike Ditka. These men, in their own way, produced results—usually in an aggressive way that left no doubt who was in charge. Many M.B.A. programs have emphasized this type of coaching, even going so far as to focusing on football coaching. Those who understand football coaching know that there are specific coaches for specific plays and that the coach of a particular play is only concerned with that play. Sound like silos?

Coaching and Sports

There are many business schools that are switching from that type of dictatorial, territorial coaching to more of a basketball approach, where coaches view the entire court and not just their particular play (Avishai, 1993). The advantage of this change to the role of the executive nurse is that the largely female profession may not be saddled with the traditional, and unfamiliar, coaching paradigm; thus, we may not have to unlearn previous behaviors. We do, however, need to focus on learning new ones.

Let's start with a definition of coaching: "Someone who cares about your dignity as a human being and your growth as a spiritual being" (Jones, 1989). There may be many who are uncomfortable with the "spiritual being" component, perhaps thinking that we are promoting a religious movement. But go back to the organizational values: Aren't those values part of the organization's and employees' spiritual growth? Aren't they part of a collective ethical construct that captures the organization's beliefs about people, health, birth, and death?

Can you think of any industry that has placed more emphasis on values than the health care industry? This has resulted in a focus on spiritual growth in our coaching. Most of us can probably think of a mentor or coach whom we admired and trusted. For most of us, that person was probably from the educational arena. What happens to coaching when we become a full-time employee?

Coaching Skills

One has to be secure and confident within the professional arena to reach out and help others grow. It can be difficult if coaching forces you to give up status, power, or span of control, particularly if your former management role model was a carbon copy of Attila the Hun!

Manager to Coach

When talking about the process used to create nursing managers, we intentionally use the word *manager* and not leader because that's how most of us started out.

Recall the staff nurse who was extremely proficient technically. What did we do? We promoted that technical star to a position where those skills weren't needed, thereby creating a duck out of water.

Historically, such conscientious (sensory) folks focused on details—*what* was being done on the unit—and not necessarily *how* things were getting done. The truly efficient manager took on many jobs, ostensibly to show how responsibly she or he could run the unit/department. Unfortunately, this was done to the detriment of staff, who were given messages such as: "Don't rock the boat." "I'll do the thinking." "There's a policy on that." "Just do your job." "Our unit is fine; it's the other ones that are a mess."

If any of these sound familiar, perhaps it's time to look at how we coach and how we can potentiate the skills and gifts of our employees. True coaching begins with a ground rule that involves how we choose to interact with each other in the work environment. Remember that ground rules are unique to each group and should be developed by the group.

Leadership Expectations

Once the ground rules have been established, it is important for the executive nurse to clearly spell out expectations of the unit or within the department. This lets employees clearly understand how you operate. It is important, at the same time, to have employees discuss their expectations of *you*. What do they need from you as their leader (intentionally using that word, as opposed to "manager")? This might be a time for you to begin your role as coach and ask how they would like recognition for their performance.

Often, the collective self-esteem among nurses is so low that they may not be able to ask for recognition. They also may have had experience with a previous manager who believed "Of course you're doing a good job; if you weren't, I'd tell you," or "You get paid, don't you? That should tell you how you're doing." Regardless of what your staff may say, they need individual and group recognition for their performance, and that's where coaching comes in.

Taking the time to meet with your staff regularly as a group, and also individually, is the first step to coaching. Discussing your values and theirs provides a climate that can launch an *organizational theme* within your own unit/department. You need to ask yourself:

- Where is this unit/department going?

- How do your vision and values mesh with the organizational theme?

- How will you implement the performance expectations within your area?

- What do your employees need in order to grow, and continue to improve, as caregivers?

Entitled Staff

Typically, nurse managers dread annual reviews. They take the onus of the review on themselves and force themselves to evaluate every performance criterion on their list. The result is a review based on the past that is usually benign and usually disappointing for both parties. There's a tendency to make everyone middle-of-the-road, with the result being "entitled staff" (Bardwick, 1991).

Entitled staff are those employees who realize that, even if they are only giving about 70 percent to their jobs, no one will say anything to them. Suddenly, a new employee comes in who's 'bright-eyed' and excited, giving 100 percent to the job. Eventually, however, the new employee figures out that nothing is happening to the 70-percent employees, nor is anything special happening to her (or him). So the new employee starts slacking off. Thus the norm of mediocrity has been established and you have entitled staff: employees who are going through the motions, who don't think much about what they do, and who are on automatic pilot. In such organizations, the self-esteem is low (after all, what's there to feel good about?), and employees describe themselves as powerless and helpless. One staff member shared that, in her hospital, "You could do anything here and you won't get fired." She was describing an organization that had low performance standards and the incident reports to support that contention. When asked how she felt, she said that she was "treated as an FTE (full-time equivalent)," someone who was just filling a position regardless of skills or talents.

Empowering Staff

A coach can revitalize entitled employees by making their expectations explicit, along with the consequences of not meeting those expectations. How many times have you heard a nurse manager complain about a nurse's behavior or attitude, and then quickly add "but she's an excellent nurse?" Is this an excellent nurse? Doesn't the concept of excellence encompass not only *what* we do, but *how* we do it? Individual coaching can provide the employee with feedback on behavior and establish the expectation that there will be a follow-up to see how things are progressing. This kind of interaction clearly establishes the expectation that a behavioral change will occur. The coach, using the first stage of the learning cycle, can ask many questions of employees that will get them both involved and invested in changing behaviors, such as "What do you need from me?" "What do you need to meet this performance expectation successfully?" You are reaching consensus, not compliance. You are also getting employees to be accountable for their own behavior.

Of course not all employees embrace the concept of autonomy. In fact, only about 50 percent of your employees will be excited about the learning cycle and their role in contributing to the organizational theme (Jones, 1983). The remaining 50 percent will need much coaching to get them comfortable with risk-taking or direct confrontation, as opposed to finger pointing. The coach can provide opportunities for employees to take on small projects, ask for help, and celebrate successes.

Having individuals or teams begin with safe projects or tasks allows them to experience success, thereby increasing their self-esteem. It is important for the coach to ask what staff need to be successful. In many instances, the following conditions may be necessary for a consensus: more education, time, dates for evaluations, sounding boards, recognition, and a renegotiation of existing responsibilities. Coaching takes one thing that most of us have little of—time. The time spent is up front, and positively impacts the long-term results. Crisis intervention, the opposite tack, has dire consequences because you are constantly putting out fires rather than preventing problems. Coaching allows you to create the environment that promotes professional growth, not stagnation.

As wonderfully rewarding as coaching is, it can also be threatening to those managers who like to control things and people. Coaching provides a transition from manager to leader; from someone who previously managed things to someone who is managing people. You can expect some other down sides to coaching. For example, people will confront you about your behavior. You may feel that you are in a fishbowl and, a, such, everything gets magnified. People are expecting you to walk the talk—to back up your words with your behavior. You may lose some employees who actively choose not to be part of the vision. You probably have already lost them mentally; they will just be leaving physically now.

Coaching Summary

The following coaching competencies may be helpful to you or to someone you are coaching:

- Take what you do, not yourself, seriously.
- Actively listen.
- Be willing to unlearn.
- Be willing to confront with dignity.
- Value the time to coach.
- Be clear about who owns the problem.
- Create the environment for self-evaluation.
- Be willing to support the employee's proposed solution or goals.
- Be willing to set follow-up dates.

Summary

This chapter explored current organizational structures and the behavioral effects of the traditional pyramidal configuration. It discussed creating a learning organization by focusing on the phases of the learning cycle: (1) questions, (2) hypotheses, (3) trial and error/experimentation, and (4) reflection.

The chapter also assessed where organizations, departments, and/or units might be currently in the use of this problem-solving process. To create a true learning organization, requires the components of an organizational theme: (1) mission, (2) vision, (3) values, and (4) behaviors.

The purpose of an organizational theme is to create an integrated approach in providing quality health care by eliminating silos and promoting achievable performance expectations throughout an organization. We explored the executive nurse's role in facilitating an integrated theme within the department or unit, and meshing nursing's theme with the overall organizational theme. Getting employees to become involved in the development and execution of an organizational theme requires the executive nurse to be a coach. In this role of coach, the nurse moves from managing things to managing people by creating an environment that not only fosters the professional and personal growth of employees but also potentiates the existing gifts of all employees. The bottom line is that "All of us are smarter than one of us" and we need each other in the form of a learning organization to propel nursing and health care well into the twenty-first century.

Discussion Questions

Please refer to the many questions within this chapter.

References

Avishai, B. (1993). Poor marks for M.B.A. programs. *Lear's*, 16–20.

Bardwick, J. (1991). *Danger in the comfort zone: Why America's job holders must renounce entitlement and earn their keep.* New York: AMACOM.

Handy, C. (1990). *The age of unreason.* Boston: Harvard Business School Press.

Jones, L. (1983). The professionalization of nursing (unpublished doctoral dissertation).

Jones, L. (1993). We need to re-expand our organizational brains. *Journal for Quality and Paricipation, 16*(3), 28–31.

Rowan, R. (1986). *The intuitive manager.* New York: Berkley Publishing Group.

Schaef, A. W., & Fassel, D. (1990). *Addictive organization: Why we overwork, cover up, pick up the pieces, please the boss, and perpetuate sick organizations.* San Francisco: Harper & Row.

Senge, P. M. (1990). *The fifth discipline: The art and practice of the learning organization.* New York: Doubleday.

Marie J. Driever
Mary Schoessler
Janice Voukidis
Arlene Austinson

CHAPTER 9

Evaluating New Organizational Models
Promoting Continual Learning

Introduction

Currently, health care organizations are redesigning care delivery processes to develop new organizational models of delivery. Developing these new models requires concerted innovation and brings profound change to the organization. In designing and implementing new models, learning occurs that in turn promotes further innovation and the understanding to put into practice improved ways to deliver care. Learning—seeing the world in a new light and acting accordingly—is necessary to redesign and improve care delivery. Integrating concepts of Garvin (1993, 80) and Senge (1990, 1), to build the learning organization requires an environment that supports and nurtures people to continually expand their patterns of thinking, create results they desire, and learn to learn together. Then an organization becomes skilled at creating, acquiring, and transferring knowledge, and modifying its behavior to reflect new knowledge and insights.

In serving as a demonstration site for the Strengthening Hospital Nursing: A Program To Improve Patient Care Project (SHNP), funded by the Robert Wood Johnson Foundation and Pew Charitable Trusts, participants at Providence Portland Medical Center (PPMC), of Portland, Oregon, have evolved a definition of organizational restructuring. Focal areas of restructuring are relationships, decision-making, and the care delivery system (Driever, 1994). In meeting the mandate of the SHNP grants to design and implement institution-wide restructuring, PPMC project participants affirmed that redesigning the way care is delivered is an organizational endeavor. The whole organization must be restructured to support both the redesign and implementation of new care delivery models. Learning is the essence of these changes.

Goals

The processes by which new organizational models are created, and the degree of organizational change that results, demand a rethinking of the approach to evaluation. In undertaking redesign and improvement, health care organizations are striving to become learning organizations and to operate in a mode of continual quality improvement. Given the new work of health care organizations, the context for evaluation has drastically changed; it demands an approach to evaluation that must respond to two needs. The first relates to the degree and comprehensiveness of the change and/or innovation to be evaluated, which then influences the degree of comprehensiveness of the evaluation; the second relates to continual reexamination of the questions guiding the evaluation design, given the emphasis on innovation and quality improvement. This chapter describes an approach to evaluation that will:

1. Generate quality data (i.e., reliable, valid data) for use in decision making across disciplines and throughout levels of the organization.

2. Promote continual learning throughout the organization at the individual, group/team, and organizational levels.

New Approach to Evaluation

Evaluation of new organizational models of care delivery must account for the new work of, and mindset about, organizations. This requires a broad definition of evaluation. **Evaluation** refers to any effort to increase human effectiveness through systematic data-based inquiry. The purpose of evaluation is to inform action, enhance decision making, and apply knowledge to solve human and societal problems (Patton, 1990, 11–12). Patton believes the challenge of evaluation is getting the best possible information to the people who need it and then getting those people to use the information in appropriate ways for intended purposes (Patton, 1990, 13).

Within a continually changing health care environment, the evaluation of effectiveness changes as well. Learning that increases individual caregiver competence and organizational effectiveness is a basic criterium for determining the success of innovations. Traditionally, evaluation has been charged with answering questions like "What difference did it make?" This question implies a circumscribed scope of evaluation. In contrast, current questions that arise in changing organizations include "What are the results in terms of care delivery?" or "Has the delivery of care been improved?" and/or "How has the innovation changed the organization?" These new questions demand a different scope of evaluation, which in turn has implications for evaluation design and methodology, as well as possible uses of the data.

Evaluation or Evaluation Research

The distinction between evaluation and research is important in determining human efectiveness. To examine and judge accomplishments and effectiveness is to evaluate (Patton, 1990, 11). When this examination of effectiveness is performed systematically and empirically through careful data collection and thoughtful analysis, the endeavor is evaluation research.

Research perspective means using the research process to strengthen the measurement needed for the evaluation (Driever, 1992). Conscious planning and use of the research process throughout the evaluation endeavor will assist all involved to design and implement their plans systematically, thereby generating quality (i.e., valid and reliable data for multiple and varied uses).

To respond to diverse evaluation questions poses a challenge of measurement, but measurement challenges exist whether the work is to be evaluation or evaluation research. A research perspective is needed to assure the generation of quality data, given the intense resources required for data collection and the major decisions data are to inform.

Rethinking Evaluation Effectiveness

A different meaning of **evaluation effectiveness** is needed based on the scope, work, and organizational impact of redesigned care delivery models. The new approach to evaluation is an integration of selected components from three earlier evaluation approaches. The merit of these approaches became evident through the authors' experience. Each of the three approaches contributes concepts and directions to meet the demands for evaluation in changing complex organizational environments.

Another issue in defining evaluation effectiveness relates to measurement of improvement that may not be directly attributable to innovations. The quality movement, with its emphasis on data as integral to the components of the problem-solving process, demands that people understand and use data. Using data provides challenges for design and implementation. Including effectiveness as part of evaluation creates a context for our approach and our designs. This context demands a variety of designs to implement an overall evaluation approach (Whyte, Greenwood, & Lazes, 1989). Organizational change, and its impact on the effectiveness of redesigned ways to deliver care, must address not only demonstrable effects but also provide a basis for engaging in a dialogue as to how changes are accomplished.

This focus is necessary, given the rapidity and extensiveness of change. In the past, there was time both to collect data before implementing a new program and to accomplish some specific change. Now, there is rarely time to do measurement either before or after a change. Change is being experienced as a process—one that evolves. Use of quantitative methodology adds to the change stress, with its demands for static "snapshots" and control of implementation. We need an evaluation approach with designs and methodologies that can capitalize on constant movement and evolution. It also needs to document the process of change, both in terms of the process and identified desired outcomes and how well the planned change fulfills criteria that are also evolving. The evaluation process needs to fit, support, and promote organizational restructuring, as well as the learning required to make organizational changes real. This new evaluation approach will be explored in terms of (1) a conceptual framework; (2) a scenario highlighting the application; (3) assumptions, principles, and methods; (4) limitations encountered; and (5) resources needed.

CONCEPTUAL MODEL

Today's health care environment demands two levels of organizational change: transformational change (Watzlawick, Weakland, & Fisch, 1974) and rapid incremental change (Watzlawick, et al., 1974). In transformational change we remake who we are as organizations by fundamentally altering our view of the world. For example, the acute-care hospital transforms itself—from the dominant arena for illness care for individuals, into a minor but important player in reestablishing the wellness care of plan member populations. This dramatic shift in self-definition requires reevaluation and realignment of all essential hospital services.

In rapid incremental change, the limits of evolutionary change are pushed by demands for faster and faster responses to stimuli, thereby shortening or eliminating a steady-state (between change) period. An example of rapid incremental change is the dramatic decrease in patients' lengths of hospital stay (LOS). At one Pacific Northwest institution, four years ago the LOS for a patient with a total hip replacement was 14 days. Three years ago, the LOS dropped to 10 days, then to 8; now, the average LOS is 5.2 days. With the first decrease in LOS, the multidisciplinary team redesigned care by improving coordination of services. With the second decrease, the team redesigned by moving presurgery care to the preadmission and physician office setting. With the third decrease, the team shifted some postoperative care to the outpatient setting, extending more care into the home. Each one of these changes triggered a ripple effect, spawning further change throughout the inpatient and outpatient system. Various structures and services were created and streamlined, while others were eliminated. Personnel were moved. Jobs were created and lost. With each decrease in LOS, the "lighter" patient days were eliminated from the inpatient system, leaving only those days when the patient required extensive nursing hours and more-expert nursing care. There was no slack time for the patient or the nurse as the pace of change continued to accelerate.

Each type of change presents unique challenges to the evaluation system. Evaluation is an important component of a learning organization; it serves as the basis of the conceptual framework. To develop this framework, we have defined and described the learning organization, discussed the implication of the processes for evaluation, identified outcomes for evaluation, and developed evaluation strategies appropriate to the intent of the process as well as to its potential applications. We sought to discover appropriate evaluation methods, frameworks and strategies for each type of change.

Components of the Learning Organization

A learning organization is composed of individuals and teams who approach work from the joint perspective of active engaged learner and co-creator of the organization (Senge, 1990). The individual and the team are simultaneously doing the work of the organization, evaluating the effectiveness of the work, and recreating the structures and processes of the organization to improve efficiency and appropriateness of care. Important attitudes and skills include: patience, creative tension, focus, the willingness to become beginners again, and intellectual honesty. Evaluation is integral to the work of the learning team because it provides a source of challenge and support, nurtures the learning team, and supports the learning process.

Patience

Patience with the ongoing process of development of self, others, and systems is a critical attitude. Patience doesn't demand perfection overnight or require that each deficit be resolved at once. Patience allows one to pace oneself and encourages both individual and team to alternate periods of activity and rest. Patience allows us to set priorities for creation and evaluation of new structures and processes.

Creative Tension

Patience is balanced with maintaining the creative tension between the current reality and one's vision of a future reality. Finding, nurturing, and maintaining this creative tension is critical to foster movement toward improvement (Senge, 1990). Evaluation can help us establish and maintain creative tension by measuring how closely the current reality approximates the vision. While the target of evaluation for incremental change is often straightforward (closer approximation to some defined level of efficiency), the target for transformational change is not.

Transformational change occurs not so much in response to a problem but in response to the envisioned opportunity created by an altered perspective. Therefore, the current evaluation information may not indicate a problem with the established process (Barker, 1989). To demonstrate the difference between the current reality and the re-visioned reality, evaluators must anticipate the re-visioned reality, identify critical factors in that reality, and create new measurement systems to highlight the differences. This requires evaluators to be involved early and continually in the discussions that will create the new perspective. Without early involvement and subsequent design of an evaluation system, evaluation information will be out of sync with transformational change.

There are several ways that evaluation can be out of sync with change. First, available information does not adequately lay the groundwork for the need to change, since the need for change comes from the new perspective, the new vision—not (necessarily) from failure of the earlier vision (Barker, 1989). Second, information is unavailable during the critical early refinement of redesigned processes. Third, information may be irrelevant to the current situation. Finally, the evaluation provides only outcome information, when both process and outcome information are required.

Focus

A third skill necessary in the learning organization is the ability to focus energies within the individual and the system (Morgan, 1993). The ability to focus energy is based on the ability to prioritize activities and identify and use the 15 percent rule. The 15 percent rule says that people have control over 15 percent of their jobs or their life (Morgan 1993); the other 85 percent is controlled by other factors or persons. Knowing this, individuals can focus their energy on the 15 percent over which they have the most control. Once this 15 percent level has been reached, individuals can begin expanding their influence outside their 15 percent boundary. As the team works together, members can add their various 15 percents to expand the rate and scope of change.

The 15 percent rule can be applied to evaluation as well. Evaluation can begin where the evaluators have the most chance of success, both in terms of performing the evaluation and in utilizing its results. Moving forward in the areas of least resistance with simple methods that will produce high-yield data is the surest way to gain support and to demonstrate the value of evaluation information.

Once the 15 percent is achieved, one can move forward into the remaining 85 percent a step at a time. Robertson (1988) refers to this as 1 + 1 stretch—incrementally adding more difficult and taxing behaviors and methodologies. A critical component of 1 + 1 stretch is finding and utilizing supports within the system (Robertson, 1988). Drawing other people and their strengths and talents into the process enhances the possibility of success, expands the evaluation effort, and invites other colleagues to join the learning team. Movement forward may occur quickly or slowly, depending on the amount of encountered resistance. Care should be taken to avoid overextending, thus falling into the trap of promising what cannot be delivered.

Beginners Again

A fourth attitude of the learning organization is the sense that we are all beginners in our learning. Barker (1989) reminds us that whenever a paradigm changes, everyone "goes back to zero." In a similar way, as incremental change occurs more and more rapidly, the constantly evolving environment challenges us with new factors every day. In this time of change, it is important to cultivate **the art of a beginner**. Beginners are actively engaged in collecting new and old information and combining the elements in new and interesting ways. The evaluation process can both facilitate and capture the information collected and the meaning constructed for study. A beginner is constantly scanning the environment for information. Some information may eventually prove irrelevant, and can be discarded without regret. Some information will be unimportant now, but may become important. Other information will prove to be critical, so that methods for obtaining it will quickly be refined. This attitude engenders a fluidity in the evaluation process and questions the value of standardized, repetitive data-sampling techniques. Repetitive data-sampling techniques assume that change in the dependent variable is due to manipulation of the independent variable and not to a change in the environment. This may not be an appropriate assumption any longer.

An integral part of being a beginner is the process of making new meaning out of old data and finding new data interesting. Clarification and elucidation of the meaning-making process occurs through narrative (Burner, 1990; Polkinghorne, 1988; Sarbin, 1986). The dominant narrative structure in Western culture is a story. The narrator introduces the people and setting, tells us the sequence of events, and steps back from the action of the story at crucial points to tell the listener why things are happening and what meaning the actors assign to the events (Paget, 1982). Since the narrative structure is learned and culturally dependent (Collins, 1985; Gee, 1985), the evaluator may need to prompt individuals to "fill out" their stories.

Narratives can be written as journals or shared in small groups as stories. The story or the journal account are data that yield rich information about how individuals view their world and life events and the sense they make of experience. Using an interpretative phenomonologic technique, the evaluator and the informant explore the meanings in the narrative (Benner, 1994; Munhall, 1994; VanManen, 1990). Exploring meanings is a process of critical thinking about experience. In the process, the informant comes to recognize what has been learned and how choices can be made to use that learning. Data may also be used to describe and document the process and outcome of the experience.

Intellectual Honesty

Intellectual honesty (Senge, 1990) refers to the ability to step back from the situation and ask questions like "What do I contribute to the problem?" "What can I contribute to a solution?" "Is there another perspective on the issue that will give me a clearer understanding?" "What does the data really show?" "Am I asking the best questions?" "Whose questions am I answering, and why?" "Whose questions are being overlooked, and why?"

Questions like these not only help us take a clearer look at ourselves but also at structures in the organization that define the sanctioned perspective. In transformational change, it is this very perspective that we seek in order to determine if the sanctioned perspective should be kept or changed. Raising assumptions for examination is a fundamental technique of critical thinking (Paul, 1992) and organizational learning (Senge, 1990).

Evaluation

Evaluation can be a potent supportive strategy for transforming perspectives. Evaluators who listen for and respond to the overlooked questions and who coach individuals and groups in obtaining and using data, provide crucial tools to those who present an alternative perspective. This is a difficult and sensitive role for evaluation. It is difficult, in that groups whose perspectives have been overlooked have often found that data generated from the currently sanctioned perspective does not help and may sometimes run counter to their perspective. As a result, some have learned to distrust the use of data. This is a sensitive issue, in that questions asked from alternate perspectives often produce data that challenge the current perspective as somewhat inadequate. The evaluator, like any change agent, must be careful to point out the discrepancies and the possibilities without vilifying anyone's accomplishments.

We must continue to honor the past and the present while looking beyond it (Bridges, 1991). Evaluation processes can help us accomplish this by continually posing questions that honor the perspectives of all stakeholders, and by reinforcing the idea that, while what we are doing today may be good, we can always do better.

Sources of Challenge and Support

Individuals and organizations engaged in learning must seek out sources of challenge and support (Daloz, 1986; Robertson, 1988). Evaluators and evaluation data can service both of these roles. Evaluators can support the questioning process by providing information, and mechanisms for obtaining that information, to ensure ongoing feedback at each stage of the change. By coaching individuals and groups in the processes of obtaining, analyzing and interpreting data, evaluators place powerful tools in the hands of stakeholders who may be new to this aspect of the learning process. Data can also provide the challenge needed to motivate individuals and groups to consider and sustain the change in the face of the turmoil that accompanies it.

Resistance is a natural product of change (Bridges, 1991). Resistance may be located in the individual or in the organization. Data can help identify areas of resistance and validate the need for change. This data must be routinely disseminated to stakeholders to reinforce the need for change, to monitor progress, and to make necessary refinements to the plan.

Nurturing the Learning Team

In order to learn from experience, individuals and groups must be committed to listening, questioning, supporting each other, challenging each other, learning from mistakes and false starts, and using data. The evaluator plays a key role in coaching the organization about generating and using data. The evaluator is responsible for creating an environment in which evaluation is part of the learning process. With no steady state, evaluation is nonlinear and interactive (Lincoln & Lincoln, 1985).

As thinking, work processes, and structures evolve, some components of the evaluation will drop away and others will assume new importance. This requires that the evaluation design maintain flexibility throughout the change period and that it must be matched to the purpose and process of the change to provide useful information. In some instances, the data will be clean and quantitative; in other instances, it will be thick and descriptive. The data should both validate and guide change, and uncover and validate new insights.

The Learning Process

The learning process is based on four interactive processes (Kolb, 1984). They are: concrete experience, reflective observation, abstract conceptualization, and active experimentation. **Concrete experience** is the real-life experience that occurs as we live our lives and enact our professional roles. Lessons embedded in that experience are about what works and what doesn't, what is important and what is not.

When we wonder about those experiences we are participating in **reflective observation**. In this process we step back and look at the experience with fresh eyes, from another perspective. We wonder about what happened and why. We ask what it means. If the experience was important enough or upsetting enough, we look for ways to understand it better or explore it further. We look for more information.

When we look to other people's experience, or to theory or data to help us understand experience, we are participating in **abstract conceptualization**. Evaluation data produced by questions targeting the experience from a variety of perspectives is used here. Evaluators are charged with the responsibility to provide valid and reliable data that as accurately as possible reflects the experience and the meanings assigned to the experience by the participants. The definitions and processes of reliability vary between quantitative and qualitative methods, and the evaluator must be comfortable describing the bases and benefits of each. The data should be useful by all stakeholders and levels in the organization.

Having reflected on experience, theory, and data, the individual or the organization can plan an experiment to do things differently. This is the process of **active experimentation**. Once the experiment is activated, new experiences are generated and the cycle begins again (Fig. 9.1).

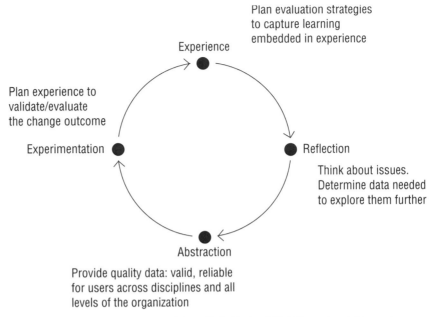

Figure 9.1   *The learning process. (Adapted from Kolb, D. A., 1984.* Experiential learning: Experiences as the source of learning and development. *Englewood Cliffs, NJ: Prentice-Hall.)*

Data and evaluation are key to this process, but only if relevant to current experience and the issue. Evaluators must keep attuned to the individuals and organization and provide data that measures or reflects the process and outcome of the experience. The evaluation process, like the learning process, is continual and interactive, providing opportunity for refining current techniques and creating new ones.

Because the evaluation is continual, interactive, and evolving, it will grow out of something and into something. It will have a history and a future. It is important and helpful to connect the form of the current evaluation to past evaluation models. Creating this link to earlier evaluation methods situates the current method as a natural evolution of already accepted processes and decreases organizational resistance to "new" methodologies. The current method of evaluation can then serve as the legitimized base for further evolution of the model. Linking the story of the evaluation with the story of the project bonds the experience of the project with the valuation of the data, thus making the data more familiar and acceptable to the stakeholders.

Evaluation for the Learning Organization

Evaluation provides data for understanding and assessing useful processes and outcomes of change. This understanding has evolved as individuals and organizations learn. By attempting to capture both the process and the outcomes of organizational change, we have been challenged to adapt evaluation strategies to capture outcomes that cannot always be fully predicted from our current understanding of the change. Our learning has resulted in a suggested framework for evaluation in a learning organization.

Evaluation as Fluid and Evolving

A fluid and evolving evaluation framework is critical. A fluid evaluation design has its roots in the individual's and organization's historical context and builds toward a more flexible and comprehensive evaluation program.

We built the project's evaluation strategy on the existing organizational history with the quality management process. The inclusion of nursing staff as stakeholders —as designers and makers of meaning around evaluation data—grew from their increasing involvement with the unit-based quality management process. As clinical nurses became more comfortable with quantitative data, we introduced qualitative methods designed to capture their own experiences and their patient's reported experiences of the care they received. This evolutionary process allows us to refine and extend the evaluation both in terms of methods and audiences served.

A fluid, evolving evaluation framework is critical during times of rapid and transformational change when anticipated outcomes of the change are only partly identifiable at the project outset. Our experience has often been one of following where the work leads. We must be prepared for people to outperform our ideas in unexpected and illuminating ways. Using strategies that capture the unanticipated is critical to documenting the processes and outcomes of the project. Qualitative methodologies (e.g., narrative analysis) can be extremely useful in capturing unanticipated events. A mixture of quantitative "snapshots" and continuing qualitative methods will help identify (1) what is happening according to plan, (2) what exceeds anticipations, and (3) what, why, and how deviations from the anticipated events occur.

Coaching for Evaluation

An evaluator in a learning organization is a learner and coach, as well as a project evaluator. As learner and coach, the evaluator learns from the stakeholders and then coaches them in the evaluation and use of data. This is an important role when stakeholder groups are not experienced with generating, using, and making meaning around data.

Look For and Ask the Unasked Questions

As new stakeholders are invited to participate in an evaluation process, the evaluators must be sensitive to the kinds of unasked questions that would give these individuals useful information within their perspective. Evaluators must also try to formulate questions from alternative perspectives in order to highlight information that will be useful in new paradigms. Often, these new data are found using previously unexplored methods in the qualitative domain. This places both the stakeholder and the evaluator in positions of stretching to learn as the project unfolds.

Use Your Fifteen Percent

The evaluation strategy should be based in an understanding of the stakeholders and their perspectives on evaluation, combined with the strengths and abilities of the evaluators. Understanding the stakeholders' and the evaluators' strengths and limitations allows the evaluation team to determine where the evaluation process will experience the most success, quickly and easily. It is important to establish a history of success early in the project, especially with those stakeholders who may be skeptical of the evaluation process.

Use 1 + 1 Stretch

The notion of 1 + 1 stretch can be applied both to the stakeholders and the evaluators. The evaluation design needs to start where the stakeholders are and invite them to participate in a way that stretches them a little beyond their comfort zone. This will help the evaluator understand how best to introduce pieces of the evaluation. For example, when a particular component of the evaluation (e.g., collection of narrative from nurses, use of patient journaling techniques) seemed too big a stretch for some units, we began using them on the units that were ready and continued to "plant seeds" for these strategies around the organization. As evaluators, it was crucial to listen to the stakeholders and reshape "our" plan to make it a mutually acceptable one. Using the 1 + 1 stretch idea, we continued to provide evidence as to when forms of evaluation provide effective and useful data and when they do not. When the current method was not as successful as it might be, we suggested alternatives and the plan was reshaped again.

As evaluators, we also participated in the 1 + 1 stretch. We began in our area of comfort—around quantitative methodologies. As we experienced both success and failure, and as we learned to expect that the nurses and administrators would outperform our expectations in learning, we searched for and included more qualitative methodologies. It was important to emphasize that we were learning as much from this process and from others as we "taught."

The following illustrates some of our learning as an organization about evaluation and how it was nurtured and supported.

LESSONS IN EVALUATION LEARNING

Two premises served as the basis for evaluation of PPMC's delivery system redesign. Evaluation was to (1) be undertaken by those doing the redesign, and (2) fit into the existing quality-monitoring process. Staff competence in quality monitoring and evaluation was gained and was combined with the two premises to guide ongoing and future work.

Developing a Readiness for Innovative Evaluation

How does an institution prepare unit staff to manage an evaluation process? For data to be valuable to the users, they must be involved in deciding the data to be collected. Preparing staff for the process required education and support to think critically and risk growing. They learned about quality monitoring, evaluation, and quality-improvement methodology and about institution-specific systems and unit-specific activity. This knowledge builds a trusting relationship. It can promote creative tensions that push the staff to new learning levels, and a sense of security in knowing there is a mechanism to acquire answers for their questions or ideas. The education process is the critical foundation, and includes determining a question to be asked, learning key elements to build a valuable data-collection tool, learning what questions to ask of the data collected in order for it to have meaning, drawing conclusions from the meaning of the data, and formulating an action plan whereby the circle of evaluation begins again: data collection, analysis, and conclusion.

Engaging Nurse Participation   *Scenario 9.1*

In 1986 the department of nursing decided to initiate a unit-based quality assurance (QA) program. This decision was made to obtain the benefits of a decentralized QA program as outlined by Schroeder and Marbush (1984) and fit with a new shared-governance structure that was to be initiated in January 1987. Although measures had been taken to involve staff in unit-based QA, that meant staff assisted with data collection only. Then in 1992, with added impetus from external review standards, staff participation in QA monitoring and analysis was required. This included identification of important aspects of care and indicators, and the collection, analysis and interpretation of data. Most managers and staff were unprepared. Traditionally, managers prepared the unit's yearly QA plan, including review of the unit's scope of practice, identification of indicators for monitoring, attempting to interpret and analyze the data, and composing quarterly reports. Historically, the indicators were formulated to monitor problem issues, including whether appropriate standards of care had been provided.

    Even though unit-based QA had been promoted, it had not been practiced. As a result, staff were not involved and frequently were uncertain as to what was being monitored or for what purpose. Since the staff had not been involved in the process, when the results of the data collection did not meet the standard, the manager was left to devise a plan of corrective action. Corrective action often occurred in the form of "notifying staff of the problem area at the next unit meeting." As could be expected, nothing more happened, and the problem continued. This cycle frustrated both the managers and the QA staff. The corrective action was not effective because staff were not involved. These were painful basic lessons. But, how could staff be encouraged and prepared to be involved in the QA process? How could we promote staff to become owners of the process? How could we implement a staff-driven QA system?

    To meet the new expectation that staff be involved in unit QA, one nurse manager requested assistance for training and educating staff. A frequently used 10-step process provided an organized method from which to begin. In the first of many sessions, QA staff assisted staff nurses to analyze their nursing scope of practice, identify the patient population they served, classify their high-risk, high-volume, problem-prone procedures, and develop indicators to monitor one or more of these areas. Scope of practice was labeled after the nurses answered these questions: For whom did they provide

Scenario 9.1
(continued)

care? What did these people have in common? What procedures and/or diagnoses did their patients experience? What were the needs of these patients? These questions led to stimulating discussions for the nurses as well as the QA staff, because the nurses had never before been encouraged to talk about patient care and reflect on the meaning of it or of their nursing actions. These sessions, which encouraged discussion about practice, demonstrated that nurses were passionate about their work and their patients. They savored the opportunity to talk about their patients, what they did for their patients, and how things were changing in nursing. With support from QA nurses, the staff nurses were able to connect the issues they identified to monitoring and to learn some principles of measurement.

Developing Quality Monitoring Skills

Discussions about nursing practice continued across the institution, and similar issues across units and patient populations were identified. The trends and issues became the basis for many subsequent planning sessions. The QA learning sessions provided a mechanism to nurture critical-thinking skills for staff nurses as they labeled and described what they did for patients beyond isolated tasks such as taking blood pressures, making a bed, and giving a bath. They identified patient issues they could influence directly that made a difference to them as nurses and to their practice. They began to see meaning and value in identifying issues for measurement that could be used to improve patient care and nursing practice.

As word traveled to other nursing units, they requested similar assistance. Each time, the same process was repeated. The dynamics of each group, the personalities of the nurses, and the unit culture flavored each of these sessions. After the first educational session, some units requested further assistance with the next steps: tallying the results of data, analyzing and interpreting data, drawing conclusions from the data, determining corrective action, and preparing a report. The staff nurses approached these new components with apprehension, as they did not have experience with analysis and interpretation of data, planning corrective actions, or preparation of quality reports. But, as had occurred earlier, the staff learned the skills necessary to take on the next steps. We learned that a one-time educational session was not enough. We had to anticipate the next steps of learning as staff became ready. Because in most cases the staff did not use the measurement information daily, when it came time for the next step (e.g., analysis), the staff again needed support. They had learned pieces of the process and now wanted encouragement to use what they had learned. They did not always remember what they had previously learned; so knowledgeable staff assisted them to recognize and use the skills they had acquired. This nurturing was essential to build confidence as they addressed the next step of the process.

Preparation for Evaluation

During the next phase, interpreting and analyzing the data, the unit staff were encouraged to examine the following questions: What did the QA data look like?

What did the actual numbers tell them? What did they think the data meant? Did everyone agree? Did everyone look at the results of the data the same way? (The staff were surprised to learn that the data meant different things to each of them.) Had the data all been collected the same way? Did the data tell them all they wanted to know? Did they have all the data they needed?

These sessions stimulated the identification of many issues. It would be the beginning of an invaluable learning process that was to have ramifications for other evaluations. Data collection tools were revised frequently as staff identified issues to improve them. The staff learned they needed to pilot a data-collection tool and to review the questions they had asked with several data collectors to assure that each person interpreted the questions the same or looked for the information in the same places. The staff learned the importance of identifying very specific criteria in their data-collection tools to ensure that the data would tell them what they wanted to know. Building an accurate data-collection tool is crucial to the evaluation process.

As the unit QA committees matured, learning from their experience, they began asking more important questions of themselves and the data they collected. They moved from asking "Did the work get done and was it done properly?" to asking "What difference does a particular intervention make to our patients?" They asked "Are the patients able to remember what we teach them?" "Are patients able to effectively use the information we provide them after they return home?" "Do we provide patients with the right information, the information that is most useful to them at home?" "Do patients have all of the information they need to successfully manage their care at home?"

This process provided the beginning work of staff teams, which was to assess and evaluate their practice together. They were learning, practicing, and utilizing critical-thinking skills to analyze data. These skills would be useful in building an evaluation process.

Redesign and Evaluation of Delivery Models

In response to rapid external changes in the managed health care environment, PPMC commissioned a number of teams to review, analyze, and evaluate the effectiveness of the nursing care delivery system. As a result of the work from these teams, recommendations were developed for the redesign of nursing care delivery.

The educational process used to prepare staff to participate in unit QI/QA activity was used in this redesign process and in its evaluation. As part of redesigning nursing care models, the staff was to determine what should be redesigned, what new interventions should be implemented, and what they as nurses would be doing differently. Labeling what was being changed and providing definitions were key not only to redesign but also to the evaluation process. After the labeling occurs, what is to be evaluated can be determined and then a question/indicator and data-collection tool can be generated.

Looking back to where these groups were before taking on the work of staff-implemented QA, it is difficult to predict whether they would have been ready to take on the work of evaluation. Many of the staff involved in the redesign teams were not directly involved in the QA teams, but the skills learned from the QA teams had spilled over to other unit staff. In most cases, as staff took on the function of coordinating and implementing their QA plan, they involved other staff from the nursing unit to collect data or to plan and implement the corrective action. Staff became accustomed to the idea that they should be involved in all quality-monitoring functions, as well as in the evaluation of their redesigned models of care delivery.

Moving On To Evaluation

Providing support to encourage, facilitate, and promote staff learning is an ongoing and ever-changing process. It is a learning process for the QA staff who provide the support and education, as well as the for staff learning to do evaluation. The QA support staff must observe the growth of the unit staff in determining the next step to take. At PPMC, the staff-driven unit QA committees, which were also taking on a quality-improvement function, had become fairly confident in determining a question, developing a data-collection tool, collecting data, analyzing the data, and drawing conclusions.

Unit staff had become almost too confident, in that some of them no longer saw value in involving QA support staff in their evaluation process. They were pleased when data appeared to demonstrate the outcome they wanted for their patients, but they had not consistently worked through the linking of patient outcomes to their redesigned process. This was because the staff was looking at the data collected based on their past level of knowledge or understanding of the data. This level of understanding would need to be challenged for staff to look at the data in a new and different way—and to learn more from the data. For example, when nurses called patients at home to ask how they were able to manage their self-care following instructions given during hospitalization, patients would describe how they were managing incisions, medication, and activity. This led the nurses to conclude that their instructions had been successful. Nurses, however, failed to recognize "other" information the patients were communicating.

The QA staff could see from the unit report an unusual trend: 50 percent of the patients reported not feeling well! The QA staff encouraged the unit staff to consider pursuing these patient reports. What additional information could they learn from their patients that would be valuable as they planned or developed patient education activities and tied these to the redesigned role of primary nurse? What did patients mean when they reported "not feeling well"? Was there a physiologic or psychologic reason for these complaints? If patients knew more about what to expect after they went home, would that make a difference?

Getting staff to the next level of questions for their model evaluation was an issue. Did the staff want to know that there is another level of questions by which they could evaluate the data? To understand each level so as to satisfy both purposes (i.e., quality monitoring and evaluation) requires time for staff and QA staff learning and growth. The challenge was how to encourage staff to see the need to move to the next level and to understand their evaluation. The interaction between the QA staff providing support and the unit staff is critical to the learning process. It would not be effective to just tell the unit staff how to look at their data. Dialogue—asking "Have you considered. . . ?"—is critical. Interaction and dialogue encourages the use of critical thinking skills and builds the learning process. This prepares the staff for the next level of questioning and learning.

Deciding What Will Be Evaluated

There are certain key issues that must be determined for evaluation of a redesign process. They are: What is the expected outcome? What will be evaluated? Will only the outcome of the redesign be evaluated? Will the implementation of the redesign plan be evaluated as well? Assuming there are different plans for implementation, does the actual plan for implementation make a difference in the results or outcome of the implementation? Does implementation over 6 months rather than 3 months affect the outcome? Did implementation of the plan occur simultaneously or in stages? These questions consider the impact of staff education, the differences in the type and amount of education, and the impact of differences in the time used to implement a plan. The answers to these questions can determine how or why plans have certain results and provide guidance to future project implementation. Issues related to redesign, such as cost, resource use, time management, and patient outcome, are of particular interest to administrators and unit staff alike.

Examples of quality indicators to monitor and evaluate redesigned care delivery are outlined in Figure 9.2. For example, medical/surgical cardiology unit staff were concerned with improving the patients' ability to remember and use their discharge instructions at home. Patients self-reported how they were feeling. The question the QA staff had was, would the staff be satisfied with the mainly positive reports of how the patients were feeling? Would the staff not be sensitive to the value of the information ("not feeling very well") and stop, because they felt successful when patients were using their discharge instructions appropriately?

In another example, the respiratory unit has a proactive, aggressive skin management program. Because this unit receives patients from critical care who have longer lengths of stay due to respiratory complications, and because their overall population has chronic respiratory problems, the patients on this unit often are at

Type of Unit	Indicator	Results
Medical and Surgical Cardiology	Effectiveness of redesigned model in meeting the discharge needs and patient outcomes of the PTCA/MI and CABG patient. (Are patients able to verbalize an understanding of their discharge instructions when called at home 48 hours after discharge?)	The first quarter's worth of data on 38 post-CABG and 21 post-PTCA patients revealed that 95% of the patients were verbalizing an accurate understanding of their medications, activity/exercise, and groin site inspection. The patient responses also revealed that among the 38 CABG patients, 50% reported that they had no complaints and felt "good," while 50% reported not feeling well, with symptoms of weakness, tiredness, nausea, soreness, and insomnia.
Respiratory Medical	Does the patient with actual skin breakdown improve or maintain skin integrity while hospitalized?	Data are currently being collected.

Figure 9.2 *Examples of indicators used to evaluate the effectiveness of nursing care.*

higher risk for skin breakdown. This unit did not identify this QA/I indicator as an evaluation method for their nursing care delivery redesign. The QA staff, however, assumed the indicator could measure their redesign based on the understanding of the coordination, collaboration, and planning that was designed to occur between primary nurses and direct-care nurses. The QA staff made the assumption that to achieve the results of intact skin would require a well-developed skin plan from the primary nurse and coordination and follow-through from the direct caregivers. If the plan was not developed or communicated well, the results of intact skin would not be achieved.

The decision on what will be evaluated, as demonstrated by these examples, often needs to evolve, to accurately frame the desired question and to account for new areas of needed data that are identified. The work of the respiratory unit provides an example of having identified a key question; however, a critical element is missing: the thinking through and devising an explanation of the way in which their redesigned model works to achieve a desired end. This learning, being able to "theorize" how the specified intervention brings about the patient outcome, is a necessary but difficult struggle for this evaluation component.

Doing the Evaluation

Evaluation of the unit-based redesign of nursing care delivery models is proceeding based on two levels, with both sets of activities following the premise of integrating evaluation activities into existing quality-monitoring processes. One level relates to documenting and examining the models across units to determine the fit of the redesign work and its implementation with the core redesign parameters. The questions for this phase of the evaluation were, what are the redesign unit models like? Do the models have the critical redesign components and fit the core redesign parameters?

To answer these questions, a review team was convened when the units had completed a first major draft of their model. Membership consisted of unit nurse managers, staff nurses, a facilitator, and the assistant director of nursing for education. The team provided peer review of the models that had been developed and guidance for future work directions, including assistance with planning for implementation. This process whereby each unit described their model in relation to the core parameters was a beginning evaluation activity. Putting together a description of their model forced each unit to document their work. Presenting their work to the review team provided an opportunity for discussion, peer review, and guidance. Feedback about unit meetings with the review team was very positive, as the units reported feeling their work was "validated" and that they had the support to proceed with implementation.

The second level relates to the monitoring at the unit level. To meet the goal of integration into existing activities, the units are in the process of developing indicators to monitor components of their model, its processes, and/or expected patient outcomes as part of their yearly QA improvement plan. The indicators in Figure 9.3 provide examples of their initial work; the work done to date was discussed earlier. The involvement of many people in developing an evaluation and using the data generated is a critical component of the proposed approach. Principles and methods for this evaluation approach will be discussed next.

Utility	A continuous focus, from planning through final report, on how to use the results of evaluation
Relevance	Evaluation process is user-oriented and tests the stakeholder's theory of action of how outcomes are achieved
Practicality	Evaluation has conceptual and instrumental applications

Figure 9.3 *Definitions of Patton's UFE: Utilization-focused evaluation. (Adapted from Patton, M.Q.* Utilization-Focused Evaluation. *Beverly Hills: Sage, 1986.)*

EVALUATION: ASSUMPTIONS, PRINCIPLES, AND METHODS

The proposed evaluation approach has three components: (a) a set of working assumptions to orient and frame the evaluation work to be done; (b) a set of principles to guide and create options in the design and implementation of evaluation; and (c) suggested methodologies. The working assumptions and principles of our proposed approach were based on thinking about evaluation from: Participatory Action Research (PAR) (Argyris & Schon, 1989; Elden & Levin, 1991; Whyte, Greenwood, & Lases, 1989; Karlsen, 1991; Morgan, 1993; Walton & Gaffney, 1989; Whyte, 1989); Fourth Generation Evaluation (FGE) (Guba and Lincoln, 1989); and Utilization-Focused Evaluation (UFE) (Patton, 1986). Each source has thinking that is complementary to the other two, providing a thorough approach for a new evaluation system.

Working Set of Assumptions

Action objectives are built into the evaluation design from the outset and learning is the driver of the process. The working assumptions of this proposed evaluation approach are:

Evaluation Is a Learning Process
Guba and Lincoln (1989) stress the teaching-learning process as a crucial aspect of this form of evaluation. All involved (including the evaluator, for whom this is a new role) are both learners and teachers as the process evolves. Evaluation is a teaching/learning process that all stakeholders teach and learn from each other about the meaning they derive from the evaluation process and the data generated from it. Evaluation is a continual, recurring, and highly divergent process, so that all meaning derived and ascribed to what is being evaluated is updated and even reformulated over time. Morgan terms participatory-action research as "action learning," and conducts the evaluation in a way to generate participant learning. All involved gain a better understanding of their problems and how to initiate appropriate actions (Morgan, 1993, 299). A PAR-based evaluation seeks to develop a "science of practice," with the aim of generating "theory and knowledge that is useful, valid, descriptive of the world and informative of how to change it" (Argyris, Putnam, Smith, 1985).

Relevant Stakeholders Must Be Involved

Relevant stakeholders must be involved in each step of the evaluation process, from inception to the use of the data for decision-making. Based on Patton's utilization-focused evaluation (UFE) (1986), inclusion of diverse stakeholders at each step of the process is a necessity. According to Argyris and Schon (1989) and Whyte (1989), practitioners are involved as both subjects and coresearchers, with action objectives built into the research design from the beginning. For advocates of PAR, such involvement can also be seen as a learning strategy to empower participants in three ways. These are (a) the specific insights, the new understandings, and the new possibilities that the participants discover in creating better explanations about their work; (b) the participation in learning how to learn; and (c) the participation in learning how to create new possibilities for action (Elden & Levin, 1989, 131).

Evaluation Data Has Specific Uses

Use of evaluation data must be kept in mind, from the critical formation of the question through actual dissemination.

To satisfy a core assumption of UFE (Patton, 1986), the focus of all decision making is on the intended use of the data by the intended users. Decisions about the content, focus, and methods are not necessarily specified in advance; the evaluator works with stakeholders to focus relevant questions, and from these questions flow the appropriate research design, methods, and data-analysis techniques (Patton, 1986). Morgan (1993) believes learning assists in the achievement of dual objectives: trying to produce useful research knowledge, and helping people involved to gain a better understanding of their situations (i.e., everyone learns by doing).

Evaluation Must Be Instructive

Organizational evaluation is not a linear, but an interactive, process that is characterized by joint collaboration and that is sensitive to diverse stakeholders' views about what is being evaluated, the process of its implementation, and the decisions about the meaning of the data.

The interactive nature is best described by PAR advocates as a continual mutual learning model. All involved, including the evaluator, are constantly challenged by events and ideas, information, and arguments posed by each participant (Whyte, et al., 1989). The nature of this new kind of collaboration can be drawn from the work of Guba and Lincoln (1989), in which they have proposed a dramatically different view of evaluation. They call for evaluation to be a joint, collaborative process, a process that aims at the "evolution of consensual constructions about what is being evaluated" (Guba & Lincoln, 1989, 253). According to Guba and Lincoln, this aim cannot be satisfied unless it is jointly pursued by all stakeholders; and, unless individual stakeholder constructions are solicited and honored, there can be no consensus.

Closely intertwined with evaluation as a collaborative process is an aspect we have all experienced; the **sociopolitical nature of evaluation** (Guba & Lincoln, 1989). Guba and Lincoln believe that social, cultural, and political aspects are integral to the process and provide meaning (Guba & Lincoln, 1989, 253). The sociopolitial factors are acknowledged as values that enhance the inquiry.

Working Set of Principles

There is a set of principles that grows out of defining evaluation. Evaluation determines the questions to be asked and the information to be collected, based on stakeholder inputs, and the inquiry carried out through stakeholder interaction and negotiation. This process creates the products of the evalution (Lincoln & Guba, 1989). A working set of principles includes the following.

Evaluation Is an Evolving Process

Evaluation is an emergent process, so the design of the evaluation evolves and includes a mix of methods. As with a more traditional evaluation perspective, the design for evaluation is essentially a plan stating what is to be measured, and when. In this type of evaluation, as the questions proposed and agreed upon by the relevant stakeholders evolve, it may become clear that there are multiple levels of questions. With levels of questions, there is often a need to use both quantitative and qualitative methods. One caution, when using differing designs for components within the overall evaluation, is to avoid narrowing the evaluation just to a pre-post design, because you may lose the evolving/emergent nature of the evaluation as a learning process.

Evaluation Is an Unpredictable Process

Evaluation is a process with unpredictable outcomes. As stakeholders learn, they achieve new insights, which in turn influence new questions to be answered and data to be identified. Raising additional questions is one measure of successful evaluation, as stakeholders identify new organizational or care delivery components requiring systematic examination and analysis before taking action.

Evaluation Is a Reality Process

Evaluation is a process that creates reality. All participants are involved in deriving meaning that can lead to shared understanding about the work they are doing, its benefits, and its outcomes.

Evaluation Is a Shared Responsibility

Evaluation is a process that results in shared responsibility. The responsibility is shared by all relevant stakeholders involved in all components of the process.

Evaluation Has Utility, Relevance, and Practicality

Evaluation is a process that fulfills criteria of utility, relevance, and practicality. These criteria are borrowed from Patton's (1986) utilization-focused evaluation. Definitions were outlined in Figure 9.3. Utility serves as an evaluation principle because it is a reminder of the core reason for doing evaluation: to use the results. In attempting to build a cohesive team of stakeholders, this principle may get blurred, as everyone tries to focus on the question (the what) and methods (the how) for data collection. To build stakeholder values and assumptions about evaluation into the work of it, the end use of the product needs to stay at the forefront.

Relevance, the second criteria, has two aspects: (1) evaluation is user oriented, and (2) evaluation must have measurement validity. The first component is met by actively including all relevant stakeholders at each step of the process. Patton's second component of relevance—validity—needs further exploration. Validity refers to the question of whether we are measuring what we think we are measuring (Kerlinger, 1993). In evaluation, stakeholders must pose questions that are not predetermined and can be answered by data. Even more important, and related to having data-answerable questions, is the view stakeholders have about the processes that lead to desired outcomes (Driever & Birenbaum, 1988). Patton (1986) termed this causal relationship the **stakeholders' theory of action**. Its application to evaluation requires that stakeholders be assisted to make explicit their assumptions and theories about the activities and processes that lead to desired outcomes. For evaluation learning to be maximally effective, understanding and testing the links between process and desired outcomes is a highly valued goal.

Patton's (1986) third criteria, practicality, refers to the ways in which evaluation processes and findings are used. He divides these ways into two kinds of evaluation uses: conceptual and instrumental. It is helpful to keep in mind (and to help other stakeholders understand) that the conceptual impact of evaluation—the insights stakeholders achieve, how they learn to see some component of their work or the organization differently—is valuable. Whether this insight leads to action or not, people have gained by deepening their understanding of how the world works. The use of findings, the instrumental component of practicality, involves using evaluation to devise concrete actions and make decisions—the traditional uses of evaluation data.

Suggested Methodology

Given these working sets of assumptions and principles, we now turn to a way of thinking about methodology. Qualitative methods are advocated by those who have developed participatory action research, utilization-focused evaluation, and fourth-generation evaluation. Guba and Lincoln (1990) focused on differences between qualitative and quantitative methods; but, after comparing these methods, Dzurec and Abraham (1986) concluded few real differences exist at the outcome level. Both quantitative and qualitative methods generate findings based in description, probability, and inference. Dzurec and Abraham (1993) highlight a critical point, that in all research, meaning is a product of (a) the researchers' perceptions, (b) their conceptualization of the research problem, (c) the theoretical/conceptual framework serving as context of the problem, and (d) the implications of the research they impose for direction of knowledge.

According to Dzurec and Abraham (1993, 75), it is apparent that although the implementation of specific techniques may be unique to a particular method, the objectives, scope, and nature of inquiry are consistent across these methods and the research paradigm they represent. Dzurec and Abraham (1993, 76) contend that the scopes and objectives of inquiry are constant across paradigms. The challenge is for researchers and practitioners to learn together the necessary ways to systematize their methods and then lend those methods to evaluation designs that will lead to understanding the transformation of organizations. Dzurec and Abraham (1993, 76) believe that, at the fundamental level, inquiry is couched in the human desire to understand and explain behavior and events—their components, antecedents, corollaries, and consequences.

We know that qualitative methods can be used to understand how organizations work, and (the new question) how they learn. As stated earlier, the purpose of the evaluation approach set forth in this chapter is to develop a framework that creates options for methodology. We have learned that an often-neglected aspect of evaluation is a way of thinking about scope and levels of questions and issues. In PPMC's experience with organizational restructuring, we needed to identify broad questions at the organizational level. To satisfy stakeholder needs for information about the models of care delivery they have redesigned, we needed to help the redesigners identify "local" questions. An addition to the cardinal rule to fit the methodology to the evaluation question, it is critical to categorize the level of question to target the needs of the various stakeholders. Methodology can and must take a variety of forms, both quantitative and qualitative. With multiple methods, there is a need to monitor with the stakeholders involved how the levels of questions fit together to meet the purposes of the overall evaluation.

This discussion of methodology is not complete without an examination of generalizability. Morgan (1993) proposed to reframe generalizability from what is commonly thought of in evaluation; Morgan's view of generalizability is based on interpretive or qualitative forms of research. Morgan advocated seeking to generalize "insights about pattern" (i.e., one solution may have relevance for understanding a similar pattern elsewhere) (304). He goes on to describe the primary aim of generalizability is to "render the rich texture of a situation and understand the patterns and processes involved so those involved may use them as key insights or key learnings" (Morgan 1993, 305). He identified two types of generalizability: the one just discussed, and the second that is comprised of strategies and tactics—learning processes through which similar problems or situations are to be captured elsewhere. For Morgan (305), this second kind of generalizability "reflects action learning's aim of creating opportunities for people to experience and see the relevance of a learning process that they can incorporate into their normal activities on an ongoing basis."

Research is a particular system of learning (Elden & Levin, 1991). For evaluation research to achieve scientific rigor, we must all learn to monitor, reframe, and fit evaluation questions to methods, and desired data to stakeholders, who can then utilize the findings of the evaluation.

EVALUATION OF NEW MODELS

"Any given design is necessarily an interplay of resources, possibilities, creativity, and personal judgement by the people involved" (Patton 1990, 13). At a minimum, an evaluation plan clarifies three aspects; evaluation questions, procedures, and cost (Stecher & Davis, 1987). Cost is often a neglected aspect. Given the evolutionary nature of this approach, one strategy is to track costs as they are incurred and build this activity into an evaluation question.

It is important to note that the design and evaluation plan presented here is a work-in-process based on PPMC participants' experience with learning. The design described is a set of suggestions on how to proceed based on principles discussed earlier.

The new evaluation approach sets an orientation for an evaluation of major scope and varied levels. Scope refers to broadness, and usually encompasses the organization as the unit of focus and analysis. The design requires working through the kinds of questions to be answered at each level of inquiry.

A qualitative methodology is recommended for the organizational level because such methods allow a detailed analysis of organizational change and dynamics. Believing that context has an influence on behavior, and vice versa, one finds evaluation questions relating to context are important. Qualitative methods provide data that give a holistic view of the situations or organization needing to be understood (Cassell & Symon, 1993, 4–5). Qualitative research has these characteristics:

> ". . . focus on interpretation rather than quantification; an emphasis on subjectivity rather than objectivity; . . . . an orientation towards process rather than outcome; a concern with context—regarding behavior and situation as inextricably linked in forming experience, and finally, an explicit recognition of the impact of the research process on the research situation." (Cassell & Symon, 1993, 7)

Qualitative methods consist of three kinds of data collection: (1) in-depth, open-ended interviews; (2) direct observation; and (3) written documents. The data from interviews consist of direct quotations from people about their experiences, opinions, feelings, and knowledge. The data from observations consist of detailed descriptions of people's activities, behaviors, actions, and the full range of interpersonal interactions and organizational processes that are part of observable human experience. Document analysis in qualitative inquiry yields excerpts, quotations, or entire passages from organizational, clinical, or program records; personal diaries; and open-ended written responses to questionnaires and surveys (Patton, 199, 10).

For more specific information on kinds of research design, see Table 9.1, on pages 176–77. It is organized to provide information on a sample of measures (i.e., survey instruments of work environment and nurse satisfaction). The list of instruments is neither comprehensive nor complete; rather it is a starting point. The goals are to provide a way to think about organizational measurement using quantitative measures and to stimulate exploration of methods and measures. For more information on varied methodologies of evaluation, particularly quantitative ones, the reader is referred to the *Program Evaluation Kit* (edited by Joan L. Herman). Critical to design for the new evaluation approach is to be aware of the varied methodologies and the merits of each.

Limitations: Creating Learning Opportunities

We have experienced limitations in developing this evaluation approach. Discussing limitations helps to clarify the process and provides suggestions for turning limitations into learning opportunities.

There are differing expectations between redesign and evaluation relating to (a) the difference of time frame and pacing of activities for each endeavor; (b) understanding concepts of measurement and the level of data quality needed for decision-making ; and (c) developing the questions that guide evaluation efforts.

Redesign participants were accustomed to an "operations" sense of time, which is to deal with the present and meet deadlines in the here and now. To accomplish redesign of their unit's care delivery model, they had to meet demanding time frames, while learning to think of care delivery over a continuum and developing a broader view of resolving issues. As well, they had to take time from redesign work to think about possible evaluation impacts their model would have on patient outcomes.

The work of both redesign and evaluation challenged them to use time differently. This use of time was complicated by the differences in the timing between redesign and evaluation. The work of redesign frequently felt overwhelming, because redesign participants had to learn a process while doing the work. They needed to learn new ways of communicating, to have constructive dialogue and group problem solving, and to develop strategies to implement their model in the midst of changing organizational goals and structures. Because redesign participants were both learning and redesigning at the same time, the work consumed much of their energy and time. While they generally agreed on the goals for the evaluation, the actual day-to-day work frequently seemed incongruent with their redesign activities. Though they knew that evaluation needed to be integrated into the work of redesign from the beginning, the actual work of evaluation was perceived as too different in focus to accomplish during the redesign process.

As health care organizations use tools and techniques of continual quality improvement, with teams becoming more data-focused in their decision making, data must become more available. This creates a need for more people to understand concepts of measurement and critieria for evaluating data. It is necessary to step back and ascertain whether the numbers generated do indeed relate to the questions posed. Also, data's reproducibility and validity need to be understood. Making information available about the data, so those involved understand the level of its quality, serves to demystify the numbers and reveal how useful the data will be. Learning to work with data requires understanding ways data will be analyzed. Interpretation of data involves attributing meaning to make it usable. Data interpretation—and the next step of using the data—require new ways of thinking and new skills.

The differences in expectations of redesigning, the day-to-day operations of care delivery, and the work of evaluation all require new approaches to timing learning skills for decision-making. We have gained awareness about these differing expectations and the understanding that participants need to overcome this limitation. We have learned of the need to establish a balance between work/action and research. Until now we dealt with this limitation by forming an evaluation committee to do two things: (a) map our evaluation questions and issues in conjunction with the work of redesign, and (b) look for opportunities to create dialogue on redesign and evaluation whenever possible. This allowed us to wait until people were ready to think about evaluation, yet still be doing useful evaluation work. Having an evaluation team lay groundwork helped create the readiness of participants to deal with evaluation. We were able to share some preliminary thinking on possible evaluation questions and methods with redesign participants. In the future, we need to continue developing strategies to help participants understand how redesign informs evaluation and vice versa; thus, we can avoid concentrating on one at the expense of the other.

Table 9.1 • Sample of Measures. *(Contributed by Darren Pennington, Ph.D.)*

Tool	Purpose of Tool	Source	Nature of Data
Charns Organizational Diagnosis Survey (CODS)	A multi-instrument survey, used to measure organizational characteristics. Was originally developed to study the components of patient care effectiveness.	Alt-White, A.C., Charns, M. & Stayer, R. (1983). Personal, organizational, and managerial factors related to nurse-physician collaboration. *Nursing Administration Quarterly, 8*(1):8–18.	Varies by instrument, mostly ordinal or nominal. Number of items varies by scale from 13 to 45. Total number of items = 191.
Collaborative Practice Scales	Two scales that assess the degree to which the interaction of nurses and physicians "enable synergistic influence on patient care."	Weiss, S.J. & Davis, J.P. (1985). Validity and reliability of the Collaborative Practice Scales. *Nursing Research, 34*:299–305.	Ordinal, 6 point Likert. 9 nurse items. 10 physician items. Higher scores suggest greater collaboration.
Nursing Autonomy Scale (NAS)	Measures professional autonomy in nurses.	Schutzenhofer, K.K. (1987). The measurement of professional autonomy. *Journal of Professional Nursing, 3*(5):278–283.	Ordinal, 4 point Likert. 35 items. Higher scores indicate higher levels of professional autonomy.
Six-Dimension Scale of Nursing Performance (6-D Scale)	Measures nurses' self-appraisals of performance.	Schwirian, P.M. (1978). Evaluating the performance of nurses: A multidimensional approach. *Nursing Research, 27*(6):347–351.	Ordinal, 4 point Likert. 52 items. Higher scores indicate greater perceived level of nursing competence.
Nurse Opinion Questionnaire (NOQ)	Nurse's perceptions of shared governance.	Porter-O'Grady, T. (1992). *Shared Governance Implementation Manual.* St. Louis: Mosby Year Book. See also: Ludemann, R. and Brown, C. (1989). Staff perceptions of shared governance. *Nursing Administration Quarterly, 13*(4):49–56.	Ordinal, 6 point Likert. 73 items. Higher scores generally indicate greater satisfaction or influence.
Index of Work Satisfaction (IWS)	Measurement of job satisfaction among nurses.	Stamps, P.L. & Piedmonte, E.B. (1986). *Nurses and Work Satisfaction: An index for measurement.* Ann Arbor, MI: Health Administration Press Perspectives.	15 "paired comparisons" (weights), otherwise ordinal, 7 point Likert. 43 questionnaire items. Higher scores suggest greater satisfaction.
McLoskey/ Mueller Satisfaction Scale (MMSS)	Measurement of job satisfaction among nurses.	Mueller, C.W. & McCloskey, J.C. (1990). Nurses' job satisfaction: A proposed measure. *Nursing Research, 39,*(2):113–117.	Ordinal, 5 point Likert. 31 items. Higher scores indicate higher levels of satisfaction.
Work Quality Index	Measures satisfaction of nurses with their work and work culture.	Whitley, M.P. & Putzier, D. (1994). Measuring nurses' satisfaction with the quality of their work and work environment. *Journal of Nursing Care Quality, 8*(3):43–51.	Ordinal, 7 point Likert. 38 items. Higher scores indicate greater work and environment satisfaction.

Table 9.1 •   *(continued)*

Tool	Subscales/Dimensions	Reliability	Administration
Charns Organizational Diagnosis Survey (CODS)	Eight instruments: Nurse Demographics, Job Inventory (4 factors), Coordination, Conflict Management (has 3 conflict situations), Influence, Quality of relations with other departments, Burnout inventory (4 subscales), Physician Opinionnaire about the unit.	Cronbach's alpha for job inventory and physician opinion are .87 and .97, respectively. Other reliability measures are not available or not appropriate.	Paper and pencil survey. Requires some changes to best reflect institution being studied.
Collaborative Practice Scales	Two distinct measures, one for nurses and one for physicians.	Cronbach's alpha reported as .80 and .84 for each scale	Paper and pencil survey.
Nursing Autonomy Scale (NAS)	None	Cronbach's alpha range reported .74 to .90.	Paper and pencil survey. Requires weighted scoring.
Six-Dimension Scale of Nursing Performance (6-D Scale)	Six: Leadership, Critical Care, Teaching/collaboration, Planning/evaluation, Interpersonal relations/communications, and Professional development.	Cronbach's alpha range from .84 to .98.	Paper and pencil survey.
Nurse Opinion Questionnaire (NOQ)	Five: Nurse demographics, Shared Governance Information, Shared Governance Feelings, Influence, and Satisfaction.	Cronbach's alpha range from .74 to .95, with the majority being above .90.	Paper and pencil survey. Requires some changes to best reflect institution being studied.
Index of Work Satisfaction (IWS)	Six: Professional Status, Task Requirements, Pay, Interaction, Organizational Policies, and Autonomy.	Cronbach's alpha ranges from .52 to .81 with a total score alpha of .82.	Paper and pencil survey. Requires calculation of weights from paired comparison data.
McLoskey/ Mueller Satisfaction Scale (MMSS)	Eight: Extrinsic Rewards, Scheduling Satisfaction, Family/Work Balance, Co-Workers, Interaction, Professional Opportunities, Praise/Recognition, and Control/Responsibility.	Cronbach's alpha range from .52 to .89. Four subscales were above .70. The total scale's Cronbach's alpha = .89.	Paper and pencil survey.
Work Quality Index	Six: Work environment, Autonomy, Work worth, Relationships, Role enactment, and Benefits.	Cronbach's alpha range from .72 to .87. The total scale's Cronbach's alpha = .94.	Paper and pencil survey.

Our proposed learning approach to evaluation has challenged people to think differently about the kinds of questions, and ways to develop them, that guide evaluation. The difference lies in the learning required.

As stated earlier, the major thesis of this chapter is that the degree of change, transformational and incremental, demands a comprehensive approach to evaluation and its design.

Yet, while it is comprehensive in scope, questions arise that can seem confusing and overwhelming. People expect systematic protocols that are rigidly followed. Our learning approach to evaluation requires different strategies. In evolving this approach, we determined two operating premises to help achieve balance among differing expectations: (a) those involved in redesign at the local/unit level must do some evaluation, and (b) evaluation activities need to fit within existing structures and activities to build on and maximize existing resources. Meeting this last premise would assure integration and continuity of evaluation; that is, it would become part of everyone's daily work.

Real-Time Evaluation

As discussed in the section on limitations, this learning approach to evaluation challenges everyone to meet real-time deadlines. While evaluation efforts are thought of as proceeding in a linear fashion, actually the planning of the evaluation and its implementation are interactive and recursive. The planning and operational needs for evaluation are similar: (a) plan to change now, (b) evaluate now, and (c) use data now to support desired changes.

There is another real-time issue that relates to the nature of change in organizational transformation. Inherent in the process of transformation is the formation of a new paradigm to guide organizational functioning. The paradigm shift required creates new demands for guiding the development of evaluation questions. While the new paradigm is taking form, it is too early for it to help with framing the evaluation questions. Once the paradigm is the commonly accepted way of viewing day-to-day reality, it feels too late to start the evaluation. Dealing with this too early–too late dichotomy calls for an evolving set of questions which were discussed in the section on Evaluation Assumptions, Principles, and Methods.

Stakeholder Development

Stakeholder development is needed in this evaluation-learning process. Some new participants think of stakeholder development as a limitation, because learning how to evaluate by this process takes time and assistance. Participants must gain knowledge and competence to make it work. Most of our staff had served on QA committees, which provided some measurement experience. This experience gave them a basis on which to build competence for the new endeavor. We discovered both redesign and evaluation depended on "revisiting." An example of "revisiting" in the scenario was where unit teams learned to do quality monitoring. At the heart of revisiting is the need for people to review the concepts they are working with, especially in light of their work experiences, and then return to them with a deeper understanding based on their level of experience and how they have used it to modify their behavior. This connection of cognitive meaning with experience contributed to our evolving definition of new ideas for redesign and evaluation.

The concept of revisiting, described by Koerner (1991, 78) helped us understand staff needs for support and reinforcement.

There is an aspect of the evaluation-learning process that is both a limitation and a strength. The continuing nature of this evaluation approach, means it has no "natural" end where some desired "truth" is known (Lincoln & Guba, 1989, 254). People do not experience desired closure; it is a strength, in that the continuing process provides a means for recurrent formulation as new information becomes known. We are still developing ways to work with this process. We have tried to maximize the data obtained at certain phases (e.g., after the redesign team's meeting with the review team). Reviewing data at this natural break in the work provided an opportunity to understand and appreciate what had been accomplished and to communicate the new forms it was taking.

Resources and Support

It is important to discuss the kinds of resources needed for an evaluation focused on learning.

Staff Meeting Time
An evaluation approach that stipulates stakeholder involvement in all phases of the process requires the resource of staff meeting time. Because it is costly to pay for staff, managers, and administrators to meet frequently, it is important to decide where to make the investment. We developed ways to modify the amount of meeting time required by building unit evaluation into their QA/I activities, which was already part of their unit responsibility. Since the evaluation-learning process is integrated with redesign, it is efficient in getting more than one job done at a time.

Staff Experience with Quality Monitoring
Staff experience and involvement in unit-based quality monitoring and evaluation is also a resource. Such experience provides staff with competence in focusing monitoring, developing and using data-collection instruments, identifying a relevant sample from the population served by their unit, working as a community of peers to analyze data, and determining how to use the data to correct or improve problematic patient care situations.

Organization of Evaluation Expertise
Evaluation is a collaborative endeavor. We formed an evaluation team with an evaluator to support the evaluation of the redesign of the unit models. While an evaluation team is not unique to this model, the team functions are. To promote collaborative decision making, the evaluation team kept unit and redesign teams thinking through evaluation issues. The evaluation team also coordinated communication and stakeholder input. In this way, the team served to develop the evaluation-learning approach to evaluation and its overall design.

Based on our experience with broad redesign and organizational change, there was a need for a team to work with the big picture and review it with the redesign team. This served as an essential monitoring function to assure there were sufficient teams of appropriate composition to do the necessary work of evaluation.

Administration-Supported, Staff-Generated Redesign Process
Providence Portland Medical Center's redesign process has two core concepts: (a) staff nurses are the generators of care delivery redesign, and (b) multilevel administrative involvement is necessary to create a context that will support innovations that result from care delivery redesign. This resource serves as environmental support for the work of evaluation. The creation of staff redesign teams, and the organization of coordinating groups such as the review team, provided a way for stakeholders to integrate evaluation with redesign activities.

Summary

The proposed approach to evaluation focuses on learning and was derived from our experiences with institution-wide redesign of care delivery. The opportunities created by the approach pose creative challenges for administrators, practitioners, and researchers to collaborate in using the research process. From the conception of an idea to the use of data, they can learn together about the effectiveness of new organizational forms of care delivery.

Discussion Questions

1. How does this evaluation approach relate to evaluations you have done?
2. What barriers would you encounter in attempting to use this evaluation approach?

References

Argyris, C., & Schon, D. (1989). Participatory action research and action science compared. *American Behavioral Scientist, 32*, 612–623.

Argyris, C., Putnam, R., & Smith, D. M. (1985). *Action science: Concepts, methods, and skills for research and intervention.* San Francisco: Jossey-Bass.

Barker, (1989). *The business of paradigms.* [Videotape].

Benner, P. (1994). *Interpretive phenomenology.* Thousand Oaks, CA: Sage.

Bethel, S., & Ridder, J. (1994). Evaluating nursing practice: Satisfaction at what cost? *Nursing Management, 25,* 41–48.

Bridges, W. (1991). *Managing transitions.* Menlo Park, CA: Addison-Wesley.

Bruner, J. (1990). *Acts of meaning.* Cambridge, MA: Harvard University Press.

Cassell, C., & Symon, G. (Eds.) (1994). *Qualitative methods in organizational research.* Thousand Oaks, CA: Sage.

Collins, J. (1985). Some problems and purposes of narrative analysis in educational research. *Journal of Education, 167* (1), 57–70.

Daloz, L. A. (1986). *Effective teaching and mentoring: realizing the transformational power of adult learning.* San Francisco: Jossey-Bass.

Driever, M. J., & Birenbaum, L. K. (1988). Patton's utilization-focused evaluation as the basis of the quality assurance process. *Journal of Nursing Quality Assurance, 2,* 45–54.

Driever, M. J. (1992). Issues in clinical nursing research: Quality assessment from a research perspective. *Western Journal of Nursing Research, 14,* 106–108.

Driever, M. J. (1994). *Project summary—overview: Where SHNP at PMC started.* (Available from Marie J. Driever, RWJ/SHNP Project Office, Providence Portland Medical Center, 4805 N.E. Glisan, Portland, Oregon, 97213.)

Dzurec, L. C., & Abraham, I. L. (1986). Analogy between phenomenology and multivariate statistical analysis. In P.L. Chinn (Ed.), *Nursing research methodology: Issues and implementation.* Gaithersburg, Maryland: Aspen Publishers.

Dzurec, L. C., & Abraham, I. L. (1993). The nature of inquiry: Linking quantitative and qualitative research. *Advances in Nursing Science, 16,* 73–79.

Elden, M., & Levin, M. (1991). Cogenerative learning: Bringing participation into action research. In W. F. Whyte (Ed.), *Participatory action research* (pp. 127–142). Newbury Park, CA: Sage.

Fitz-Gibbon, C. T., & Morris, L. L. (1987). *How to design a program evaluation.* Newbury Park, CA: Sage.

Garvin, D. A. (1993). Building a learning organization. *Harvard Business Review,* pp. 78–91.

Gee, J. P. (1985). The narrativization of experience in the oral style. *Journal of Education, 167* (1), 9–35.

Guba, E. G., & Lincoln, Y. (1989). *Fourth-generation evaluation.* Newbury Park, CA: Sage.

Karlsen, J. I. (1991). Action research as method: Reflections from a program for developing methods and competence. In W. F. Whyte (Ed.), *Participatory action research* (pp. 143–158). Newbury Park, CA: Sage.

Kerliner, F. N. (1973). *Foundations of behavioral research.* San Francisco: Holt, Rinehart & Winston.

Koerner, J. (1991). Building on shared governance: The Sioux Valley hospital experience. In I. E. Goertzen (Ed.), *Differentiating nursing practice: Into the twenty-first century.* Kansas City: American Academy of Nursing.

Kolb, D. A. (1984). *Experiential learning: Experiences as the source of learning and development.* Englewood Cliffs, NJ: Prentice-Hall.

Lincoln, Y., & Guba E. (1985). *Naturalistic inquiry.* Newbury Park, CA: Sage.

Mishler, E. (1990). Validation in inquiry-guided research: The role of exemplars in narrative studies. *Harvard Educational Review, 60* (4), 415–441.

Morgan, G. (1993). *Imaginization: The art of creative management.* Newbury Park, CA: Sage.

Munhall, P. (1994). *Revisioning phenomenology.* Newbury Park, CA: Sage.

Packer, M., & Addison, R. (1989). *Entering the circle: Hermeneutic investigation in psychology.* New York: State University of New York.

Paget, M. (1982). Your son is cured now, you may take him home. *Culture, Medicine and Psychiatry, 6,* 237–259.

Patton, M. Q. (1990). *Qualitative evaluation and research methods* (2nd ed.). Newbury Park, CA: Sage.

Paul, R. (1992). *Critical thinking.* Foundation for Critical Thinking. Sonoma, CA: Sonoma State University.

Polkinghorne, D. (1988). *Narrative knowing and the human sciences.* New York: State University of New York Press.

Robertson, D. L. (1988). *Self-directed growth.* Munci, IN: Accelerated Development.

Sarbin, T. R. (1986). *Narrative psychology: The storied nature of human conduct.* New York: Praeger Special Studies.

Schroeder, P. S., & Maibusch, R. M. (Eds.) (1984). *Nursing quality assurance: A unit-based approach.* Gaithersburg, MD: Aspen Publishers.

Senge, P. (1990). *The fifth discipline: The art and practice of the learning organization.* New York: Doubleday/Currency.

Senge, P. (1990). The leader's new work: Building learning organizations. *Sloan Management Review, 32* (1), 7–23.

Stecher, B. M., & Davis, W. A. (1987). *How to focus an evaluation.* Newbury Park, CA: Sage.

Van Manen, M. (1990). *Researching lived experience.* New York: State University of New York.

Walton, R., & Gaffney, M. (1989). Research, action, and participation: The merchant shipping case. *American Behavioral Scientist, 32,* 582–611.

Watzlawick, P., Weakland, S., & Fisch, R. (1974). *Change: Principles of problem formulation and problem resolution.* New York: W. W. Norton.

Woods, N. F., & Catanzaro, M. (Eds.) (1988). *Nursing research: theory and practice.* Washington: Mosby.

Whyte, W. F., Greenwood, D. J., & Lazes, P. (1989). Participatory action research: Through practice to science in social research. *American Behavioral Scientist, 32,* 513–551.

PREPARING FOR THE FUTURE

PART III

CHAPTER **10**   *Harriet V. Coeling*

Organizational Subcultures
Where the Rubber Meets the Road

Introduction

In Chapter 4, Taft identified various levels of organizational culture, ranging from the culture of the corporate leaders to that of specific work groups such as nursing units. Taft focuses on culture at the corporate level and identifies the need for nurse executives to understand corporate culture and how it relates to the organization's mission and strategic plan, as well as its internal and external environment.

Although it is essential for the executive nurse to be cognizant of organizational culture at the upper organizational levels, this knowledge is not sufficient of itself. Rather, the executive nurse must also appreciate the differing cultures of various work groups within the organization, for it is at this work-group level that organizational change occurs. Within the nursing division, it is at the unit level where the "rubber meets the road"—where the mission statement is enacted and the strategic plan is implemented. Failure to consider culture at both the corporate and work-group level will block the health care reforms so necessary to the survival of every health care agency.

This chapter is designed to increase the executive nurse's appreciation of the importance of work-group subcultures. It will do so by defining cultures as unique patterns of behaviors, describing strategies to assess these cultures, documenting subcultures at various organizational levels, discussing the relationships among these different cultural levels, and identifying sources of these cultural differences. The chapter will then apply these insights to research data to illustrate how knowledge about a specific work group's culture, specifically the group's decision-making preferences, can be used to facilitate organizational hiring, merging, innovating, and team building—activities essential for today's health care reforms and organizational survival. The term *units* is used in many examples and is intended to be inclusive of work-group subcultures found in any health care setting, not just the acute care facility.

DEFINITIONS

Before beginning our examination of unit subcultures, it is important to clarify the terms used here.

Organizational Culture

Organizational culture is a concept derived from the discipline of anthropology and applied to organizational settings. Organizational culture at the corporate level is generally called the corporate, or the official, culture (Jermier, et al., 1991). In contrast, organizational cultures of various subgroups are called **work-group cultures**. Anthropologists characterize **culture** as a unique, dynamic yet stable, holistic pattern of assumptions and behaviors. Organizational culture will be explained by discussing the relevance of each of these characteristics for the executive nurse.

Of utmost importance in understanding culture is the realization that each culture is unique. We have come to understand, and even celebrate, the fact that each individual is unique. One evidence of this uniqueness is the fact that all individuals have their own fingerprints, unique patterns of lines that are different from those of any other person. Studies of group behavior now suggest that, just as each individual is unique, so is each group. In a sense, the culture of the group could be described as the fingerprint of that group. The executive nurse who appreciates the uniqueness of each work group will recognize the need to treat each work group differently when hiring for the group, merging the group, innovating work patterns, or facilitating teamwork within the group.

The fingerprint metaphor does break down in that, while a fingerprint remains the same throughout a lifetime, the culture of a group changes over time. Although cultures resist sudden changes, they are constantly evolving in response to internal and external forces. A culture resists sudden changes because, as Taft notes in Chapter 4, it is a survival strategy. We hesitate to let go of anything seen as essential for survival. Yet, because culture is a response that enables individuals to survive in their environment, and because our environment is constantly changing, culture is also continually changing. An awareness of the dynamic yet stable nature of culture enables the executive nurse to have an attitude of patient expectation regarding organizational change. Change will occur, but it tends not to occur as quickly as the executive nurse would like it to.

Culture scholars also emphasize the pattern, or holistic nature, of culture. Ott (1989) explains that trying to think about organizational culture in a reductionist way is like trying to appreciate a painting by analyzing its stroke patterns or its chemical content. Pacanowsky and O'Donnell-Trujillo (1983) add that organizational culture is not something an organization *has*; rather a culture is something an organization *is*. Lessem (1990) uses phrases such as "integral whole," "interwoven," and "total pattern of human behavior" to describe culture. Lessem also seeks to avoid reducing culture to its parts, striving instead to offer what he calls a rich diet that, he adds, may be difficult to digest. Yet digest it executive nurses must if they are to understand organizational culture in its total complexity.

Part of the complexity of culture relates to its all-inclusive nature. Various authors describe a culture as consisting of assumptions, beliefs, values, knowledge, meanings, symbols, language, artifacts, norms, rules, customs, and behaviors. The components of culture include both what goes on inside of peoples' minds and what they do. Much, if not most, of organizational work, then, is cultural in nature (Ott, 1989). As executive nurses come to understand the all-encompassing, holistic nature of a work group's culture, they can better appreciate that what appears to them to be a small change in organizational behavior may become a large change in the eyes of a work-group member. This is because the behavioral change may be very tightly interwoven with a variety of other behaviors, all of which must change to bring about the initial, small change.

Groups obtain identity from their unique pattern of assumptions and behaviors. In organizational settings, this group identity grows stronger over time as the pattern is constantly reinforced by employees who, seeking both to be faithful members of the group and to survive, use the same behaviors over and over again. This identity is an essential element of work-group behavior because it promotes a sense of purpose and harmony (Lessem, 1990).

Another defining characteristic of the concept of culture is that of **pattern**. Martha E. Rogers (1992) describes human beings as having pattern. Rogers uses such adjectives as "irreducible," "indivisible," and "pandimensional" to describe human beings, noting that humans are identified by pattern, manifesting characteristics that are specific to the whole and which cannot be predicted from knowledge of the parts. Although Rogers herself does not go on to describe groups, she comments that the science of unitary human beings who are manifested by patterns is as applicable to groups as it is to individuals.

As noted, culture consists of both assumptions and behaviors. Schein (1985) focuses on an organization's values and assumptions. He defines organizational culture as the pattern of basic assumptions that a given group has invented, discovered, or developed in learning to survive by coping with its problems of external adaptation and internal integration. He encourages us to seek to understand the basic assumptions of the organization in order truly to appreciate the organization's culture.

Other organizational scholars, however, emphasize the importance of looking at the actions of organizational members. Their definitions reflect a more behavioral orientation. Van Maanen and Barley (1985) define organizational culture as a set of solutions devised by a group of people to meet specific problems posed by the situations they face in common. Those who favor focusing on behaviors argue that behaviors are more readily identifiable and accessible to study than are assumptions. They add that behaviors do not always correspond to our basic assumptions because competing desires or behaviors may force a person to choose between two important values. Depending on the circumstances, one behavior may win out on one occasion, while another behavior may dominate under differing circumstances. The relevance of this debate to the executive nurse will be addressed more fully in the corporate and the work-group culture section.

Organizational Climate

It is important for the executive nurse to differentiate the concept of culture from similar concepts. The concept with which organizational culture is most often confused is the concept of **organizational climate**. Denison (1990) notes the following four similarities between culture and climate:

1. Both focus on organizational behavior and, specifically, study organizational units as the level of analysis.

2. Both cover a very wide range of phenomena.

3. Both try to explain the way in which the behavioral characteristics of a system affect the behavior of individuals, while at the same time explaining the way in which the behavior of individuals continually recreates the system.

4. Both include mental perceptions and physical behaviors.

Because these concepts are so similar, it is not surprising to find they are often confused. Nor is it surprising to find that the variables addressed by each concept are often the same. Items measured in social climate scales are similar to those addressed in a cultural assessment.

Climate versus Culture

However, there is a difference between climate and culture (Flarey, 1993). Climate takes a more individual point of view, whereas culture takes a more group-oriented view. James, James, and Ashe (1990) note that climate reflects a personal orientation, being a function of personal values, whereas culture reflects an organizational orientation, being a product of group values and norms. Climate is generally conceived of as the perceptions or feelings about an organization, whereas culture consists of common beliefs and expected behaviors (Thomas, et al., 1990). Reichers and Schneider (1990) add that climate is a more specific construct that has a particular referent, as in the climate for service, whereas culture is a more general, and probably deeper, less consciously held set of meanings that specifies a common understanding of the group's goals and practices.

Another difference between the two concepts, notes Denison (1990), is a difference in the manner in which each concept has been studied. Climate researchers have tended to use questionnaires to characterize specific organizational dimensions and principles. In contrast, organizational culture researchers, like anthropologists, have favored qualitative research in seeking to understand the meaning the culture has for organizational functioning. These differing methodologies may relate at least in part to the era in which each concept blossomed. Climate research emerged in the 1970s, a period in which quantitative research was at a high point. In contrast, culture research emerged in the 1980s, when qualitative research was coming into its own.

The goals of the executive nurse in assessing the two phenomena also differ. Social climate is generally studied to assist the manager in creating an environment that will increase social functioning, worker satisfaction, and productivity by identifying problems contributing to worker dissatisfaction and poor performance (Flarey, 1991). Culture, on the other hand, is studied to enable organizational members to understand and predict how the organization or work group will behave when a change is introduced (Ott, 1989).

Denison (1990) observes that, historically, organizational climate has had two different meanings. Although climate was originally described as a perception, it later came to include a set of conditions or characteristics of the social system. In a sense, this latter connotation reflects what is now called organizational culture. Denison (1993) summarizes the distinction between climate and culture, noting they differ primarily in their interpretation, with climate being an individual perspective and culture a group perspective, rather than in the underlying phenomena they study.

ASSESSMENT

Organizational culture is a very powerful force in the life of a work group. Hence it is essential that executive nurses know how to assess the cultures of their various work groups. Culture is difficult to assess because it operates on an unconscious and implicit level (Hughes, 1990). Different circumstances call for different assessment strategies.

Cultural Patterns

Early cultural researchers utilized ethnographic and other qualitative approaches to describe the cultures of various organizations. Caroselli (1992) recommends these qualitative approaches, noting the best way to assess a culture is to observe the members as they go about their daily activities, listening to what they say and, from time to time, asking them to explain what a situation means to them. In doing this, the researcher can identify what the group values by noting how they spend their time, what they speak highly of, and what they look down on or criticize. Specific behaviors to observe and questions to ask while observing a group, so as to better understand its culture, are presented elsewhere (Caroselli, 1992; Coeling & Wilcox, 1988; Ramirez, 1990).

Although qualitative observations provide the richest information about a culture, the executive nurse must recognize that they do require skill and time on the part of the assessor. Skill is needed because culture is such a subtle force, a force that operates on an unconscious and implicit level. Generally, group members themselves are not aware of their cultural behaviors or why these behaviors are important to them. The observer must first identify the common behaviors and then make sense of these activities in order to interpret a culture. Time is required, because the researcher must observe for the repetition of behaviors on many occasions before being sure they are typical cultural responses.

Recently, to facilitate cultural assessment by organizational members, some researchers have begun to develop quantitative tools to assess culture. A variety of these tools are described elsewhere (Coeling & Simms, 1993). Although ease of administration and scoring make the quantitative tools attractive to the executive nurse, the qualitative approaches are more in line with the definition of culture as a unique, dynamic, holistic pattern of assumptions and behaviors. Cultures are unique; it is difficult to bring out this uniqueness using tools that seek to reduce culture to a

*...*es are also complex, interwoven patterns of behavior; it is dif-
*...*ne interwoven complexity of behavioral patterns using numbers.
*...*courages the researcher to use the research methodology that best
... of the phenomena being investigated. This advice is important to con-
*...*essing cultures. However, the executive nurse needs to consider the re-
*...*ailable. Often, using qualitative and quantitative measures together will
... the best picture of group culture in the most economical manner.

Cultural Factors

A popular definition of organizational culture comes from the early work of Deal
and Kennedy (1982), who describe it as "how we do things around here." To make
the concept more tangible, and hence easier to assess, it is necessary to pull out
from this broad concept the important elements of culture. Coeling, Simms, and
Price (1993) have identified important elements of nursing unit work-group culture through a factor analysis of 607 responses to the Nursing Unit Cultural
Assessment Tool (see Appendix). This tool is easy to use yet qualitative in nature,
in that it elicits the unique cultural themes of a specific nursing unit (Coeling &
Simms, 1993). This varimax factor analysis yielded ten cultural factors relevant to
practicing nurses (based on the Scree test and factors having eigenvalues above
1.17). These ten factors are listed in Table 10.1, along with several behaviors included in each factor.

Table 10.1 • Ten Cultural Factors Relevant to Nurses*

1. Following orders:
   - Following policies and procedures
   - Following the organizational chain of command
   - Attending in-service meetings
2. Growing professionally:
   - Seeking promotions
   - Attending college
   - Discussing new nursing-care ideas
3. Valuing technical skills:
   - Handling emergencies competently
   - Working efficiently
   - Making patients comfortable
4. Using professional judgment:
   - Using individual judgment
   - Understanding patient's feelings
   - Being creative in providing nursing care
5. Preferring one's own way:
   - Trying to change someone's behavior by joking about it
   - Telling a peer how they should do a certain procedure
   - Competing with co-workers

6. Caring for co-workers:
   - Offering to help others
   - Providing emotional support for co-workers
   - Socializing with co-workers outside of the agency
7. Maintaining traditions:
   - Going along with peer pressure
   - Maintaining life when death is inevitable
   - Preferring old ways of doing things
8. Communicating directly:
   - Trying to change behavior indirectly
   - Asking for help directly
9. Working under difficult conditions:
   - Calling in sick when physically ill
   - Calling in sick when one needs a day off to rest
10. Assuming responsibility:
    - Having one nurse, rather than many nurses, develop the plan of care
    - Documenting what you have done

Based on the Scree text and factors having eigenvalues above 1.17.

ORGANIZATIONAL CULTURE LEVELS

Early scholars of organizational culture believed that a unitary culture characterized an entire organization. Peters and Waterman (1982, p. 75) wrote that "without exception the dominance and coherence of culture proved to be an essential quality of the excellent companies." Their landmark study consisted of identifying the dominant cultural themes of ten "best-run" companies. Other early researchers, too, looked only for unitary cultures within organizations (Deetz, 1982; Wilkins & Ouchi, 1983). This early belief in a unitary culture very likely came from researchers who identified the organizational culture based on descriptions given by key executives, and assumed that the executives' descriptions applied throughout the organization (Donnelly, 1984). Initially, then, the term *organizational culture* was synonymous with that of corporate culture.

Group Level

In 1985, however, Van Maanen and Barley questioned the idea of a unitary culture. They wrote that even the "best-run" companies are comprised of a variety of cultures. Van Maanen and Barley went on to suggest that, if we wish to discover where the cultural action lies in organizational life, we must discard presumptions about unitary or organizational culture and move to the group level of analysis. It is at the group level that organizational members discover, create, and use culture; they judge their organization against this background.

European scholars of organizational culture (Hofstede, et al., 1990), too, have faulted U.S. scholars for failing to distinguish between the values of founders and significant leaders and the values of the bulk of the organization's members. They suggest that at the work-group level, action is dominated by traditional responses and habits, rather than by overriding organizational values.

The following research review will respond to this critique by citing U.S. scholars who have distinguished, through research, various subcultures within organizations. This review is presented here to increase executive nurses' awareness of the variety of differing subgroup cultures.

Subcultures

Subcultures have been identified at the following organizational levels:

- The division,
- The type of job or profession,
- The unit, and
- Any group that interacts together for any reason.

In the executive nurse's health care setting, this could translate to organizational subcultures at the departmental level (e.g., direct patient-care services contrasting with financial services), the discipline or occupational level (i.e., nursing as compared to medicine), the nursing-unit level (where one nursing unit differs from another), and the shift level (the day shift that differs from the night shift).

Organizational culture research documents cultural differences based on the division level. Deal and Kennedy (1982) early on reported four departmental sub-cultures. They described that within most companies:

- The marketing department reflects the tough-guy culture (individualists who take risks and get quick feedback);

- Sales and manufacturing are characterized by working and playing hard (both with quick feedback);

- Research and development typify the "bet-your-company" culture (cultures with big stakes and slow feedback); and

- The accounting section is more process-oriented, where limited feedback results in concentrating on how the work is done.

Schall (1983) compared an information-systems division with an investment division. The information-division workers built alliances to increase resource control and valued the seeking and sharing of information, whereas the investment-division employees increased resource control by personal involvement in the day-to-day operations. The investment division built fences around individuals and subgroups to contain the information sought and shared, thus restricting information flow.

Research has identified cultural differences at the occupational or professional level. Gregory (1983) described differences between computer scientists and software engineers. The computer scientists were interested in the academic aspects of computers. Lengthy written descriptions of their work fit their style. In contrast, the software engineers were more hands-on and enjoyed building and producing a useful product. Faules and Bullis (1990) compared pilots, assessors, and scientists. They found that pilots and assessors rated high on group allegiance, whereas scientists came off as very individualistic, goal-oriented, and career conscious. Scientists reported lower levels of regulation via policy than pilots or assessors, placing more emphasis on independence and the opportunity to work hard as an individual choice. Scientists were motivated by a desire to get the project done, pilots by the physical and emotional experience of flying, and assessors by doing the job according to the rules. Within the health care field, Coeling and Wilcox (1991) identified cultural differences among different health care professionals within a hospital. They reported physicians focused on maintaining life, nurses emphasized individualizing patient care, and respiratory therapists were most concerned with getting oxygen into the cells.

Research is beginning to explore cultural differences among work groups within the same department and/or profession. Short and Ferratt (1984) reported differing types of work-group cultures in industrial settings, while Coeling and Wilcox (1988) described two very different nursing unit cultures within the same hospital.

Subsequent research by Coeling and Simms (1990) has documented a variety of cultural norms among different nursing units. Examples of these differing unit norms are presented in Figures 10.1 and 10.2, where unit scores for 33 different units are presented for ten behaviors, one behavior typifying each of the ten cultural factors described above. Of special interest to the executive nurse is the observation that the average scores for each hospital are very similar to each other,

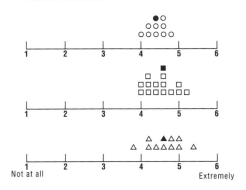

1a. BEHAVIOR FROM FACTOR 1
How important is it to follow the organizational
chain of command?

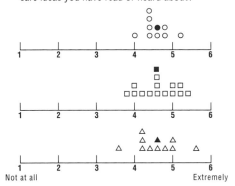

1b. BEHAVIOR FROM FACTOR 2
How acceptable is it to discuss new nursing
care ideas you have read or heard about?

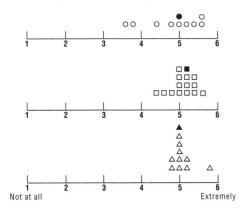

1c. BEHAVIOR FROM FACTOR 3
How important is it to make patients comfortable?

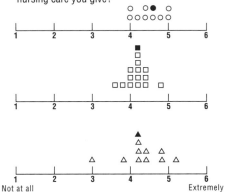

1d. BEHAVIOR FROM FACTOR 4
How important is it to be creative in the
nursing care you give?

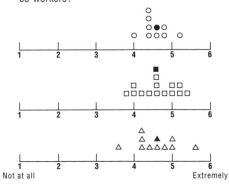

1e. BEHAVIOR FROM FACTOR 5
How acceptable is it to compete with your
co-workers?

KEY

△ Mean unit score for a unit in Hospital A
○ Mean unit score for a unit in Hospital B
□ Mean unit score for a unit in Hospital C

▲ Mean hospital score for Hospital A
● Mean hospital score for Hospital B
■ Mean hospital score for Hospital C

SCALE   1 = not at all   4 = quite
        2 = slightly   5 = very
        3 = somewhat   6 = extremely

Figure 10.1 *Mean unit scores of 33 units illustrating behaviors from factors 1–5.*

2a. BEHAVIOR FROM FACTOR 6
How important is it to offer to help others
even before they ask for help?

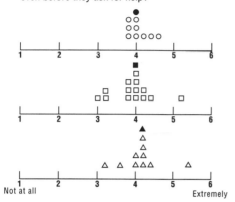

2b. BEHAVIOR FROM FACTOR 7
How acceptable is it to focus on maintaining
life, rather than enabling death to be
comfortable, when death is inevitable?

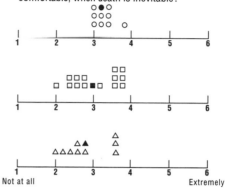

2c. BEHAVIOR FROM FACTOR 8
How acceptable is it to tell someone directly,
rather than indirectly, that you dislike their
behavior?

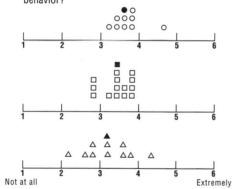

2d. BEHAVIOR FROM FACTOR 9
How important is it to call in sick when you need
a day off to rest up?

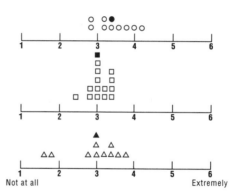

2e. BEHAVIOR FROM FACTOR 10
How important is it to have one person, rather
than the whole group, decide what nursing care
is needed for a particular patient?

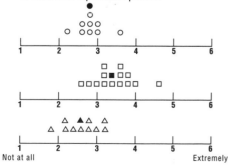

KEY	
△	Mean unit score for a unit in Hospital A
○	Mean unit score for a unit in Hospital B
□	Mean unit score for a unit in Hospital C
▲	Mean hospital score for Hospital A
●	Mean hospital score for Hospital B
■	Mean hospital score for Hospital C

SCALE		
1 = not at all	4 = quite
2 = slightly	5 = very
3 = somewhat	6 = extremely

Figure 10.2   *Mean unit scores of 33 units illustrating behaviors from factors 6–10.*

while there is considerable diversity in the scores for the different units within a given hospital. This data suggests that when behaviors relevant to practicing nurses are analyzed, there is a greater difference between units than there is between hospitals. This finding adds support to Van Maanen and Barley's (1985) comment that if one wants to study culture where the action is, one should give serious attention to studying culture at the work-group level.

Anecdotal information suggests that cultural differences exist even within a given work group. Nurses report, for example, that the day shift is very different from the night shift. In fact, after studying the day-shift culture on one nursing unit, the author was asked to come back and study the culture of the night shift so that the nurses could understand why there was so much conflict between the two shifts. Conversations with nurses who have begun to understand the culture of their units also suggest that, on larger units, even within a particular shift, there are different cliques that may represent differing cultures.

CORPORATE AND WORK-GROUP CULTURES

Researchers and executive nurses alike are now asking "What is the relationship between the corporate culture and that of the organizational subcultures?" "Are they similar to each other, do they conflict with each other, or do they exist independently of each other?"

Similarities

Coeling (1994) found that cultures of two nursing units in the same medical center were similar to that of the corporate culture but differed in emphasis. Three important corporate values of this medical center included innovation, teamwork, and a feeling of family. Although both nursing units embraced these values, the groups differed in the emphasis given to the behaviors that reflected these values. Group A was relatively less concerned with innovation and more inclined to emphasize teamwork and a sense of family than was Group B. In contrast, Group B spent a considerable amount of time innovating, but less time promoting teamwork and a sense of family. Although the culture of the work groups did not conflict with corporate-level cultural elements, the emphasis given to different behaviors varied between these groups within the organization.

Differences

Jermier, Slocum, Fry, and Gaines (1991), however, compared and contrasted an organization's official culture with that of its subcultures and found considerable conflict between the official culture and four of the five subcultures. In this large police department, only one of the five work groups matched the official culture of a "crime-fighting, command bureaucracy." The other four cultures were described as "crime-fighting street professionals," "peace-keeping moral entrepreneurs," "ass-covering legalists," and "anti-military social workers." These resistance subcultures substantially modified or rejected top management's dictates.

Independent Cultures

Yet others have found corporate and work-group culture to be quite independent of each other. Curran and Miller (1990) suggest there may not be a strong connection between the corporate culture and that of a nursing unit. They write that most staff nurses become acutely aware of issues related to the corporate culture of their organizations only when there is a change in administration at the top level. Morley and Shockley-Zalabak (1991) also studied the degree to which corporate culture penetrated down the hierarchy. They reported that the organizational founders perceived the corporate culture to be much stronger than did the workers.

Bullis (1990) compared corporate and professional cultures. She assessed the correspondence between cultural values of the U.S. Forest Service and those of three disciplines within this service—professional foresters, engineers, and biologists—after a change in the organizational mission statement. Her findings caused her to question whether a change in an organizational mission statement resulted in a meaningful change toward a common culture. In this study, the organizational mission changed in a manner that diverged from the forester's professional values. After the change, articulated values of the foresters tended to remain consistent with their professional values and became less consistent with the organization's overall values. In analyzing these findings, Bullis concluded that mission statements, or transcendent values, are not necessarily followed by consistent concrete values, which are relied on in the decision situations and which determine behaviors. She observed that a difference in the type of work at the corporate level versus the type of work at the professional level seemed to relate to differences in culture at these levels.

These comparisons between the corporate and work-group cultures have been discussed in light of the different nature of the work at each organizational level. When Riley (1983) compared two organizational cultures, she found one culture to be much more rule-governed than the other. She noted that the members of the rule-governed firm viewed organizational life according to the specific, behavioral rules and exhibited little insight into the political, or nonrational, side of the organization, until they moved to a higher level of the organization where the tasks were more ambiguous. Then they became less specific in applying the rules. Riley (1983) explains this by noting that work at the corporate level is different from work at the level of the typical employee, in that corporate-level work is more abstract and more ambiguous. Hofstede, Neuijen, Ohayv, and Sanders (1990), report a similar finding regarding the difference between corporate and worker levels, in that corporate leaders were more concerned with general values while the workers were more concerned with specific behaviors. Shockley-Zalabak and Morley (1994) reported that management's cultural values had a much stronger impact on employee values than on employee behaviors.

Work at the corporate level must transcend the entire organization because the corporate level is broad and inclusive. Hence, it is often more general, more abstract, than work at the unit level. Early on, we noted that one debate in organizational culture related to the merits of looking at cultural values versus cultural behaviors. These research studies, analyzing the relationship between the corporate culture and the work-group culture, suggest to the executive nurse that, at the corporate level, basic assumptions and values may play a larger role, whereas at the work group (nursing unit) level, the way these assumptions are acted out in specific behaviors may be more important. This conclusion underlines the importance that the executive nurse be cognizant not only of organizational values at the corporate level but also of the cultural behaviors of various subgroups, noting the differing ways in which these values play out at the work-group (unit) level.

SOURCES OF CULTURAL DIFFERENCES

The executive nurse might question how work groups in the same organization, and often work groups in the same division representing the same discipline, can develop such different cultures. Three main sources of culture have been suggested: (a) early and current group leaders, (b) the group members themselves, and (c) the technology or nature of the work.

Group Leaders

Schein (1983) early on emphasized the role of the founder in creating organizational (corporate) culture. He explains that cultures are usually created because someone takes a leadership role in seeing how the concerted action of a number of people could accomplish something that would be impossible through individual action alone. For example, companies are created by entrepreneurs who have a vision of how a concerted effort could create a new product or service in the marketplace. Early group members follow the lead of the founder and new group members follow in their steps as they join the group.

A similar process occurs in a health care setting when a new unit opens. In this scenario, the executive nurse appoints a leader and gives this person the responsibility of determining how the nurses can best work together to accomplish the goal of the new unit. The early leader's challenge is to determine what styles of control, role relationships, and work practices will best meet the needs of the new unit. Behavioral patterns that are found to work are reinforced, or altered somewhat, as new leaders assume authority. What these leaders pay attention to, how they react to crises, and what they reward, all help to shape the culture (Schein, 1985).

Group Members

Even though group leaders are very important, no leader can impose a culture on unwilling followers. Thus, group members too play an important role in determining the culture. Rousseau (1978) studied the characteristics of departments, positions, and individuals, and found that individual worker characteristics are related highly to attitudes and behavior in work situations. She notes the need for more research to explain the reciprocal relationships between individuals and their jobs.

One ethnographic study reported a nursing unit on which seven nurses all graduated together from the same class. They also joined the unit at the same time, bought new cars, married, and began raising children in the same year. Many years later, the culture of that unit strongly reflected the values and behaviors this group of nurses had learned in school (Coeling, 1987).

Technology

The technology of the work group can also influence the group's culture. This influence is recognized when nurses make comments like "It's a typical critical care unit" or "Isn't that just what you would expect on a psych unit?" A study using the Nursing Unit Cultural Assessment Tool to compare 25 nursing units, reflecting five major technologies (surgical, medical, psychiatric, rehabilitation, and critical care units) showed that psychiatric units were the most significantly different from the other units. On the psychiatric units, it was more important to follow orders, demonstrate professional growth, provide individualized care, demonstrate concern for peers, and be assertive. In contrast, the critical-care units were significantly more likely to focus on technical skills and emergencies, insist things be done in a certain way, and calling off duty was absent. Medical units were least likely to follow traditions, and rehabilitation units were most likely to document and take personal credit for their decisions. However, it should be pointed out that, out of 100 possible significant differences between units based on technology, only 40 differences were noted. Furthermore, each unit demonstrated some behaviors more typical of other technologies than their own technology, and technologies showed very different patterns of clustering together, depending on the specific cultural behavior considered. The researchers concluded that support was indeed found for some of our common stereotypes of different specialty units. However, many cultural behaviors did not vary by technology (Coeling, Simms, & Price, 1993). Hence, the executive nurse will do well to assess each unit individually in order to predict the differing impact of a given change on each unit.

Additional Sources

Other factors that impact on the culture include group tolerance for members who do not conform to the culture, critical incidents, the physical layout of the unit, and the culture of the surrounding community. When executive nurses consider the many forces influencing a work group's culture, they become less surprised to realize that, just as all individuals have their own fingerprint, each work group, over time, also develops its own unique culture.

CULTURAL DIFFERENCES BETWEEN UNITS

We now turn to an examination of the ways in which work groups express their cultural differences.

Decision Making

Nurse decision making is complex because of the multiple sources from which nurses receive directives to guide nursing care. The directives can come from the health care agency (policies and procedures), from the nurse's knowledge (nurse's independent judgment), from the physician (medical orders), and from the nurse's professional peers (suggestions regarding nursing care).

Throughout the history of nursing, the primary source of directives to guide nursing care has varied. Before the 1890s, nurses practiced relatively autonomously in the community. Early in the twentieth century, the nursing profession began to lose professional independence as nurse training schools were organized within newly developed hospital settings. There physicians and administrators limited the autonomy and decision-making authority of the nurses, who were no longer expected to make independent decisions. Rather, nurses were provided with rules to tell them what to do when. Nurse leaders did not agree with relinquishing power over nursing practice, but they felt compelled to do so because they were dependent upon the hospital administrators to provide nursing students with room, board, and education (Porter-O'Grady & Finnigan, 1984). Although nursing today is still limited in autonomy and independent decision making, the nursing profession is striving to increase professional autonomy.

Thus, a renewed emphasis is being placed on independent nursing judgment as a basis for nursing care. Yet the presence and the power of other sources will not disappear overnight—nor should they. Nurses will continue to make decisions on the basis of policies and procedures as employees of health care institutions (themselves accountable to the public), and on the basis of physicians' orders as long as nurses care for patients who require medical care by physicians (who are accountable to the public for their own right to practice). Also, group norms will always exert pressure for conformity (Schein, 1985). Thus, the executive nurse will find a variety of power-relationship patterns on various nursing units; and nursing units will differ in the relative importance attached to various sources of decision making.

Recent attempts to increase nursing autonomy have met with varied results (Blake, 1990; Schwartz, 1990). These differing cultural preferences for sources of decision making may explain the varied results obtained from research on a variety of delivery systems and governance structures.

Sources of Decision Making

The following paragraphs report a research study identifying a variety of cultural preferences for sources of decision making. In this study, 478 registered nurses representing 33 different units in three midwestern hospitals were asked to describe their primary source of directives for nursing care (Coeling, 1991). They were presented with a list of four sources of directives:

- Policies and procedures
- Individual nurse's judgment
- Physician's orders
- Peer pressure

They were then asked to rate them from 1 (most important in guiding the nursing care in their group) to 4 (the least important item). They were asked to do the same to indicate their preferred source of directives. Findings presented in Figure 10.3 suggest that policies and procedures, individual nurse's judgment, and physician's orders were all important sources of direction for nursing care. Twenty-three percent said policies and procedures were the most important source of directives; 35 percent indicated individual judgment was their most important guide; and 39 percent said physicians were their primary source of directives. Peer

Source	Current group norm	Norm preferred by individual nurse
Policies and procedures	23%	22%
Individual judgement	35%	49%
Physician's orders	39%	28%
Peer Pressure	4%	1%

Figure 10.3 *Most important source of directives.*

	Unit A C	Unit A P	Unit B C	Unit B P	Unit C C	Unit C P	Unit D C	Unit D P
Policies and procedures	50%	25%	25%	25%	13%	4%	46%	46%
Individual judgement	25	75	25	25	44	57	23	46
Physician's orders	25		50	50	39	35	31	8
Peer pressure					4	4		

	Unit E C	Unit E P	Unit F C	Unit F P	Unit G C	Unit G P	Unit H C	Unit H P
Policies and procedures	13%	27%	30%	35%	13%	18%	5%	5%
Individual judgement	47	40	25	40	36	51	73	90
Physician's orders	40	33	35	25	49	29	11	5
Peer pressure			10		2	2	11	

C = Current first-ranked source of directives   P = Preferred first-ranked source of directives

Figure 10.4 *Current and preferred first-ranked sources of directives.*

pressure ranked low in all areas. This is probably because peer pressure is a reflection of group culture and the culture defines a group's preference for the other three sources. As Figure 10.3 shows, although 49 percent of the nurses preferred that their individual judgment be the most important source of directives, 50 percent preferred policies and procedures or physicians' orders. Figure 10.4 shows how these preferences differed markedly as a function of the different units. Implications of these differences for the executive nurse will be discussed here to illustrate the importance of understanding cultural differences.

Since culture is a pattern, norms other than those related to decision making also interact with these decision-making preferences. These particular decision-making behaviors were pulled out to illustrate the need to understand work-group cultures, but the perceptive executive nurse will recognize that the manner in which decision-making preferences interact with the unit's many other cultural behaviors determines the overall culture of a given unit.

USING AN UNDERSTANDING OF CULTURAL DIFFERENCES

Hiring

The culture of a nursing unit is an important consideration when hiring personnel. Nurses who fit in with the culture of their group are more likely to have a longer tenure on the unit, both because they enjoy the way the unit "does things" and because they feel accepted there (Carlson, 1992; Coeling, 1990; O'Reilly III, Chatman, & Caldwell, 1991). Research suggests that in nursing, close matches in preferences for group support, helping each other, growing professionally, decision making, and activity level are especially important in a nurse's length of stay on a given unit (Coeling, 1992).

The reason workers do not feel accepted on the unit relates to the way in which culture is taught to newcomers by the more tenured workers. This teaching occurs informally as experienced workers show newcomers how to do things. Much of this teaching occurs as experienced workers praise newcomers for doing things "our way" and cast judgment on newcomers who do not conform.

Most often these judgmental cues are sent nonverbally, through the rolling of eyes, shrugging of shoulders, heavy sighs, and raised eyebrows. Most newcomers quickly learn to read these signs and adjust their behavior accordingly. However, some workers do not adjust their behavior; they choose not to adapt to the unit's culture. Others lack the skill to read these signs. Those lacking this skill continually feel judged and cannot understand why. When this judgmental attitude becomes intolerable, they seek to leave the unit for a more comfortable situation. Some nurses who have difficulty reading cultural cues move from unit to unit, always looking for the "right place."

Whether a worker who does not conform to the unit culture will "work out" depends on both the unit and the worker. Some units have a high tolerance for nonconformity and accept workers who do not do things their way. And, some units will accept a cultural nonconformist because that person has other characteristics that meet a special need on that unit, such as a willingness to work permanent nights. Also, some people are able to work in situations where they are not totally accepted. Those with a high tolerance for partial group acceptance are able to continue working on a unit even though they might not quite fit in. Some nurses are willing to do this for personal reasons because the unit meets a special need for them.

The fact that different personnel have different cultural preferences has several implications for the hiring process. First, it is important that the person interviewing the potential employee have a feel for the culture of the group to which this employee will be assigned. Most experienced nursing managers intuitively have a feel for the culture of their unit; as they interview, they compare the candidate with the unit culture. Assisting nursing-unit managers to become even more "culture conscious" can improve this intuitive process.

It is recommended that at least two people be available to interview applicants. As noted, it is essential that a person close to the unit, one who knows the culture well, be available for interviews. However, in addition, it is useful if someone who has knowledge about the culture of a variety of units interview the applicant—so that, if it becomes clear the applicant would not match very closely with one unit, a unit that has a different culture can be offered as an alternative job site. If the applicant is qualified for both jobs, though, the choice of job sites is up to the candidate. A possible cultural mismatch is not grounds for denying a person a job.

It is recommended that the executive nurse facilitate the development of policies and allow transfer to another unit soon after being hired if it becomes obvious the newcomer is not fitting in with one culture and there is a suitable job opening available elsewhere. Numerous nurses have told this author that they can tell within a week whether a new nurse will make a good adjustment to the unit. If both orientee and unit members feel the orientee will not adjust to the prevailing culture, there is little to be gained by insisting the newcomer remain on an assigned unit for a given period of time, especially if there are openings on units where the person would fit better. There is much to be lost in terms of lowered productivity and emotional stress for all involved when the employee is forced to stay on a unit under difficult conditions.

Figure 10.4 can be used to illustrate how knowledge of a unit's culture and knowledge of an applicant's cultural preferences can facilitate assigning the nurse to the right unit. Nurses on Unit A currently do not feel they are able to use their individual judgment in making nursing-care decisions. However, the majority of them desire to do so. Suppose an applicant was a nurse who wanted a job that allowed independent nursing judgment. This nurse may well enjoy the challenge of working with Unit A nurses as they move toward increasing their autonomy, but would probably be frustrated by working on Unit B, where the nurses show very little desire for increased autonomy.

The above suggestions also pertain to the hiring of nursing-unit managers. Often the person selected as the new manager for a unit is someone who has shown leadership ability on another unit without consideration of the type of culture in which this person functions best. Consider, for example, a unit manager who sees the enforcing of policies and procedures as an important part of the manager role. Such a manager would probably have difficulty as manager on Unit G, where the nurses do not draw heavily upon policies and procedures to make nursing decisions, but prefer using their individual judgment to guide their nursing care. All other things being equal, this manager would fit better on Unit D, where nurses value policies and procedures more highly.

Merging

Another situation in which the executive nurse's awareness of a nursing unit culture can facilitate management outcomes is that of mergers. In this era of cost-containment, more and more hospitals are merging two smaller units into one large unit in an attempt to cut overhead administrative costs. Frequently, these mergers are based on similarity of technology. However, as noted above, similarity of culture does not necessarily follow from similarity of technology. Merging two nursing units with different cultures can be frustrating for managers and workers alike. If Unit H (see Figure 10.4), which rates individual judgment highly, were to merge with Unit D, which bases considerably fewer of their nursing care decisions on individual judgment, but has much higher regard for policies and procedures, a cultural clash is to be expected. When nurses from Unit H would disregard standard protocols in favor of their personal judgment about what is best for a given patient, nurses from Unit D would probably accuse these nurses of giving poor nursing care.

When two hospitals merge, it is often assumed that it will be easy to put, say, the two dialysis units together at one site and the two obstetrical units together at the other site. Again, this may or may not prove to be a smooth merger, depending on the cultural differences that exist between the units. If the cultures are similar, they can expect an easy transition, all other things being equal; but if there are considerable cultural differences, tension between the two groups can be expected as each group perceives the other to be either inadequate or uncaring.

Innovating

Almost all significant changes involve some cultural changes and the work-group culture is an important consideration. As Deal (1990, p. 25) notes in his discussion of cultural change, "A lot of money has been wasted and a number of promising careers have been busted because executives did not take the time to learn the lay of the land before taking action." Change occurs most readily when a group's cultural values and behaviors are allowed to remain at least somewhat intact. Most employees do not object to changing their ways if they are allowed to maintain those behaviors that are very important to them. What they object to in the change process is giving up their cherished values and behaviors. Adapting the change to the culture is important because culture is a stronger force in the lives of most employees than is the desire for the change. DeLisi (1990) notes that the basic assumptions held by a group affect the change more fundamentally than the proposed change affects the culture. Organizational change, he explains, must fit the existing organizational culture.

When change is mandated, the creative executive nurse preserves a group's cherished values and behaviors by adapting the change to the culture as much as possible. An example is a unit in a health care agency (e.g., Unit B, of Figure 10.4) that has made the decision to move toward shared governance. This move involves independent nursing judgment. On a unit like Unit B, which is low in a desire to use independent judgment but high in a desire to follow physicians' orders, the executive nurse could enlist physician support and perhaps even ask the physicians to encourage nursing judgment and/or be actively involved in establishing new governance policies. In this way, these nurses would be holding on to their cherished mode of operating (i.e., following the physicians' orders), while learning new behaviors that reflect a higher level of professional performance. They will accept this new behavior more readily if they do not have to do what they consider "wrong" in the process.

This concept of adapting a change to a given culture is relatively new in organizational literature. Denison (1990) explains that change is often described in organizational literature as a conversion process, initiated by a top leader and then transmitted throughout the organization. In this model, an enlightened leader changes his or her mind and change in the organization follows. Denison writes that his work in organizational culture presents a different picture. This is because existing cultures have considerable inertia; after all, maintaining the culture is seen by group members as essential for survival. Changes that do occur, do so slowly, as responses to changes in the external environment. Cultural change will occur most readily when it is not a drastic change from workers' cherished values and behaviors and when they see the change as essential for survival. As Thompson and Luthans (1990) note, however, this process can be greatly enhanced by the organization's rewarding the new behaviors they desire. Rewarding new behaviors will increase the organization's chance of survival in a rapidly changing environment.

Team Building

An understanding of the work-group culture is useful when facilitating team building on a particular unit. Group culture is closely related to group identity, or self-concept. A group that knows what it stands for and where it wants to go is in a better position to move forward than a group that lacks an identity and is aimless.

Forward movement occurs as a group seeks to enhance its identity by building on its strengths. Pinderhughes (1989), in discussing helpful interventions for clients with ethnic backgrounds different from that of mainstream America, emphasizes focusing on strengths that build on client assets.

The above strategy, a reverse of traditional approaches focusing on weakness or pathology, can be applied to working with a group. Developing those skills that a work group already values and that work well for the group may be the most efficient way to improve performance. To do this, first determine, through a cultural assessment, what the unit values and what behaviors it might want to change.

Referring again to Figure 10.5, the executive nurse would note that Unit E values and wants more emphasis on following policies and procedures. Perhaps on this unit errors have occurred, or were perceived to occur, because some workers did not pay close enough attention to existing procedures. In contrast, they would prefer less emphasis on medical directives. This unit might be strengthened by the development of policies and procedures that would allow for less direction from physicians, especially in regard to nursing care procedures. Developing protocols unique to this unit would both enhance the nurses' sense of identity and their sense that their unit is distinct from any other unit in the agency and hence "special," thus motivating them to follow their new guidelines, build team spirit, and improve the quality of care.

RESPECTING CULTURAL DIFFERENCES

Although a given culture may be more or less appropriate for a given goal, there is no one overall best culture and units should be allowed to emphasize their valued behaviors. Morgan (1986) warns against seeing cultures as right or wrong. He encourages organizational leaders to help a group understand its culture, but not to tell it what culture to have. Early organizational-culture literature emphasized an organization's having the "right" culture. More recent scholarship has focused on the need to assess and understand a given culture. The organizational goal is achieving a specific outcome or product. This achievement can be enhanced by recognizing the uniqueness of each work group's culture and working within that culture to achieve the organization's desired outcome.

Summary

Culture represents a group's unique, dynamic, holistic pattern of responses to the environment at a given time. Increasingly culture is viewed not as an outcome variable (i.e., a specific goal to attain), but as a unique pattern of behavior. Cultural behaviors at both the corporate and work-group level influence organizational processes and must be taken into account by the executive nurse in organizational activities such as hiring, merging, innovating, and team building. The executive nurse will want to assist each unique work group, especially in this era of delivery system changes, to define and redefine the culture that best enables that group to achieve the outcomes for which the work group and organization exist.

Discussion Questions

1. Describe the ideal nursing group culture.
2. How does your group culture impact nursing care and patient outcomes?

References

Blake, C. M. (1990). Selected measurements of pain intensity and nursing response in the orthopedic patient receiving patient-controlled analgesia. Unpublished manuscript, Kent State University School of Nursing.

Bullis, C. (1990). Organizational transformation through values: A comparison of unitary and pluralist perspectives. Paper presented at the annual convention of the International Communication Association, Dublin, Ireland.

Carlson, K. (1992). Family issues: Organization issues. *Journal of Post Anesthesia Nursing, 7*(1), 77–78.

Caroselli, C. (1992). Assessment of organizational culture: A tool for professional success. *Orthopaedic Nursing, 11*(3), 57–63.

Coeling, H. V. (1987). A comparison of work group rules on two nursing units. *Dissertation Abstracts International. 48*, Issue 6, Section A. (University Microfilms No. 87-20-063.)

Coeling, H. V. (1990). Organizational culture: Helping new graduates adjust. *Nurse Educator, 15*(2), 26–30.

Coeling, H. V. (1991). Multiple sources of directives for nursing care. Paper presented at the Fourth National Conference on Nursing Administration Research, The University of Iowa College of Nursing, Iowa City.

Coeling H. V. (1992). Fitting in on the unit: Work culture is the key. *Nursing 92, 22*(7), 74–76.

Coeling, H. V. (1994). Organizational culture. In L. M. Simms, S. A. Price, N. E. Ervin (Eds.), *The professional practice of nursing administration* (2nd ed.). Albany, NY: Delmar.

Coeling, H. V., Simms, L. M. (1993). Facilitating innovation at the nursing unit level through cultural assessment, Part I. *Journal of Nursing Administration, 23*(4), 46–53.

Coeling, H. V., Simms, L. M., Price S. A. (1993). Work group technology and cultures: Is there a link? Paper presented at the Fifth National Conference on Nursing Administration Research, The University of North Carolina School of Nursing, Chapel Hill.

Coeling, H. V., Simms, L. M. (1990). Preventing nurse turnover. Unpublished research, Partly funded by Kent State University Research Council.

Coeling, H. V., Wilcox, J. R. (1988). Understanding organizational culture: A key to management decision-making. *Journal of Nursing Administration, 18*(11), 16–24.

Coeling, H. V., Wilcox, J. R. (1991). Professional recognition and high-quality patient care through collaboration: Two sides of the same coin. *Focus on Critical Care, 18,* 230–237.

Curran, C. R., Miller, N. (1990). The impact of corporate culture on nurse retention. *Nursing Clinics of North America, 25*(3), 537–549.

Deal, T. E. (1990). Healthcare executives as symbolic leaders. *Healthcare Executive, 6*(3), 24–27.

Deal, T. E., Kennedy, A. A. (1982). *Corporate cultures.* Reading, MA: Addison-Wesley.

Deetz, S. A. (1982). Critical interpretive research in organizational communication. *The Western Journal of Speech Communication, 46,* 131–149.

DeLisi, P. S. (1990). Lessons from the steel axe: Culture, technology, and organizational change. *Sloan Management Review. 32*(1), 83–93.

Denison, D. R. (1990). *Corporate culture and organizational effectiveness.* New York: Wiley.

Denison, D. R. (1993). What IS the difference between organizational culture and organizational climate? A native's point of view on a decade of paradigm wars. Paper presented at the School of Business Administration July Seminar, The University of Michigan, Ann Arbor.

Donnelly, R. M. (1984). The interrelationship of planning with corporate culture in the creation of shared values. *Managerial Planning, 32*(6), 8–12.

Faules, D. F., Bullis, C. (1990). Cultural constraints and the relationship between social and symbolic orders. Paper presented at the 40th Annual Conference of the International Communication Association, Dublin,Ireland.

Flarey, D. L. (1991). The social climate scale: A tool for organizational change and development. *Journal of Nursing Administration, 21*(4), 37–44.

Flarey, D. L. (1993). The social climate of work environments. *Journal of Nursing Administration, 23*(6), 9–15.

Gregory, K. L. ((1983). Native-view paradigms: Multiple cultures and culture conflicts in organizations. *Administrative Science Quarterly, 28,* 359–376.

Hofstede, G., Neuijen, B., Ohayv, D. D., Sanders, G. (1990). Measuring organizational cultures: A qualitative and quantitative study across twenty cases. *Administrative Science Quarterly, 35,*286–316.

Hughes, L. (1990). Assessing organizational culture: Strategies for the external consultant. *Nursing Forum, 25*(1), 15–19.

James, L. R., James, L. A., Ashe, D. K. (1990). The meaning of organizations: The role of cognition and values. In B. Schneider (Ed.) *Organizational climate and culture* (pp. 40–84). San Francisco: Jossey-Bass.

Jermier, J. M., Slocum Jr., J. W., Fry, L. W., Gaines, J. (1991). Organizational subcultures in a soft bureaucracy: Resistance behind the myth and facade of an official culture. *Organization Science, 2*(2),170–194.

Lessem, R. (1990). *Managing corporate culture.* Brookfield, VT: Gower.

Morgan, G. (1986). *Images of organizations.* Beverly Hills: Sage.

Morley, D. D., Shockley-Zalabak, P. (1991). An examination of the influence of organizational founders' value. *Management Communication Quarterly, 4*, 422–449.

O'Reilly III, C. A., Chatman, J., Caldwell, D. R. (1991). People and organizational culture: A profile comparison approach to assessing person-organization fit. *Academy of Management Journal, 34*(3), 487–516.

Ott, J. S. (1989). *The organizational culture perspective.* Chicago: Dorsey.

Pacanowsky, M. E., O'Donnell-Trujillo, N. (1983). Organizational communication as cultural performance. *Communication Monographs, 50*, 126–147.

Peters, T. J., Waterman Jr., R. H. (1982). *In search of excellence.* New York: Harper & Row.

Pinderhughes, E. (1989). *Understanding race, ethnicity, and power.* New York: Macmillan.

Porter-O'Grady, T., Finnigan, S. (1984). *Shared governance for nursing: A creative approach to professional accountability.* Rockville, MD: Aspen.

Ramirez, D. C. (1990). Culture in a nursing service organization. *Nursing Management, 21*(1), 14–17.

Reichers, A. E., Schneider, B. (1990). Climate and culture: An evolution of constructs. In B. Schneider (Ed.), *Organizational climate and culture* (pp.5–40). San Francisco: Jossey-Bass.

Rogers, M. E. (1992). Nursing science and the space age. *Nursing Science Quarterly, 5*(1), 27–34.

Riley, P. (1983). A structurationist account of political culture. *Administrative Science Quarterly, 28*, 414–437.

Rousseau, D. M. (1978). Characteristics of departments, positions, and individuals: Contexts for attitudes and behavior. *Administrative Science Quarterly, 23*, 521–538.

Schall, M. S. (1983). A communication-rules approach to organizational culture. *Administration Science Quarterly, 28*, 557–581.

Schwartz, R. H. (1990). Nurse decision-making influence: A discrepancy between the nursing and hospital literatures. *Journal of Nursing Administration, 20*(6), 35–39.

Schein, E. H. (1983). The role of the founder in creating organizational culture. *Organizational Dynamics, 12*(Summer), 13–28.

Schein, E. H. (1985). *Organizational culture and leadership.* San Francisco: Jossey-Bass.

Shockley-Zalabak, P., Morley, D. D. (1994). Creating a culture. *Human Communication Research, 20*(3), 334–355.

Short, L. E., Ferratt, T. W. (1984). Work unit culture: Strategic starting point in building organizational change. *Management Review, 73*(8), 15–19.

Thomas, C., Ward, M., Chorba, C., Kumiega, A. (1990). Measuring and interpreting organizational culture. *Journal of Nursing Administration, 20*(6), 17–29.

Thompson, K. R., Luthans, F. (1990). Organizational culture: A behavioral perspective. In B. Schneider (Ed.), *Organizational climate and culture* (pp. 319–44). San Francisco: Jossey-Bass.

Van Maanen, J., Barley, S. R. (1985). Cultural organization: Fragments of a theory. In P. J. Frost, et al. (Eds.) *Organizational culture* (pp. 31–53). Beverly Hills: Sage.

Wilkins, A. L, Ouchi, W. G. (1983). Efficient cultures: Exploring the relationship between culture and organizational performance. *Administrative Science Quarterly, 28*, 468–481.

Wolfer, J. (1993). Aspects of "reality" and ways of knowing in nursing : In search of an integrating paradigm. *IMAGE:The Journal of Nursing Scholarship, 25*, 1941–1946.

Mary Jane Reinhart

CHAPTER 11

Power in Your Hands

Introduction

Power in the hands of the executive nurse is a major determinant of nursing practice outcomes within health care organizations. It is also a characteristic of the executive nurse's leadership success or failure within any health care setting. The exercise of power is even more critical at present because executive nurses are frequently viewed as powerless and as abandoning nurses. For example, the current concentration on health care costs is resulting in staff mix changes in most delivery systems. These changes are perceived to be within the power of the executive nurse and felt to be negative by many professional nurses.

These practice and leadership outcomes may range from catastrophic through somniferous to awesome. The nursing profession is more interested in outcomes that are awesome than catastrophic. Therefore, it is necessary to examine the concept of power to better understand the mechanism of achieving desired outcomes. The intent of this chapter is to review the basic concepts of power so as to encourage executive nurses in all health care settings to refocus on their power to shape a new health care delivery system. Executive nurses today must understand and use their power to further the goals of quality health care.

POWER DEFINED AND DESCRIBED

Myriad definitions or descriptions have been presented in the general literature for the concept of power. The descriptions of power tend to circumvent the actual definition and concentrate on describing behaviors inherent in power expenditure, often reflecting an individual's ability to influence another person's behavior. French and Raven (1959) described power in terms of five social bases of power:

reward power, coercive power, legitimate power, referent power, and expert power. This view reflects a person-to-person perspective, with the assumption that one person has influence over another. In 1975, Adams described power in terms of the amount of control over valued resources, reflecting a view of legitimate power. Goldberg, Cavanaugh, and Larson (1983) described five theoretical power orientation constructs: power as good, power as resource dependency, power as instinctive drive, power as political, power as charisma, and power as control and autonomy. These power orientation constructs reflect the awareness that the power arises within the individual, regardless of social base.

Reinhart (1988) described power in terms of the expenditure of an energy commodity that resides within an individual who in turn exists within a social and resource-filled environment. In this way, the definition of power becomes the potential to achieve desired outcomes. Assuming the desired outcome is control, the individual thus has the potential to control decisions that affect the self, other people, and the distribution and use of valuable resources. The magnitude of an individual's power is dependent on the degree of potential power energy inherent in a particular social base of power. The expenditure of power may be influenced by the individual's power orientation or attitude.

Hage (1980) explained power in the context of the organization where an individual is employed. Organizational power resides where the decisions are made that determine desired outcomes. These outcomes reflect control over other people's behaviors, control over the individual decision maker's behaviors, and the distribution and use of valuable resources. Hage described these organizational structures as centralization power, formalization power, and stratification power. Each structure has related functions. Merging Hage's description of power within the organization with Reinhart's definition of an individual's power, the definition of organizational power becomes the potential to achieve desired outcomes within the employing organization.

The top executive nurse in an organization presumably has the greatest amount of power among all the nurses employed in the organization. Therefore, the accountability for achieving desired professional nursing outcomes within the organization becomes an immense responsibility for the executive nurse. An assumption may be made that the top executive nurse has the inherent ability to make deliberate decisions.

POWER STRUCTURES AND FUNCTIONS

The nature of decisions made that govern other nurses' behaviors, the executive nurse's own behavior, and the distribution and use of valuable resources warrant examination using the framework of Hage's 1980 organizational power structures and functions. Table 11.1 illustrates the three structures with notations of related functional areas.

Centralization Power

Perhaps the highest level of organizational power exists in the arena of centralization power. The potential to make and act on decisions that govern the actions of others has widespread ramifications. An organization takes on a personality as well

Table 11.1 • **Organizational Structures and Functions of Power**

Centralization Power	Formalization Power	Stratification Power
Definition: Hierarchical authority that reflects the level and degree of participation in making strategic decisions that govern the involvement and behaviors of individuals throughout the organization (Hage, 1980).	*Definition:* The degree of rules, regulations, and restrictions placed on an individual that govern the degree of organizational involvement and daily behaviors (Hage, 1980).	*Definition:* A positional status system that reflects the level of position, pay, benefits, rewards, and privileges (Hage, 1980).
Functions within the structure include making decisions that: • Hire, fire, and promote workers • Establish new rules, regulations, and policies • Change existing rules, regulations, and policies • Establish new programs or discontinue old programs • Actually *allocate* funds	Functions within the structure involve an individual's level of *autonomy*. A high level of formalization power indicates a high level of autonomy.	Functions within the structure involve the status and reward systems granted by the organization to individuals relative to all other workers. Upward mobility is a key component.

as a reputation based on the actions, attitudes, and outputs of its employees. The organizational personality involving nurses' actions and attitudes is often a reflection of the leadership style of the executive nurse. It reflects the power decisions made. For example, the executive nurse may decide to develop a policy to decentralize authority. The sharing of governmental decisions means allowing some centralization power decisions to be made by the people most involved in the situations. Examples are the shared governance model, quality circles, and total quality management. It may seem that the executive nurse has given away power, when in actuality, power (the potential to achieve desired outcomes) has been increased through insightful situation assessments and appropriate problem resolution. A careful examination of decisions made by shared government groups is warranted, because the tendency may be to limit the decisions to day-to-day operational problems rather than to focus on strategic policy matters. A decision to paint the lounge pink or to have fried chicken at the organization's summer picnic is not a strategic policy decision. The decision to encourage and support others in their nursing-practice decision making demonstrates the decentralization of power.

It is only within relatively recent years that nurses have been involved in the preparation of organization or unit budgets. Preparing a budget gives the illusion of power. However, it is the potential to allocate (not ask for) funds that indicates true centralization power. The degree of an executive nurse's centralization fiscal power is indicated by the degree to which financial allocation control is present in the position. Fiscal power is important for the executive nurse so that the human and material resources needed for the delivery of quality nursing care can be obtained.

Formalization Power

Formalization power is autonomy power, also frequently thought of as behavioral empowerment. When centralization power is expended by administrators to control the actions of employees through strict rules, regulations, and restrictions, autonomy of the worker is acutely limited. In this situation, the individual has a low level of formalization power. Traditionally, nurses have experienced low levels of formalization power. As health care changes occur throughout the 1990s, higher levels of formalization power may be granted to advanced-practice nurses, while the average staff nurse may experience lower formalization power by sharing patient care with ancillary employees in a redesigned organization. Higher formalization power may be seen when the nurse is accountable for other health care providers and is recognized accordingly.

The executive nurse must decide how to handle the issue of nursing autonomy and empowerment within the formalization of power. Potential levels of differentiated practice of nurses must not hinder the delivery of care and the contributions to health care by nurses. There are unfortunate splits within nursing around nursing education and the role of advanced practitioners that can create difficult governing issues for the executive nurse.

Stratification Power

Stratification power is reflected by the degree of one's status and rewards in relation to others in the organization. The status and reward system of an organization is reminiscent of certain concepts in the classical motivation-hygiene theory of satisfiers and dissatisfiers proposed by Herzberg (Herzberg, Mauser, & Snyderman, 1959). Satisfiers (motivation factors) include the opportunity to achieve, advance, and be recognized for achievement in the organization. Dissatisfiers (hygiene factors) are those job conditions that result in dissatisfaction when not present to an acceptable degree. Examples of dissatisfiers include pay, fringe benefits, and privileges. To have a high level of stratification power is to possess high levels of motivators and hygiene factors relative to others in the organization. Currently, stratification power is being framed within organizations around teams, total quality management, and case management. The executive nurse must decide what stratification levels to grant the various nurses in the organization to achieve desired outcomes.

STRATEGIES AND OUTCOMES

When making organizational power decisions, the executive nurse must decide what management strategy to use. Three basic strategies include the use of control, empowerment, and evolution (Table 11.2).

Control

The strategy of control reflects an autocratic style of leadership. Decisions are generally made by the executive nurse with little input from other nurses. All suggestions and recommendations must be approved before action occurs. Rules and regulations are strictly enforced. Rewards are limited to a selected few individuals.

Table 11.2 • **Comparison of Strategies and Outcomes of Power Decisions**

Power Expenditure		Behavioral Outcome
Strategy used	**Structural/functional aspects**	**Indicators**
Control Delegation of tasks with only responsibility granted	*Centralization power* Must approve all recommendations before taking action *Formalization power* Use of rules and regulations to achieve desired outcomes; may have to ask someone higher before action; use of supervisors to enforce rules *Stratification power* Use of limited rewards given to a select few	Innovation by a selected few; few incentives for workers to be willing to risk trying changes; moderate-to-low esprit de corps; presence of complicated political system among workers competing for selected status; high turnover of workers; short-term achievement of desired outcomes, but effect does not last over time
Empowerment Delegation of tasks with both responsibility and authority granted. Extrinsic and/or intrinsic empowerment may be used in all three structures	*Centralization power* Policy decisions made and implemented by those close to the problems *Formalization power* Workers have high level of autonomy over daily operations *Stratification power* Many intrinsic as well as tangible rewards experienced by workers; presence of upward mobility	High level of innovation; high esprit de corps; low turnover among workers; attraction of highly talented workers; high achievement of lasting desired organizational outcomes
Evolution No particular delegation or direction used	*Centralization power* Few new policies; status quo; new policies may be set by non-nurses *Formalization Power* Rules and regulations may be set by non-nurses; enforcement of rules through mediators *Stratification power* Rewards focused on pay; few intrinsic rewards	Low innovation; low esprit de corps; collective power may be used by workers to make desired changes or gain recognition; outcomes may not be desired

An executive nurse who has relatively low legitimate power within the administration of a health care agency may be compelled to use control to enact the decisions of those with higher legitimate power. In times of exigency, control may be the appropriate strategy for quick action. When used as a strategy over time, outcomes among employees include low levels of innovation, low morale, increased competition, and high turnover.

Empowerment

Effective use of inherent position power enjoyed by the executive nurse entails the expenditure of empowerment. Simply stated, empowerment is the movement of "decision and responsibility down the chain of command" (Smitley & Scott, 1994, p. 40). Empowerment requires the delegation of both responsibility and authority. The executive nurse must decide to what extent, and to whom, empowerment will be granted and what the qualifications of the individuals must be. Moving decision making and responsibility to lower levels of employees necessitates a reformed organizational structure and altered expectations, posing a risk the executive nurse must be willing to take.

Two forms of empowerment are necessary to unlock the potential found in an organization's work force (Table 11.3). Smitley and Scott (1994) described these two forms as extrinsic empowerment and intrinsic empowerment. An assumption in both extrinsic and intrinsic empowerment is that the employee will make decisions that will enhance the success of the organization. This means the executive

Table 11.3 • **Extrinsic and Intrinsic Empowerment**

Type of Empowerment	Characteristics	Outcomes
Extrinsic empowerment	• Protocols establish specific parameters of decision making • Specific outcome expectations are stated • Independent decisions may not exceed parameters of empowerment	• Control is maintained by persons in higher authority • Outcomes are predictable • Creativity is limited • Innovative changes are not encouraged • Individuals are free to make decisions within set parameters without asking permission
Intrinsic empowerment	• Responsibility and authority are granted to individuals to solve organizational problems through creativity and innovation • Empowered individuals are free to set situation parameters within the boundaries of the organization • Risk taking is encouraged • Implementation of innovative changes is endorsed by administration	• Outcomes may be different from, or surpass, expected outcomes • Failures are not treated as doom but as an opportunity to try again • Implementation is flexible, adapting to improvements during the pilot trial change process • The organization attracts and retains highly creative workers • The executive nurse shares in the reputation and benefits of the empowerment

nurse must clearly and accurately communicate the organization's mission and goals to enable employees to contribute to organizational success.

Extrinsic empowerment originates outside the employee, bestowing a given position with responsibility and authority to make certain organizational decisions. Extrinsic empowerment can be further defined and measured by outlining specific processes and outcomes expected. A certain mechanistic flavor and an exertion of external control exists in this type of empowerment. Guidelines and protocols may be established beyond which the empowered individual may not stray.

On the other hand, the executive nurse may choose to extend intrinsic as well as extrinsic empowerment. Smitley and Scott (1994) described intrinsic empowerment as the condition whereby an individual is granted the power to make creative decisions to solve problems and establish innovative changes in the organization. Such innovations are based on active listening, responding to situations, exploring possibilities, adapting to parameters, and taking the initiative to lead the change. The executive nurse, in granting intrinsic empowerment, would encourage risk taking and foster the enhancement of the individual's human potential. The executive nurse has the opportunity to further intrinsic empowerment in the current wave of system reengineering.

With either extrinsic or intrinsic empowerment, employee autonomy is increased, and daily operational decisions may be made by the practitioner to whom the task has been delegated. A sense of task ownership develops and the employee has the power to plan and achieve desired outcomes within the parameters of the task. With successful task achievement, the willingness to be innovative and the spirit of morale increase. Turnover of employees is decreased because work satisfaction is increased.

The executive nurse may find the delegation of responsibilities and authority without close supervision to be a threatening concept. On the surface, it appears that the executive's power is given away. In reality, the executive's power is expanded and enhanced, largely reflecting the employees' achievement of desired outcomes (which are assumed to be congruent with the organization's desired outcomes).

Along with decisions of empowerment, the executive nurse must be willing to take risks, willing to risk failure. Failure in this case is used as a basis to build, to try again in a different way. Pilot trials of projects and programs are typical in intrinsic empowerment. If the pilot trial does not achieve desired outcomes, the involved individual or group is empowered to develop and implement a new method. Many examples are seen in nursing, primarily related to staffing mix and scheduling, such as primary nursing, 10- and 12-hour shifts, case management, and weekend options. The individual's desire to be innovative and grow is truly enhanced through intrinsic empowerment.

Evolution

The executive nurse may choose to use evolution in making decisions. In this manner, decisions are delayed or sent to committees who debate, and may table, issues. Changes will usually occur through the normal course of organizational events rather than by deliberate decisions on the part of the executive nurse. Actual outcomes seldom resemble desired outcomes. Other administrators may make the decisions in lieu of action by the executive nurse. Few new policies are developed. Inaction on the part of the executive nurse may lead unit nurses to seek/force changes through mediators. In the guise of organizational stability, status quo prevails. As a result of decision by evolution, staff nurses may have little sense of direction, low morale, and high turnover rates. Because little is achieved, few rewards are evident. The concept of collective nursing-staff power may arise in an effort to force desired rewards. The following exercise includes an example in which a hypothetical, though realistic, scenario is presented. From the scenario description, information found in Table 11.1 was used to discuss the dynamics of the situation. The discussion does not presume to solve the problems found. There are many pathways executive nurses may choose to problem solve, all dependent on the choice of desired outcomes and the manner of power expenditure.

Scenario 11.1   **Challenges of a Home Care Agency**

Things aren't going well at XYZ Home Care Agency. The agency began as a small independent health care agency through the entrepreneurial efforts of two close friends who were registered nurses. Everything went well in the beginning when the case load was relatively small. Four other RNs were hired, and the six professional friends did all the home-care work as well as the office work. Problems were tackled together and decisions made at round-table discussions. The agency functioned like a real team.

Word spread that XYZ Home Care provided excellent service at reasonable prices. The home-visiting nurses had effectively filled a niche created when more and more patients were being sent home from hospital stays "sicker and quicker." The practice grew rapidly. Clerical staff were hired to tend office functions. More nurses were hired, as well as a cadre of unlicensed home health aids. The facility became crowded, necessitating shared desks and telephones. Everyone was busy and the round-table discussions became fewer and fewer. Indeed, the table itself was no longer large enough to seat all workers, so a selected few began to meet to solve problems, develop rules, delineate procedures, and establish policies. The two RN agency owners found themselves in the roles of joint chief executive officers of the business. They became too busy running the mushrooming business to carry a caseload themselves. Myriad health-insurance carriers imposed an increasing overload of complicated paperwork and coverage problems. And still the business grew . . .

Grumbling among staff members began, first at a murmur and then at a roar. The two nurse executives found themselves seated alone at the round table making all the business decisions. Everyone else was busy with patient care or paperwork. It became obvious that things weren't going well at XYZ. Few of the nurses and clerical staff were speaking to one another. Absenteeism was rampant, making staffing very difficult. Turnover of staff had increased, as evidenced by the fact that orientation of new staff was an ongoing activity. In a benevolent attempt to smooth over staff complaints, the two busy executive nurses would send out memos to the staff about new trouble-shooting decisions and policies. To boost morale, a staff-member-of-the-month was given a little fuzzy bunny to stick on the name tag.

When the problems continued, a consultant was called in. Together with the two executive nurses, the consultant conducted an employee survey to learn more about the nature of staff problems and to discern employees' perceptions regarding the organization's strengths and weaknesses. Results of the survey revealed that the XYZ Home Care Agency had a body of workers who were extremely dedicated to the mission of the agency and were proud to be identified as XYZ employees. However, the workers documented their perceptions that they had definite problems in the following areas:

- They had little or no input in making company policy decisions.

- They did not get enough information about how well their respective departments were doing. The only feedback they got was negative.

- XYZ was not recognizing or rewarding the quality of work they were doing.

- There were too many rules and regulations that were constantly changing without explanations for the changes. Not everyone knew about the changes until they made an error.

- When they did get a job performance evaluation, they did not have any input.

- They didn't feel secure in their jobs. If they tried to be creative in their work, it might go against the rules and they would be fired.

- Each department thought favoritism was shown to other departments. Co-operation between departments was minimal.

- Paperwork was overwhelming and usually had to be done after the scheduled and recorded working hours. Workers did not record extra hours of work time spent in paperwork because overtime was frowned on. Excessive overtime led to being fired for mismanagement of time.

- They weren't sure whether they were paid adequately for the work they did.

- Retirement benefits might not be adequate for their needs when the time of retirement occurred.

Using the information found in Table 11.1, we can examine the structures and functions of power in the XYZ Home Care Agency as it had evolved since the beginning of the organization. When the two nurses began the business, the centralization power functions were shared among the staff during actual round-table discussions. In a highly decentralized manner, joint decisions about such matters as hiring and establishing policies were made by the whole staff. By the time of the employee survey, a highly centralized administration had evolved, with the two executive nurses making practically all the strategic decisions. To add to their centralization power, they used a benevolent autocratic leadership style with little extrinsic or intrinsic empowerment of workers.

The organization operated around a highly formalized structure with many rules and regulations. As the number and complexity of staff members grew, worker autonomy lessened. The two executive nurses believed that everyone should use common procedures and follow common rules if the standard of care was to be maintained. This belief placed restrictions on workers' daily behaviors, hence decreasing autonomy and eliminating creativity. To complicate matters, outside influences such as health care insurance companies' changing policies necessitated frequent alterations in paperwork and procedures. Sometimes a new documentation form was added without the old one being eliminated.

Stratification power of the worker was at a low level. Shared desks and telephones led to little or no privacy when workers wished to call patients or client families. Because governance was conducted by the two nurse executives without a middle-management layer, there was no chance of upward job mobility. Little fuzzy bunnies weren't sufficient rewards for work well done. Workers harbored considerable uncertainty regarding whether their pay and benefits were adequate and commensurate with their work output and complexity.

The saving grace for XYZ Home Care Agency was that the workers still held high standards, practicing quality patient care. How long this quality could endure is uncertain. Without a working environment that fosters and facilitates decentralization of decision making (centralization power), autonomy and creativity in daily practice (formalization power), and an adequate reward system (stratification power), even typically altruistic nurses may falter. The two nurse executives have a pressing need to decide what changes in the organization's power structure they need to make if they continue to seek high quality patient care as a desired outcome.

IMPLICATIONS FOR NURSING EDUCATION

The time to learn about power and its use is before the nurse begins the ascent to an executive level. The implication for nursing education is that educational programs must incorporate the concept of power in all levels of nursing curriculum. If nurses are to achieve desired outcomes in clinical practice, they need to have an adequate understanding about the power potential. As nurses rise through the clinical ranks, increasing levels of legitimate organizational power will be granted to them. Successful use of this increasing power enhances further upward mobility. By the time the nurse becomes an executive, great talent in power expenditure should have been adequately developed, enabling the executive nurse to assist nurses in their professional quests for excellence in health care. With the position as executive nurse comes the responsibility of mentoring the next generation of executive nurses. Through this emphasis on successfully and appropriately expending the inherent potential an executive nurse has to achieve desired outcomes, the future of professional nursing is bright.

Summary

There are basically three options for the executive nurse regarding the expenditure of power inherent in the position. First, power potential may be used to take the risks necessary to preserve and promote the professional role of nurses as health care administrators redesign their organizations to use increased numbers of "cost-effective" ancillary helpers in direct patient care. Second, power may be used to assist (or coerce) professional nurses to change their professional roles to fit the organization's redesigned health care system. A third option, which is unfortunate for the nursing profession, involves the decision that executive power may be used to further the executive's career goals by bypassing the role as nurse champion and assuming characteristics of non-nurse executives who have as a basic goal the acquisition of profits and/or glory.

As nurses experience changes in health care provision, a vulnerable balance of power exists. The executive nurse is instrumental in deciding which way the balance of power will tilt. Nurses either will gain or lose their potential to achieve desired professional outcomes, largely dependent on the decisions of an executive nurse. It is the responsibility of every executive nurse to examine carefully the options available and the decisions to be made in the expenditure of power. Future nursing positions and traditions will be shaped by power decisions that are made and carried out in the provision of health care.

Discussion Questions

1. Describe how executive nurses or nurse managers could exercise power to achieve quality patient care.
2. Describe how total quality managment, restructuring health systems, and the elimination of nursing management positions change the power in organizations.

References

Adams, R. (1975). *Energy and structure: A theory of social power.* Austin, TX: University of Texas.

French, J. R., Jr., Raven, B. (1959). "The bases of social power." In D. Cartwright (Ed.), *Studies in social power* (pp. 150–167). Ann Arbor: University of Michigan.

Hage, J. (1980). *Theories of organizations: Form, process, and transformation.* New York: Wiley.

Herzberg, F., Mauser, B., Snyderman, B. (1959). *The motivation to work* (2nd ed.). New York: Wiley.

Reinhart, M. J. (1988). Nurses' perceptions of organizational power in relation to educational preparation. (Doctoral dissertation, Indiana University, 1988.) *Dissertation Abstracts International,* DAI-B 50/07, p. 2848, Jan 1990.

Smitley, W., Scott, D. (1994, August). Empowerment: Unlocking the potential of your work force. *Quality Digest, 14,* 40–46.

Donna Brown   CHAPTER **12**

Consultant: Friend or Foe?

Introduction

At some point in an executive nurse's career, there may need to be a decision about using a consultant's services. To avoid the many misconceptions about consultants and to use consultants effectively to achieve the desired targeted results, it is important to approach the use of a consultant as a process; doing this can determine whether a consultant becomes friend or foe. Being aware of the issues, asking probing questions, and structuring the professional relationship between the executive nurse and consultant from the beginning can dispel misconceptions of both parties and ensure a positive and effective experience. This chapter addresses issues and methods for determining a need for a consultant, the selection process itself, and the actual consultant-client relationship (Fig. 12.1).

DETERMINING THE NEED

The executive nurse may be confronted with considering the use of a consultant for a variety of reasons. The executive may be approached by a consultant with a service that sounds desirable, may be feeling a need for a third party's objective input, or may be needing a skill or process that is not within the division's repertoire of skills, talents, or time constraints.

Why, What, and How

One of the first steps in determining the need for a consultant is to determine the desired outcomes. Stephen R. Covey (1989) identifies "beginning with the end in mind" as a key to effectiveness. In terms of hiring a consultant, beginning with the end in mind provides direction for the selection process and ensures the selection

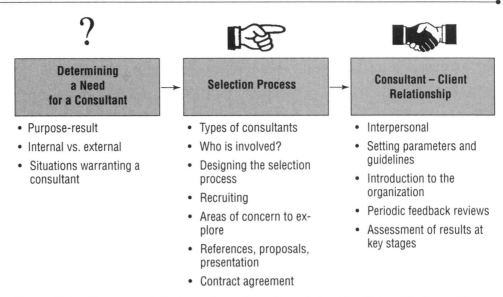

Figure 12.1   *The process of selection and consultant-client relationship. (Designed by Donna K. Brown, Oak Wood Associates.)*

of a consultant with the necessary capabilities, experience, and role understanding to ensure success for the entire project.

After the executive nurse asks what the consultant is to accomplish, three questions must be addressed. The *what* has been addressed in determining the desired outcome. The *how* is addressed by answering the following three questions.

The first question is whether the consultant will provide the actual service needed. Some examples of a consultant providing the actual service would be developing a personnel manual or designing a special computer database. The project would have a starting and ending date, with a specific function to be accomplished solely by the consultant.

The second question involves determining if the consultant should perform the task or if it is more desirable to train staff members so that they can function independently in the future. Clarification of the consultant's role as trainer rather than "doer" of the task is critical in the initial planning stages of using a consultant. Clarifying everyone's roles and responsibilities is also critical at this stage. For example, who internally is the contact person for the consultant? What are the expectations and roles for the consultant and for staff members involved in the project?

Many disappointing results occur when these issues are not clarified. For example, in one account, a CEO hired a computer consultant for $55,000 for the year to put a software program into operation. The consultant did so, but afterward, no one in the organization was able to operate the software program. Too many assumptions and not enough direction sabotaged the project!

If an executive nurse is unable to answer the first two questions, it may be because the root causes of the problem have not been identified or the need is not clearly defined. Hiring a consultant may assist the executive nurse in problem identification and need definition. In fact, this may be the purpose for using the consultant. The consultant assisting in this task may not necessarily be the one to implement the recommendations, and it is important to choose the appropriate consultant for this preliminary work. Examples of this type of consulting might include looking at high turnover, low morale, or a department in continual crisis. It may be apparent to everyone that a certain condition exists, but the root causes are not always obvious.

Advantages

There are many advantages to approaching the use of a consultant as a process. For example, hiring a consultant to train staff rather than registering for a seminar may be more cost-effective, since the consultant can compress the knowledge and skills staff needs to know for the particular situation. In addition, the skills can be taught at the level and learning style which best meet the needs of the staff member.

A consultant is not hindered by day-to-day operations and can keep a steady, consistent pace on the change and/or process efforts. Purchasing the consultant's time may appear expensive on first glance; however, in terms of completing the project, the overall effects of a completed task, without taking the executive nurse's time away from other projects, may justify the expense as a cost-effective alternative.

A consultant, due to wide experience with other organizations and the role as an external observer, can assist in identifying problems and needs. Staff closest to the problem may be too close for problem identification.

In addition, hiring a consultant adds expertise to a staff on a temporary basis without extra employee benefit costs. It also resolves the concern about hiring a full-time employee when there may be no need for the services when the task is completed. Thus, the consultant is hired based on a need for a specific window of time.

Initially, it is important to determine if a consultant is needed to provide the service, if staff members can be trained to accomplish the service independently, and/or if the executive nurse needs to assist in identifying the problem. When this differentiation is not made at the onset of a consulting contract, an organization, department, or individual may become consultant-dependent. The consultant delivers the service, yet no one internally has learned to maintain the service; so, every time the service is needed, an external consultant is required.

Pitfalls to Avoid

When using a consultant, several pitfalls can occur if the process is not managed properly by the executive nurse. We have already looked at the pitfall of staff being consultant-dependent.

A second pitfall can occur if the aim of the project is not made clear and then attached to very specific outcomes: the consultant may develop a personal agenda, and the executive nurse may end up far from the desired final outcomes. It might have been an interesting journey, but after expenditures of time, money, and energy, the initial need still exists.

A third pitfall is hiring a consultant without the necessary skills to proceed effectively as the scope and needs of the project change. Often, as a project progresses, it may veer from the original need. For example, a consultant may be hired to identify the reason for a high turnover rate in a department. The consultant may be very skilled in diagnostic assessment but not in the training and development needed to deal with the identified cause. It is important for the executive nurse to continually assess the needs and activities of the project as it progresses. It is also important to arrive at agreements with the consultant as to the contingencies should such change occur. For example, will the consultant be able to provide other associates or resources to assist in the progression of the project?

A fourth, and extremely dangerous, pitfall is hiring a consultant who cannot deliver the desired results. Many consultants are good talkers about what needs to be done and what they can do, and yet they prove unable to get the job done. As corporations downsize, many people are going out on their own as "consultants," believing that because they performed a certain task within an organization, they can consult in that area. Performing a task in an organization requires a different set of skills than performing the task as an external consultant, or leading members of an organization to perform the task themselves. Some consultants make this transition and get results for their clients; other consultants do not succeed. The client can become very frustrated with the time and money wasted.

Internal versus External Consultants

In choosing between an external and internal consultant, the executive nurse must first assess if there is anyone within the organization who has the skills and capabilities to fill the consulting needs. In large health care organizations, the executive nurse may be faced with the option of engaging an internal consultant from a different department (i.e., human resources, organizational development, computer services).

Besides having the skills and abilities, it is important that an internal consultant be at a relevant level of the organizational structure to ensure the success of the project. Selecting a staff person to do consulting and attitudinal changes with the top management team would be futile, as well as intimidating for the staff chosen. If an internal consultant is to be effective, the selected employee must be viewed by the target individual or group with a high degree of trust and confidence. The internal consultant must have support from all administrative levels to make sure the project receives the appropriate attention. Typically, if an internal consultant is subordinate to the group she is working with, she may not be as effective as an external consultant.

The internal consultant should be relieved of other responsibilities in order to give full attention to this project. Broad organizational projects, or collaborative projects, lend themselves to internal consultants.

Situations Warranting a Consultant

Certain situations may trigger consideration of using a consultant. These general areas include sensitive issues, unbiased-third party needs, facilitation needs, lack of time, lack of skills in a particular area, and sounding-board assistance.

One such situation is created when the issue is of a very sensitive nature. It may involve job coaching a manager or a vice president. There may be a need to deal with confidential information that management does not want disseminated among the general employees at that particular time. Dealing with conflict among various departments or individuals can necessitate the need for an unbiased, objective third party.

A second area that may warrant a consultant arises in situations in which an impartial perspective, without any prior knowledge of the situation, can enhance the process. This can involve a conflict resolution. It can involve a technical problem that the staff has worked on continually without gaining a clear perspective or a solution. An outside perspective can give the problem solvers a new way to approach the situation.

A third area is the use of the consultant to facilitate a meeting so that the executive nurse can participate in the process with staff, as opposed to being the facilitator of the process. It is very difficult to facilitate a meeting while still trying to contribute ideas. Having a facilitator design and direct the meeting so that the executive nurse can be free to brainstorm and problem solve with staff as an equal can be of great benefit to the executive. Examples of meeting situations that could be facilitated by a consultant include strategic thinking forums, operational planning sessions, and problem solving a departmental or cross-departmental issue.

A fourth situation involves gathering employees' candid perceptions about a particular problem or event. Employees may not share as openly with their supervisors as with an unbiased third party—not necessarily because employees avoid the truth, but because they may skirt an issue or protect their supervisor from issues that the supervisor should know about to be more effective. Employees are often afraid to share the feedback with the executive nurse because they do not want to engender hurt feelings or because they fear retaliation. An impartial third party, trained in feedback analysis, can gather straightforward feedback from all involved parties and through an analysis obtain for the executive nurse a clear perception of the current situation.

A fifth situation that may create a need for hiring a consultant is one in which the executive nurse lacks the time to perform the task. The executive nurse has multiple priorities and must continually assess which of these priorities should be delegated. As mentioned earlier, it may be more cost-effective to hire someone to perform certain tasks (e.g., research, gathering information, collecting pros and cons on an issue). Other tasks might include developing a salary schedule or some type of management tool, revising a personnel manual, or developing drafts of policies. These are tasks that consume a great deal of time. Even with the best of intentions, such tasks are often shuffled to the bottom of the priorities list. However, some of these tasks, if completed, can eliminate the brushfires that consume time on a daily basis.

A sixth, and usually obvious, area that may create a need for a consultant is when the skills needed are out of the executive nurse's area of expertise. Based on the need, a specific area of expertise may be required, such as computer skills for the development of computer software or organizing data. It might include training in a particular area for staff. The executive nurse needs to conduct an honest self-assessment of skills and abilities matched against the desired results to determine if there is a match. An effective manager knows personal strengths and weaknesses and knows how to compensate for them. So, engaging a consultant is one method of compensating for an area outside of the executive nurse's expertise.

The final situation addressed in this chapter that may warrant the hiring of a consultant is when the executive nurse needs an impartial sounding board before taking action, or for assistance in planning strategy or problem solving. The executive nurse remains the implementor; however, the consultant serves as an advisor to challenge thinking, to brainstorm with, and to ensure that everything needed to obtain results in a particular strategy is in place.

In summary, before hiring a consultant, it is important first to determine if a consultant is really necessary. What does the executive nurse want the consultant to do? The executive can list the pros and cons of hiring a consultant for the particular situation, keeping in mind the situations mentioned in this chapter that might warrant either an external or internal consultant. Doing this thinking process before moving to the selection process actually lays the foundation for the activities of the selection process.

THE SELECTION PROCESS

Many people call themselves consultants. Consultants have a wide variety of skills and training in myriad diverse subjects. Again it is important first to determine the situation that warrants a consultant and to clearly define the outcomes. Once the situation and desired results are clearly defined, the executive nurse can begin to filter through the ocean of people hanging out shingles, calling themselves consultants.

Types of Consultants

Checking the consultant's background and credentials is extremely important in ensuring that the consultant has background skills and experiences which match the desired outcomes. The skills, competencies, approach, and focus of a consultant should be explored in detail. One way to achieve this is obtain opinions from current or former clients.

It is important to review both the positions held by the consultant before becoming a consultant, and the results achieved in that particular field. Many consultants are no longer in the same field as when they held a job within an organization, but field is not as relevant in most cases as is the consultant's ability to gain results in an effective and efficient manner.

Who Is Involved?

The selection process for hiring a consultant varies from organization to organization. The process is dependent upon how widely the consultant is going to be used and for what purpose. If the individual will be a personal consultant to the executive nurse, the selection process may be exclusively the executive's choice. However, the degree of influence of the project within the organization will determine the types of positions and number of staff who need to be involved in the process. A project span of influence and type determines if the selection process is best implemented by an individual, or by a team who have a vested interest in the project. In most cases, the hiring of a consultant should be a team approach. For example, in dealing with a culture change, where developing a great deal of trust between management and union is critical, both parties should have a part in the selection process and in the final choice of the consultant. Joint involvement helps establish trust.

If a consultant is brought in to begin building trust between union and management (or between two departments) and management selects the consultant without anyone else's input, the consultant has a much more difficult time building trust with all parties concerned. The consultant must reassure the participants that management has no ulterior motives in terms of the selection. It is strongly recommended that when a consultant is to be used between individuals or departments, representation from all those involved be involved in the selection process and final choice of the consultant.

Designing the Selection Process

Individually or through a group process (depending upon the number of representatives), the selection team outlines in writing each step of the selection process. Stages include:

- Recruiting
- Screening
- Interviewing
- Credentials/results reviews
- References
- Critique of proposal and presentation
- Sample of skills

The following expands upon each of the stages of the selection process.

Recruiting

Once the types of skills and competencies required of the consultant are identified, the executive nurse and/or selection team approach other organizations, hospitals, and professional consulting organizations. At this stage, the type of consulting firm desired should be defined (i.e., large versus small, national versus local, famous versus well-known). The decision may be to recruit consultants from each type of firm; however, it wastes time and energy to recruit only local or national, and then later decide to start screening the other type of firm. The type of consulting firm to be approached needs to be determined early in the process.

Talking to other professionals will minimize the screening efforts required. Sources for various types of consultants include:

- Professional organizations for the particular type of consultant (e.g., accounting professionals for accounting, computer specialists for computer) and level of consultant (e.g., national, state, or local)
- Professional organizations within the executive nurse's technical or manage-

ment field (e.g., hospital associations, medical associations, at the national, state, or local levels)

- A business with a well-respected department of the type of consultant needed (e.g., the marketing department for a marketing consultant); professionals within a department usually know of consultants within their own field

- Universities, colleges, and technical colleges

- Chambers of commerce, offices of economic development, or other similar business groups

- Professional consulting organizations

After the recruiting efforts yield the names of consultants who appear to have the skills and competencies designated for the project, the selection team interviews the consultants using standardized interview questions prepared by the screening team (assuming it is a team approach). The interviews are conducted by the selection team to obtain a sample of the consultant's style—in terms of responding to questions, dialoguing, and listening. The following section includes general questions that can be adapted or expanded upon for any selection team's interviewing process.

Areas of Concern
There are many questions to ask a consultant who is under consideration. These questions vary with the situation and need. The following is a sample interview agenda compiled by a consultant from the experiences of being interviewed by numerous organizations.

1. Before asking questions, inform the consultant what created the need, what the needs are, and what has already been tried, as well as what areas need help. The only exception to this is if a consultant is being hired to determine what the problem is. In this case, the current situation is described for the consultant to respond to in terms of direction that might be recommended.

2. Develop and ask questions to determine if the consultant understands the implications of the need explained by the selection team.

3. Develop a situation, including the people the consultant would be working with, and present a scenario to the consultant. Have the consultant sit down with the designated group and work through an issue during the interview process. Observe the consultant's interactions with the staff. Debrief staff at a later time (without the consultant present) to discover their perceptions.

4. Ask how the consultant would work with the executive nurse and/or staff. Share the executive nurse/staff's perception with the consultant to assess if the consultant's perceptions of the needs, project, and approach mesh.

5. In asking a consultant to share a proposal, request that the following questions be addressed:
   - What are the outcomes?
   - What does the implementation process look like?
   - What does it mean in terms of time, dollars, and other resources?

6. Get to know the consultant.

   - Discuss past and present projects in terms of successes and failures.

   - What was the reason for failure or success?

   - Has the consultant ever been terminated from a contract? (Most good ones have.) Why?

7. Ask for concrete results with the type of clients and projects the consultant has served.

8. Toward the end of the interview, after sharing your situation with the consultant, ask for the consultant's assessment of the project and the critical steps the team may have missed or been unaware of.

9. Ask the consultant how to get the appropriate people on staff to accept what she is proposing.

10. Ask the consultant:

    - How do you see the project beginning?

    - How will you know when it is time for you to exit?

    - How will you prepare us for the exit?

    - Will there be certain skills you will teach us? What are these skills?

11. What are the tie-ins for sustaining the change created by the consultant, so that the results will last after the consultant leaves? In other words, what is the consultant going to do to ensure that you do not become consultant-dependent?

The executive nurse, her staff, and whoever else is working to hire the consultant should develop a list of questions to ask of the consultant's references and clients, so that the process is standardized and the comments from references can be compared. Interviewing the consultant's clients is as important as interviewing the consultant. Conversations with the consultant's references assist in confirming the consultant's effectiveness.

References, Proposal, and Presentation
Screening for a consultant can become an expensive activity in terms of time, based on the number of people involved in the process. Reading proposals is extremely time consuming. Developing a proposal is expensive for a consultant. To save everyone time, after identifying several consultants who appear to have the necessary credentials, contact their references and use the data to help narrow the field. When asking a particular consultant for a proposal, the selection team should be feeling very confident about that consultant; the team should not request numerous proposals. At the proposal stage, consultants should be narrowed down to two or three.

Key Aspects of the Proposal
When requesting a proposal, it is important to specify the criteria needed to make a final decision. However, if the criteria are specified without a requested format, the team has an opportunity to assess the consultant's organization, attention to detail, knowledge base, and ability to communicate in writing. These critical skills will be necessary during the project.

Beyond the obvious review of the proposal in terms of its general appearance and content, reasons for this process include:

- Note the timeliness in which the proposal's deadline was met. Did the consultant meet the required time lines?

- Did the candidate make additional contacts to gather and collect pertinent information or did the proposal develop only from the interview data?

- Does the process look and sound reasonable? Is it spelled out specifically enough?

- Are there additional people who might be helping her? Does the client have a say in terms of who comes in and who does not? (For example, many consulting firms will bring in a more experienced consultant to land the sale. The person who actually consults may be a junior consultant with only two or three years' experience.)

The selection team should be certain there is a clear understanding in the proposal of who is going to be doing what action (the consultant, staff, or executive nurse). If additional consultants are coming in to assist, how will this occur? If additional consultants are going to be brought in, their resumes should be included in the proposal's appendix so there is familiarity with the entire team of consultants. Support consultants may be requested to attend the interview even if it is not certain they will be used during the project. This enables the team to become familiar enough with them to assess their effectiveness—not after one consultant is hired, and others are needed.

The proposal should contain a cost summary that outlines both costs of the stages and the overall proposal. No proposal, no matter what it is for, should be an open-ended type of commitment with a surprise dollar amount. If the project is so creative that it is difficult to calculate the dollar amount, various stages and monetary caps should be set. As the work progresses, there are checkpoints where assessment of the project and mutual agreement about how to proceed occur, so the client maintains control over the process, results, and cost.

A professional consultant rarely mails a proposal; generally there is a request to present it in person at a specified date and time. If the candidate does not request a presentation, the selection team should. It is critical to observe the style and manner in which the consultant presents materials and interacts with the selection team. This process provides an indication of how the consultant will function within the organization.

Finally, once the consultant is selected, a written contract is developed and signed. Consulting work should never be done on a handshake. Everyone involved in the project must begin with the same understanding and perceptions of roles, events, purpose, and outcomes.

Consulting is a professional business function and a contract should address the following:

- Purpose
- Desired outcomes
- Responsibilities

- What is being agreed upon

- The phases and stages of the project

- The cost

- How the invoicing is going to occur (retainer, hourly, project)

- Whether there is a commitment fee and, if so, whether that fee is going to be applied to the overall invoicing, or whether it is above and beyond the costs (a commitment fee is similar to a deposit)

- How the hourly rates are designated in terms of consultants (for example, a hospital hired a consultant at $150 an hour for two weeks; however, four consultants an hour were brought in, and the total invoicing for each day was $4,800!)

In addition, the use and cost of any extra materials (e.g., videos, manuals) should be outlined. Are they included in the cost? Is the consultant working on a daily rate that includes preparation and follow-up time, or are preparation and follow-up time additional? What constitutes a day rate, versus a seminar rate, versus a half-day? Is a seminar rate a flat rate, or is it dependent upon the number of participants? (For example, a seminar may be $2,400 for the day for 15 participants plus the $40 per participant over the limit of 15, or the seminar may be $2,400 for the day regardless of participants.) Is telephone time with the consultant invoiced?

As the contract is developed with the consultant, additional items should be agreed upon:

- What if a date has to be changed?

- What if there is a cancellation? Will there be a charge for the changed date, with or without sufficient notice?

- How are travel and meal expenses for the consultant handled? (Some charge a daily rate plus travel and meal expenses and, with long-distance consultants, a full-day charge may occur for a partial day.)

A contract assists the consulting relationship so that both parties are clear as to expectations and roles. This prevents conflicts from arising in the middle of the project that could be detrimental to its success.

CONSULTANT-CLIENT RELATIONSHIP

It is important to develop a solid relationship with the consultant selected. This begins with defining and clarifying the relationship between the consultant and executive nurse and/or staff involved in the project. The following are questions to clarify among the executive nurse/team and consultant:

- What is the purpose and mission of the project?

- Who is responsible for what?

- How is conflict resolved when it occurs?

- How are feedback and input gained?

- How are problems worked through?

- How does the project interface with other groups or individuals?
- How should the consultant interface with the executive nurse's supervisor and under what circumstances, if any?
- What are the needs of each member involved in the project ?
- What are additional ground rules for working together (e.g., scheduling, refreshments at meetings, consultant relationships with others outside the project)?

Fostering Rapport

It is important to set parameters and guidelines within the consultant-client relationship. Without guidelines, a consultant may overstep the authority of the executive nurse. In human-resource circles, there is a story of a human-resource director who hired an external consultant. The human-resource director gave the consultant a broad overview of what was needed and left him alone. The human-resource director never had time to meet with the consultant during the project. Several months later, the human-resource director was terminated and the consultant became the new human-resource director! This was obviously not the human-resource director's desired outcome.

Consultants are usually not after anyone's job. However, if a consultant's project is not managed by the executive nurse to demonstrate her or his leadership and command of the situation, it may be perceived as a weakness, and the project may veer off course.

Clear direction, paired with effort in establishing genuine rapport with the consultant, provides a winning combination for success. The more time the executive nurse or staff spends in developing a relationship with the consultant, the stronger the foundation is for working together.

In establishing rapport, the executive nurse should think about including consultants at staff parties, sending them a thank-you note, or taking them out to lunch occasionally. This effort assists in developing a committed relationship. Consultants are like any other supplier—the more the consultant feels part of the organization, the more commitment and loyalty will develop. Commitment and loyalty breed increased effort, which results in better service.

Ongoing Assessment

It is important for the executive nurse to set down parameters, guidelines, and periodic feedback sessions with the consultant; this enables the consultant to report on activities, give views on progress, and share perceptions of what is needed in the future. There should be a time schedule of events in place so that the executive nurse knows what is occurring on a timely basis. The executive nurse should also share perceptions of the project and views on the progress. If discrepancies exist between the perceptions of the consultant and the executive nurse, they need to be analyzed and resolved at these meetings.

In addition to these periodic feedback sessions, the consultant's performance and end results should be assessed by the executive nurse or team to evaluate success and to justify costs. This should not be left until the end of the project; rather, the project should be periodically reviewed in terms of short-term results at various stages. This gives both the executive nurse and the consultant opportunity to make changes if results are not occurring to ensure future success.

Consultant Introduction to the Organization

The consultant's introduction into the organization begins with sharing information on the organizational structure, the employees, and the persons in the key positions with whom she will be working. If any employee has negative feelings toward the project or the consultant, this should be discussed openly so that a strategy can be agreed upon as to how to work with, or around, that particular individual.

The executive nurse or team should be quite familiar with the consultant by this point; however, a short welcoming meeting on the first scheduled day would be appropriate. In addition, those persons affected indirectly by the consultant should be briefed on the project and given an opportunity to meet within the first few days or weeks. Depending on how widespread the work of the consultant is, staff meetings at various levels of the organization may be effective in communicating to employees the role of the consultant and the project. A hospital newsletter may be an effective vehicle to explain who the new face is and what the consultant's role will be.

Those employees most involved in the project should hear a very strong message of support for the project and consultant from the executive nurse. A consultant's success is nurtured by the strong backing of management. Although a consultant must establish rapport with employees, visible support of management helps foster this rapport more rapidly.

In conclusion, it is important to develop a consultant-client relationship that is based on a clear understanding of the mission of the project, the parameters, and the ground rules, in an open atmosphere based on trust. The executive nurse should initiate routine feedback periodic reviews to assess progress, direction, and outcomes. Fostering rapport with the consultant by establishing a genuine relationship is a critical foundation for that open, honest relationship based on trust. The executive nurse, in introducing the consultant to the organization, must evidence strong support of the consultant and the project. This message must be continually reinforced in the relationship with the consultant, so that others will be inspired to follow.

Summary

The use of a consultant can be a helpful tool for an executive nurse in all health care settings. Having the experience of working with a consultant can develop into a relationship of either friend or foe. If the executive nurse approaches the use of a consultant as a process, there is much more likelihood of success.

Before hiring a consultant, the executive nurse determines if a consultant is necessary and, if so, whether there is a need for an external consultant, an internal consultant, or both. There are certain situations that warrant an external consultant; in others, an internal consultant will be the better choice.

The second phase of the process is the actual selection. When searching for a consultant, the executive nurse should be aware that there are many types of consultants. It is important to check backgrounds and credentials to determine the skills, competencies, approach, and focus of the consultant. The selection process should be outlined so that there is a match between the consultant and the identified needs. To make an effective selection, the proposal, presentation, backgrounds, and credentials of consultants should be analyzed. Once a consultant is selected, a written contract with the consultant should be developed.

The third phase, after the consultant is selected, involves establishing the consultant-client relationship. To work most effectively with a consultant, the executive nurse should spend time developing an open, honest, candid relationship. Parameters, guidelines, and ground rules are set. Consistent, periodic feedback reviews should be scheduled so that the consultant and executive nurse can share perceptions of the project's progress to keep the project on course. Assessment of the consultant's performance and end results should be determined at the outset of the project.

Following the process and guidelines outlined will assist the executive nurse in working with a consultant and help make the experience both effective and rewarding. The consulting process can actually strengthen the executive nurse's leadership skills, which will transfer into her dealings with other professionals and colleagues. Since this process is similar to a typical problem-solving process (identifying the problem, defining the causes, generating solutions, developing an action plan, assessing and monitoring the plan, making adjustments as needed, and standardizing the results), continued implementation of the consulting process can sharpen the executive nurse's skills in each of the problem-solving areas. In addition, working with a consultant and picking up leadership, change agentry, and technical skills can be an education in itself.

Discussion Questions

1. Identify specific situations, or one area, for improvement in your health care setting that would benefit from the assistance of an internal or external consultant.

2. How would you introduce an external consultant to the organization?

Reference

Covey, S. R. (1989). *The seven habits of highly effective people.* New York: Simon & Schuster.

Kathleeen M. Driscoll
Julie M. Brightwell

CHAPTER 13

Legal and Ethical Issues

Introduction

This chapter explores the legal and ethical concerns of executive nurses in the changing health care system. First, the chapter presents frameworks that executive nurses can use as a foundation for raising legal and ethical concerns. Second, the chapter examines actual and potential competing legal and ethical perspectives in the highlighted areas of the above executive nurse concerns.

Throughout, the chapter suggests a three-pronged executive nurse/nurse manager/staff approach to dealing with these areas of concern. First, executive, management, and staff must educate themselves about the economic, sociopolitical, and cultural forces driving ongoing and prospective health care change. Second, management and staff should discuss the possibilities for nursing's contributions to health care. From that discussion they should arrive at a shared vision of nursing's role that can guide nursing practice. Organizations and society will remain in constant flux, creating a need for reconfigured visions and new responses; thus, omnipresent change dictates the third prong to be maintenance of continuing dialogue.

OVERVIEW OF LAW AND ETHICS

In the sea of economic, sociopolitical, and cultural change, what is the role of law and ethics? Both draw attention to values. Law formally embodies the recognized values of a society. Law focuses on ordering relationships in society. Ethics asks under what framework those relationships are rightly ordered. Ethics strives systematically to reconcile conflicting values so that what *ought* to be done in any situation can be determined. Schemas for analyzing situations from an ethical perspective emphasize recognition of all parties related to a concern. Existing law can be in conflict with, or reflective of, various approaches to resolution of ethical dilemmas.

Law

In today's populous, technologically complex, and socially stratified U.S. society, health care law attempts to order relationships among providers, consumers, and payers. Existing laws affecting these relationships are today's health care policy; issues related to laws affecting health care law that are discussed today become tomorrow's health care policy. Today, a concern is the extent to which antitrust law influences the nature and scope of relationships among hospitals, other health care facilities, and provider groups. Evolving case law and Department of Justice stance on pursuit of antitrust suits will affect future policy.

For executive nurses, this area of health care law has potential for affecting the scope of their management responsibility. Executive nurses will be responsible for nursing and other consumer care services across formerly separate institutions. Formerly acute-care settings will vertically integrate nursing and other patient care services across a continuum of care. Primary care, home health, and long-term care facilities will legally relate through merger, affiliation, or payer. Antitrust law will permit large market share, but not monopolies. More familiar areas of law will continue to receive emphasis in health care.

Types of Law

Statutory, Case, and Administrative Law
Statutory law, case law, and administrative law are the three *sources* of law. They do not stand alone. They relate to each other. Congress generates federal statutory law; state legislatures generate state statutory law; courts are the source of case law. Negligence law is an example. The legal elements that must be demonstrated for a finding of negligence derive from case law. Executive agencies of the federal and state government develop regulations that are the source of administrative law. Counties and cities create laws depending on the degree of home rule provided for by the state. A no-smoking ordinance may be a local law.

Civil and Criminal Law
Law divides additionally into civil and criminal law. Nurses and other health care providers have potential for involvement with both. Acting fraudently in seeking reimbursement can involve both levels. Civil law achieves redress through payment of damages. Criminal law achieves redress through deprivation of liberty by imprisonment or probation.

Substantive and Procedural Law
Law also divides into substantive and procedural law. Substantive law addresses the area of the law under which controversy between/among provider, consumer, or payer should proceed. For example, is the question a matter of tort or a matter of contract law? Negligence, a form of tort law, asks whether the duty of care was breached and whether harm resulted from the breach. Was the medication error

the source of harm to the consumer? In a dispute under contract law, a question might be whether or not a duty was carried out. Did the third-party payer fulfill its responsibility to pay the provider under the terms of its contract with the consumer?

Procedural law establishes the rules for legal argument. These include the proper court in which to bring the case, time frames for bringing suit, and what evidence may be presented.

Ethics

Ethics asks what relationships among providers, consumers, and payers achieves good. Executive nurses recognize a dilemma when they ask whether discharge of the consumer from an acute-care facility is in the consumer's best interest. Early discharge reduces the opportunity for acquisition of a nosocomial infection. But is the likelihood of wound infection equally present if the consumer remains weak and has no personal or financial support system to provide for dressing changes at home? What about access to an adequate diet to ward off infection?

A research study might answer this dilemma. Thus, the dilemma could be clinical rather than ethical in nature. Equal likelihood of infection makes either choice a good choice. Lesser risk in either situation argues for choosing that alternative.

Changing the facts slightly makes the situation an ethical dilemma. Now the consumer wants to leave the acute-care facility against medical advice. Short of forcible restraint, which would violate the law, what nursing administration effort is sufficient to convince the consumer to stay? A conflict arises of consumer right versus provider duty. The nurse may be less persuasive regarding continuing stay if the consumer is well educated. The nurse may assume that person can manage self-care at home. The nurse may be more persuasive with a consumer from a lower socioeconomic group who has less education. Even though the nurse meets the legal standard of a reasonable, prudent nurse's response to the consumer, will the nurse be comfortable with the words chosen? Chances are the nurse will not be comfortable.

Why? Because, provider beneficence is in conflict with consumer autonomy. Put differently, provider duty conflicts with consumer right. There seems no clear course that will serve as a consistent intervention for all consumers.

Ethical Decision Making

In the consumer-provider-payer triad, and with nurse managers and staff, the executive nurse meets constant ethical decision-making challenges. How might the executive nurse conceptualize ethical decision making? Five approaches can serve as categories. These approaches are duty-oriented, rights-oriented, goal-oriented, case-oriented, and principle-oriented.

Duty-Oriented Approach
A duty-oriented approach assumes certain duties. In the above scenario the duty-oriented nurse might use equally persuasive language with all consumers. But nurses might differ with respect to the value of continued stay and the influence of education on capability for self-care. Thus, the problem with a duty-oriented

approach is difficulty in achieving agreement on values. Lack of agreement precludes similar actions by all nurses.

Rights-Oriented Approach

Using a rights-oriented approach and viewing the right as belonging to the nurse, the nurse might even argue a right to interfere with consumer decision making that extends to physical restraint. Rights *ranking* is the problem with the rights-oriented approach. In the illustration, the right of the nurse to provide care conflicts with the right of the consumer to refuse care. Which of the two rights should rank higher?

Goal-Oriented Approach

Goal-oriented frameworks select rights and duties of providers and consumers based on whatever maximizes happiness. Here happiness occurs with the choice that creates the greatest good in a society. In the example, the agreed-upon goal may be the consumer's health. But provider or consumer rights would suffer, depending on the whose right prevails—consumer or nurse. Overriding of rights is thus the problem with the goal-oriented approach.

Case-Oriented Approach

A case-oriented (casuist, intuitionist, or relativistic approach) looks at the particular provider and consumer situation. Goals, rights, and duties may be ignored because there is no set framework to follow. The consumer could experience various nurse responses to the desire to leave the facility.

Principle-Oriented Approach

The principle-oriented approach examines ethical dilemmas for health care providers, using generally recognized ethical principles. These include beneficence, nonmaleficence, autonomy, justice, fidelity, veracity, and confidentiality. Ethical dilemmas can be viewed as conflicts among the principles. In the earlier scenario, autonomy conflicts with beneficence. Fidelity—keeping a professional commitment to care—might also be viewed as in conflict with consumer autonomy. None of the approaches fully meets the characteristics of consistency, coherence, and comprehensiveness required by an ethical theory. So, like other disciplines, ethics struggles to agree on theory. There is agreement, however, that ethical dilemmas should be systematically addressed. Any framework for decision-making includes several steps. Problem identification, players, options, ethical theories, law, shared decision making, resolution, and action is one model of these steps. There is general agreement that shared decision-making among providers and consumers is the best approach. Payers should not be exempt from the process.

SOCIETAL HEALTH CARE NEEDS

Executive nurses need to be conscious of both their ethical and legal professional responsibilities as they participate in decision making regarding the consumer market their facility will target. Vulnerable to being overlooked in an increasingly competition-oriented health care market are members of low socioeconomic groups and persons requiring high-cost care.

Two statements of the *American Nurses' Association Code for Nurses* are relevant. The first statement directs that "The nurse provides services with respect for human dignity and the uniqueness of the client unrestricted by consideration of social or economic status, personal attributes, or the nature of the health problems" (ANA Code for Nurses with Interpretive Statements, 1985). The last statement of the Code obligates that the nurse ". . . works with members of the health professions and other citizens in promoting community and national efforts to meet the health needs of the public."

Curiously, physicians are not similarly obligated. The *American Medical Association Principles of Medical Ethics* permits physicians to choose whom to serve except in cases of emergency. This leaves the nurse administrator in the role of consumer advocate. The role of advocate is not enviable, because assuming advocacy pits executive nurses against traditionally more powerful groups like physicians, hospital administrators, and payers.

In the 1993–1994 battle for health care reform, nursing earned professional recognition from Congress for its efforts. Nursing's message to politicians focused on wellness and preventive care, increasing access to primary care, and outcome measurement. Congress balked at the Clinton plan and all alternatives when none balanced public and private responsibility in a proportion to satisfy a congressional majority.

The American cultural fear of government involvement in industry has deep roots. The Founding Fathers based the Constitution on a set of values that included government restraint in private affairs. Although the late 1960s Great Society laws welcomed government as payer in the Medicare and Medicaid programs, current dissatisfaction with the increasing cost of these programs has created a more traditional political climate chary of government as payer. Health care is once more regarded as a private-sector affair.

Of congressional proposals for health care reform, none sufficiently balanced the self-interest needs of the more powerful professional and political players. Increasingly powerful in the health care lobby are the insurance companies, who act as both provider and payer of care. Immune from even state reform efforts are self-insured companies, protected from any government encroachment on their health care plans through the 1974 Employee Retirement Income Security Act (ERISA).

The aftermath of this stalemate is increasing requests for state Medicaid reform waivers. Many of those efforts are aimed at bringing managed care to this population. However, even approved waivers are currently on hold as Congress wrestles with Medicaid reform as part of fiscal year 1996 budget-reduction efforts (GAO, 1995). Furthermore, despite widespread belief that managed care will reduce health care costs, the jury is still out on the cost-effectiveness of this approach (GAO, 1993).

How then does the newfound professional reputation of nursing, as champions of access to care, wellness and prevention programs, and outcome measures, link to ethical responsibilities of executive nurses? There is opportunity for entrepreneurship to fill gaps in access, attend to wellness and prevention, and develop outcome measures. Executive nurses can promote development of contracts to staff managed-care systems' wellness and prevention programs. Opportunities are not confined to executive nurses based in hospital settings. Deans of academic institutions can develop contacts with staff wellness and prevention programs while concurrently providing experiences for their students. Public hospitals formerly meeting the needs of populations vulnerable because of their low socioeconomic status through clinics have the opportunity to transfer their skill to managed-care settings serving this population. Measurable outcomes for wellness and prevention programs include increasing positive health behaviors. Outcomes for managing chronic illness includes impacting consumer behaviors to reduce the rate of complications.

While the nation continues to struggle with creating a more systematic health care system, executive nurses have an opportunity to assume leadership. Executive nurses have the opportunity to create legal arrangements for delivery of care that are ethically accountable with respect to the goals of society and the rights and duties of consumers, nurses, and other providers of care. An outcome orientation has the potential for adding value to society's health.

REDESIGNING NURSING CARE DELIVERY

Payers expect economic value for their investment in health care. This goal is achievable when structure and process yield satisfactory outcomes of care. But producing outcomes laden with ethical values that are within the law is central to the success of the current redesign of nursing care delivery.

Although cycles of reorganization in nursing management are a frequent occurrence, reorganization of nursing care delivery has historically occurred only at longer intervals. From the 1960s through the mid-1970s, team nursing was the method of patient care delivery. The late 1970s and 1980s saw a transition to primary nursing. Primary nursing put the registered nurse totally in charge of the patient. The nurse carried out every patient care activity from personal hygiene to titrating dosages of narrow therapeutic range medications. In many geographic areas, all-RN staffs became the norm. During this period, delegation received only passing reference in nursing education. Any discussion of the notion of teamwork has been limited. Physicians and other providers, nurse, and patient have been the focus triad. Other potential team members have not been viewed as essential to consumer care.

Both these modes of delivery had shortcomings. With team nursing, the focus of care tended to be tasks. In primary nursing, the nurse at the bedside did *all* care. But if nurses do all the care, what is the role of the professional nurse?

Once again in the 1990s nurse administrators find themselves in the throes of nursing care delivery change. This time, unlike team nursing, the focus of care is on consumer, not task. This time, unlike primary nursing, the role of the professional nurse is clear. He or she no longer provides all care, but is responsible for using nursing judgment to determine the level of nursing-care provider the consumer needs. The ability to delegate care appropriately becomes a prerequisite for the professional practice of nursing.

While change is always disruptive, maintaining a steady course through the implementation and evaluation phases of this cycle seems especially challenging. One barrier to smooth sailing is the almost 15 years of nursing graduates raised in the primary-care mode. Furthermore, for all nurses practicing in acute-care settings, primary care has become the accustomed approach. Certainly no one ever thought of cross-training the water boy to become a linebacker.

Societal influences drive the development of professions. The driving force in health care delivery is cost control. This economic force, and arguably nurses' sociological status as employees, has directly affected the 1990's changes in nursing care delivery. New configurations of personnel demand that new professional conceptual models emerge and be integrated in the individual's professional self-image. For the profession and the individual nurse, that revised sense of self must be satisfying in both a legal and ethical sense. Nurses must be comfortable with delegation of nursing care and still maintain their unique place among the health profession disciplines.

What legal and ethical questions must be raised and addressed to develop that revised sense of professional self? Executive nurses need to create administrative climates where staff and administration can, without fear of loss of job, begin to address these questions. They include the following:

- Does the legal duty of care (the standard of care) match the ethical duty of care?

- Is the consumer more at risk for an adverse outcome with a change in the mode of delivery of nursing care?

- What is the relationship of nursing care delivery system change to licensing laws?

There are not now, and probably never will be, definitive answers to these questions. But, they must be addressed.

The Standard of Care

What, exactly, is the standard of care for nurses? First, it is not a singular concept. The question really is, what is the standard of care in a particular situation? Stated another way, the standard of care is the duty of a nurse to provide care that an ordinary reasonable, prudent nurse of similar education and experience would provide in a similar situation. Implied in this standard is the nurse's obligation to avoid reasonably foreseeable risks to consumers of care. *In this changing nursing care delivery system, meeting the standard of care means the nurse is accountable for delegating care reasonably and with prudence so that the consumer can rely on continuing to receive safe care.*

For nurses whose total professional experience has been in primary nursing, this responsibility will seem weighty. The nurse must know the education and experience of the team members. The executive nurse must oversee the development of policy that assures this information about team members is available. In malpractice litigation, the standard of care for delegation will be at issue not only for the individual nurse but also for the executive nurse with respect to guidelines for delegation in the nursing delivery system. Health care case law early on established this corporate responsibility (Darling v. Charleston Memorial Hospital, 1965).

Staff Education and Evaluation

Redesigns of nursing care delivery that increase delegation call for education of staff. Education, however, is necessary but insufficient to making change. Evaluation of the effectiveness of the educational process as it transfers to safe practice is critical.

If a nursing system permits nursing staff to delegate observation of consumer response to care, the delegee must know when to consult with the nurse and when to take personal action.

Scenario 13.1	**Housekeeper or Nurse?**

Housekeeping staff are on the patient care team. Part of their job description includes meeting consumer requests for care. The consumer complains of chilling. The housekeeper obtains an extra blanket for the consumer and does not report the request. Actually the consumer is receiving a blood transfusion and experiencing an adverse reaction.

What education would the housekeeper and nursing staff need to receive to avoid this well-meaning but potentially adverse response to the consumer's concern? Clearly, where a housekeeper is cross-trained to provide assistance to consumers, parameters of practice for such unlicensed assistive personnel (UAPs) need to be set. In this instance the housekeeper needs to know that all consumer concerns must be reported to the nurse. Judgment calls about the cause of the chilling belong to nurses. Lack of knowledge may have triggered this adverse event. Personal counseling with the housekeeper will be helpful, but change in the content of the educational programs socializing both housekeepers and staff to the changed delivery system is also in order. The situation has triggered program evaluation; legal accountability calls for this revision.

At the same time, creation of a truly team-oriented approach to consumer care means the information provided by the housekeeper must be valued. Valuing the housekeeper's input includes valuing that person's speculation about the cause of the chilling. For example, the housekeeper might report chilling occurred after the consumer complained of feeling nauseous and the housekeeper wonders if the person is experiencing an infection resulting from drinking a fast-food shake that a relative brought.

Even though a reasonable prudent nurse would still stop the blood transfusion, the housekeeper's input offers an alternative explanation, should tests show the blood transfusion compatible. Respect for the person in this scenario, the housekeeper, by valuing her contribution to the team, demonstrates ethical accountability of nursing staff.

Adverse Outcomes

Because nurses have brought their concerns about use of UAPs to Congress, state legislatures, local governing bodies, and the public through mass media coverage, adverse events involving UAPs will be closely scrutinized (Himali, 1995). While zero risk of an adverse event is impossible to achieve, three risk-reduction measures are imperative. These are alluded to under the discussion of standard of care but deserve reiteration. First, there must be clear job descriptions; second, there must be training programs highly specific in their content; and third, there must be ongoing evaluation of both.

Executive nurses are ultimately responsible for making prudent choices about the care that can be delegated to UAPs. Insuring that those decisions are prudent occurs best when staff, executive nurses, and nurse managers have input into the design of the job description and the education programs for nursing staff and UAPs. The job description should include UAP task responsibility. Relationships with nursing staff are also a key component of the job description. Conversely, nursing staff require a job description that outlines their responsibilities for care and their relationship with UAPs. Records of content and nursing and UAP staff attendance will be sought by plaintiff attorneys in lawsuits where delegation is an issue.

Education programs for UAPs must be carefully developed to reflect content necessary to assist nursing staff. Models from long-term care are a good beginning. In acute-care settings, however, UAPs will have to have some understanding of high-tech equipment as well as the ability to meet basic needs such as mobility, rest, and nutrition.

The pool of persons identified as the source of UAPs may be a source of risk. Persons who have never worked in health care, and persons without high-school diplomas, differ in their learning foundation from RNs, LPNs, and perhaps other health care workers who were displaced from their positions and seek the UAP role as an avenue for staying in health care. These differences suggest creation of various curricula depending on foundational knowledge. Level of RN education is one of the explanatory variables suggested for examination in the American Nurses Association proposed report card for acute-care settings (American Nurses Association [ANA], 1995). Level of education of UAPs also needs to be examined.

Change in nursing care delivery should be considered a continuous process rather than a one-time bend in the road. The bend may be too sharp and need straightening. Hence, raising education and experience requirements may be dictated by an evaluation process. Revising job description and training programs may also be suggested. A one-time review is not sufficient. An annual schedule of review is a reasonable standard for an executive nurse to set. Executive nurses have a responsibility to keep abreast of research, examining not only preparation issues but all questions relating to use of unlicensed assistive personnel.

An interesting legal question is raised when RNs and LPNs find themselves in UAP positions. Are they held to the standard of care for RNs and LPNs or to the standard of care for UAPs? The answer is arguably yes for RNs if the RN has experience comparable to the delegating nurse. The answer may be no if more weight is given to consideration of the UAP role the RN is now occupying. A variation of the question occurs when the RN is a recent graduate who has passed state boards but is unable to obtain a registered-nurse position (the experience is missing but the credential is present).

Change and Adverse Outcomes

Based on the preceding question, should executive nurses limit the pool of UAP applicants? Probably not in this initial period of change. Should they examine the outcomes of care considering variation in educational background of UAPs? Certainly, yes. What outcomes of care are appropriate to address? One would be the number of adverse events that occur in the inpatient setting and across settings where care occurs in a vertically integrated system. Studies using valid and reliable measures permit comparison of adverse events only when the only variable is change in nursing care delivery. A concurrent introduction of a program emphasizing risk management would bias results. A second outcome would be functional outcomes across the continuum of care. Are they better or worse after introduction of a changed nursing-care delivery system?

Measuring outcomes is an infant area of health services research. The Lewin-VHI report to the ANA (and summarized by the ANA) looked at structure, process, and outcome indicators of nursing quality. The evaluators found lack of data to support many of the indicators. Additionally, the evaluators noted the indicators lacked specificity to nursing (American Nurses Association [ANA], 1995).

Ordinary reasonable, prudent executive nurses will want skilled researchers on board their management team who can design, carry out, analyze, and report outcome data to the professional and public communities. Who intervenes and what differences occur must be known. In addition to nursing personnel other providers make a difference in outcome. The total configuration of providers must be examined to know what makes a fiscal and consumer outcome difference in a given set of consumer circumstances. Society needs to know, and will ask, what percent of variability in these outcomes is accounted for by each provider's contribution to care. Because all providers will function in a number of care communities (e. g., acute care, home care, long-term care, rehabilitative care, schools, community centers), the interventions associated with positive changes will need to occur within and among these care communities. Payers will examine outcomes within and across care communities and pay only for those outcomes that are cost effective.

Cost of care has driven the choice to redesign care. Another change in the care team may be necessary to achieve both cost reduction and optimal outcomes. When lawsuits occur, attorneys will be quick to ask whether a different configuration of personnel would have avoided an adverse outcome.

Licensure

When state legislatures enact licensing laws, boundaries are set on a field of human service. The concept of licensure is distinct from that of registration, professional recognition that comes from completing a state-recognized educational program preparing a person for a field of human service. **Registration**, often called *permissive licensure*, was nursing's first form of government recognition. Licensure, as closing boundaries on a field of practice, developed in nursing with the advent of practical-nurse programs. Registered nursing required differentiation from practical nursing if both were to be licensed areas of practice within the profession of nursing (Bullough, 1980).

Today the National Council of State Boards of Nursing takes the position that advanced nursing practice should also be a licensed area within the profession of nursing (1993). The American Nurses Association differs, preferring to recognize advanced nursing practice through specialty certification (1981). **Certification** is simply a process of professional recognition generally contingent upon educational prerequisites, defined areas of practice experience, and examination (Inglis & Kjervik, 1993). Licensed plumbers create plumbing systems and fix leaky pipes. Licensed cosmetologists are in the business of grooming people. Persons without licenses do the same. Licensed nurses deal with human responses to actual and potential health problems. Persons without licenses do the same. They include family members, who are generally exempted in practice acts from charges of practicing without a license. But arguably they also include teachers, priests and ministers, and persons responding to fire and police calls. The boundaries of nursing are not as clear as those of other professions.

Thus, nurses have a problem. Many definitions of nursing in licensure laws are broad-based—indeed, best characterized as ambiguous—and apply, at least in part, to a number of health and human service care providers. Thus nursing, in addition to carving up its own turf with various levels of licensure, has one of two problems. Either other providers are encroaching on nursing's turf or nursing is encroaching on other health care providers' turf. Examples are abundant. The nurse walks a consumer with a hip replacement down the hall. Is the nurse acting as a nurse assisting the consumer to respond with activity to the health problem? Or is the nurse acting as a physical therapist? Conversely, is the physical therapist acting as a nurse in assisting to increase the activity level of this consumer? These questions lead to one of two conclusions. Legally, nursing needs either to better define its sphere of practice or to enforce licensure as turf control. Otherwise, licensure in health care professions is simply a myth.

Perhaps, however, the ambiguity of nursing's definition in licensure laws is an advantage to the profession. Perhaps, instead of carving out turf, licensure for all health care workers ought to be conceived differently. First, the knowledge and skills of licensees ought to be directed to the roles they play in the care of the consumer, even though these may vary by setting. For example, the nurse may function in a co-ordinator or case-manager role in the delivery of home health care, while largely acting as assistant to the physician in a critical-care unit or in some nurse-practitioner positions. Neither case manager nor physician assistant role is unique to nursing.

Second, with respect to persons with actual health-care problems, the nurse should be the expert in identifying the consumer's management of the problem and, where positive responses to that problem are not existent, to assist the person to cope with that problem in the holistic sense. This perspective supports a sort of Venn-diagram view of health and human service care providers that has the consumer at the center and providers arranged around the edge. This Venn-diagram perspective allows the state to continue to recognize graduates of nursing programs by awarding them the privilege to practice nursing so long as they practice competently and conduct themselves in a manner to earn the public's trust. This same view permits flexible use of health care providers in care settings through not only responsible delegation of care but also sharing of care responsibilities among health care providers.

Unlike the Venn-diagram view, the profession of medicine still views itself as the delegator of any wellness or illness interventions to anyone (Hadley, 1989). Because nurses work so closely with physicians, nursing seems the profession most prone to have the capabilities of its practitioners not fully implemented because of arguments from medicine. This is particularly true in the areas of medical diagnosis and prescriptive authority. For the advanced-practice nurse, authority with respect to medical diagnoses and follow-up care for chronic illnesses (e. g., diabetes, hypertension) may range from dependency on protocols to independence across a full range of diagnoses. Prescriptive authority is different from state to state. In one state (Alaska), nurses are unhampered by formulary, protocol, or other professional board surveillance (Bertholf, 1986). In other states, nurses may prescribe only from formularies or for certain classifications of drugs, with prescriptive authority under the purview of the medical or pharmacy board. In these areas of nursing clinical specialty, crossovers to medicine are omnipresent and it is difficult to tell where nursing begins and medicine ends.

As health care moves toward acceptance of primary-care practitioners as gatekeepers to specialty services, nurses' primary-care roles will be partly dependent on existing practice acts. Major determinants of the sociopolitical climate for expansion will be the number of available physician primary-care practitioners, willingness of nurses to move to and serve disadvantaged populations, availability of reimbursement, and community acceptance of nurse primary-care providers. In the meantime, executive nurses need to assure that advanced-practice nurses, particularly those delivering primary care, practice within the scope of their state's law. Executive nurses should also work to develop a market for the unique aspects of nurses' contributions to health care in the areas of both health promotion and prevention and to enhance the capabilities of consumer and family to cope with illness.

The Venn-diagram perspective offers opportunity for uniqueness and delegation of care by each profession. Physicians can delegate diagnostic and prescriptive power to nurses. Professional nurses can delegate nursing care to technical nurses and licensed practical nurses.

Questions remain. Can physicians delegate nursing care to licensed practical nurses or can physicians only delegate strictly medical acts? Can a nurse practitioner delegate medical acts? Are nurses responsible for foreseeing the same potential harm that may come to a consumer as a physician when nurses are making diagnoses and writing prescriptions? Will liability accrue to a team of health care providers or continue to rest with the deep pockets of physicians and health care facilities? Executive nurses practice in an arena where professional awareness must include legal questions affecting scope of practice.

Risk Management Strategies

In today's climate of practice, every health care provider must be continually aware of risk management.

Societal and Professional   Licensure and certification may be regarded as necessary but insufficient as risk management strategies for executive nurses. Relevant continuing education on new technology and application of nursing research will continue to be essential risk management strategies. Not all states have mandatory continuing education, but continuing education remains professionally necessary to provide evidence that practice standards are current.

Institutional The nurse administrator needs to be aware of, and employ, risk management strategies in all settings. Risk management divides into four areas. First, identifying areas of risk includes determining areas of risk through a survey of departments and consumers. Second, estimating loss includes a review of past and current claims as well as risk potential to purchase insurance or self-insure against claims. Third, risk prevention includes sound policy and procedure development, hiring and developing qualified staff, and continuing to review incident reports to determine new or changing patterns of risk. Fourth, controlling risk occurs when damages for adverse events are kept to a minimum. Practices such as acknowledging when adverse events have occurred and offering to pay health care bills resulting from these events are examples of controlling risk.

CONSUMER AUTONOMY VERSUS PROVIDER OBLIGATION

Informed consent, use of life-sustaining measures, and assisted suicide have created ethical dilemmas and generated legal responses. Each presents an ethical dilemma because the "good" goal of the provider may conflict with the "good" goal of the consumer of care. In turn, this differentiates how provider and consumer view the rights and duties of each. From a principle-oriented perspective, the conflict is between parentalism and autonomy. Legally, autonomy has prevailed with informed consent and use of life-sustaining measures. Requirements for informed consent for invasive procedures and public policy encouraging use of advance directives represent the legal responses. Assisted suicide continues to create uneasiness in both legal and ethical arenas.

Consent

An early case addressing the concept of consent to care was the 1914 case of Schloendorff v. Society of New York Hospital. This New York Court of Appeals opinion noted the right of "every human being of adult years and sound mind . . . to determine what shall be done with his own body" and, in fact, extended the right to individuals no longer capable of expressing their wishes but who had previously done so. The case involved a surgical procedure where physicians extended their treatment beyond the scope of the person's consent. Informed-consent processes and advance directives are contemporary embodiment of this right to consent or refuse treatment.

The formal process of informed consent should be distinguished from the general consent to care. Routine noninvasive care may fall under general consents to treatment in health care facilities. Blood tests and routine care addressing elimination and mobility needs are examples of care falling under general consents. Can a person refuse this care at any time? Yes! Touching a person capable of decision-making who refuses ordinary care could constitute battery or unwanted touching. Ensuing litigation would complain of an intentional tort. Intentional actions are not covered by malpractice insurance. The facility, or person's, resources would be at risk in such litigation.

On the other hand, the formal process of informed consent involves explanation of *invasive* procedures, and the risks, benefits, and alternatives (including no treatment) to the procedure. Legal responsibility for obtaining consent rests with the physician. The nurse's legal role is generally limited to obtaining the person's signature on a consent form and signing the form as a witness to the person's signature. Preferred practice would assign even the witness responsibility to the physician, because the physician acting as witness to the person's signature can be evidence that both were together with opportunity to discuss the procedure.

What if the person raises questions about the procedure when a nurse seeks their signature on the consent form? For information not within the nurse's scope of practice, the nurse then has an ethical responsibility, and arguably also a legal responsibility, to alert the physician so the person gains the information required to make an informed consent.

There is another consent arena of concern to executive nurses. Researchers hold responsibility for obtaining the consent of their subjects. Executive nurses should assure that any research studies using their facility to obtain subjects have undergone review for consumer risk. For federally funded studies, this includes Institutional Review Board scrutiny by the sponsoring facility—either academic or health care. Executive nurses will also want a procedure for objective review of the research proposal for their facility conducted by a facility committee, nursing committee, or risk manager. Informed consent forms deserve particular examination. Forms should be simple so that every subject can understand their contents with respect to the risks and benefits of participation in the research.

What additional implications does the concept of consent have for the work of executive nurses? Both orientation and ongoing education of staff are relevant activities for the executive nurse to support. In most facilities, risk managers can assume the educator role in orientation. Beyond orientation, however, a wise executive will encourage unit staff discussion of resolution of concerns about consent. How was the situation handled when a postoperative consumer refused to walk? What information was necessary to resolve the consumer's concerns about the invasive procedure? What verbal and written communication techniques did the staff employ? Was the approach persuasive, that is, respectful of the rights of both person and staff? On the other hand, was it manipulative or coercive, that is, demeaning of the rights of the consumer? If there have been problems with a research study, was the investigator notified? Opportunity to debrief when such situations arise fosters staff professional growth.

Use of Life-Sustaining Measures

Use of life-sustaining measures raises complex ethical and legal questions. Executive nurses should be particularly sensitive to these because they touch the heart and soul of human existence and the nature of our society.

Legally, many statutes provide that advance directives be invoked only when persons no longer capable of decision making are also terminally ill. But what about the comatose quadriplegic whose wife and holder of his durable power of attorney states he wants the respirator discontinued even though there is the possibility of returning to a cognitive state? From an ethical perspective, this approach awards a higher level of personhood in terms of choice making to the cognitively capable (persons who are cognitively capable can refuse even beneficial treatment) and demeans the personhood of the incompetent person. This approach seems a departure from the rights orientation of the nation's culture. On the other hand, this approach can be viewed as consistent with the "death denying" bent of our culture that supports life until on nature's course there are no more forks in the road. Daniel Callahan (1987) has suggested we set limits on entitlements to use of these costly measures.

Ten years elapsed from Quinlan (1976) to Brophy (1986), in which courts have moved from withdrawal of respirators to withdrawal of nutrition. Ohio's durable power of attorney for health care statute required amending to permit withdrawal of feeding tubes for persons in persistent vegetative states (1991). The need to revise the statute reflects the ethical tension felt by the legislature. The statute permits withdrawal from persons in vegetative states (PVS) only after a year elapses following the precipitating event. This time frame is inconsistent with medical standards for making the PVS diagnosis. Again, persons incapable of decision making, even with a durable power of attorney, might be viewed as having a lower level of personhood in terms of choice making. Nurses also have difficulty with withdrawal of feeding tubes. Like the Ohio legislature, nurses' discomfort also stems from ethical tension.

From 1982 to 1986 the nation frequently saw legal updates in the media on the use of life-sustaining measures for infants. The Indiana Baby Doe case spawned the controversy. In that case, parents of an infant with Down syndrome and a tracheoesophageal fistula refused consent for the fistula's surgical repair. The Reagan administration was outraged. The controversy led to federal rules requiring posting notices in delivery, maternity, pediatric, and nursery units stating "Discriminatory failure to feed and care for handicapped infants in this facility is prohibited by federal law" (47 Federal Register 26,027, 1982). This rule, in turn, outraged the health provider community who viewed the rule as an indictment alleging provider lack of concern for handicapped infants. Following the Department of Health and Human Services' losing a number of legal battles on the rules, Congress passed a compromise amendment to the Child Abuse Prevention and Treatment Act. That legislation led to rules that define child abuse, with respect to withholding medically indicated treatment, as the failure to respond to the infant's life-threatening conditions by providing treatment (including appropriate nutrition, hydration, and medication) that in the treating physician or physicians' reasonable medical judgments will be most likely to be effective in ameliorating or correcting conditions (45 Code of Federal Regulations S 1340.15 (b) (2), 1985). Three categories of infants were exempted from the provisions. These included (a) infants who are chronically and irreversibly comatose; (b) infants when provision of treatment would merely prolong their dying, not be effective in ameliorating or correcting all life-threatening conditions, or otherwise be futile in terms of infant survival; or (c) infants for whom providing such treatment would be virtually futile in terms of survival and the treatment itself would be inhumane (45 Code of Federal Regulations S 1340.15 (b) (2) 1985). These provisions clearly obligate the treatment of very-low-birthweight infants except in situations where brain hemorrhage results in a chronic and irreversibly comatose state. While we are unable to pose a legal question, an ethical question can be raised. Given multiple adverse outcomes in many of these cases, are we ethically obligated to treat very-low-birthweight infants? Parents free to refuse even beneficial treatment for themselves are not free to refuse questionable treatment for infants. Further adding to the complexity of questions about low-birthweight infants is the lack of certainty in prognosis. In this situation no individual has autonomy in decision making. Society has chosen a totally parentalistic approach.

Assisted Suicide

Recurring front-page coverage of Dr. Jack Kevorkian's physician-assisted suicides has brought this legal and ethical issue to the nation's attention. Suicide is not proscribed by law. Assisted suicide, however, is a crime in most states, but not all. Michigan, Kevorkian's state of residence, lacked a statute. A statute passed later was found constitutional, thus making Kevorkian's continuation of assistance with suicides a violation of the law (Marzen, 1995). Assisted suicide is generally defined as an individual providing the means and guidance to take one's own life. The choice to die and conduct of the act of dying remains with the individual requesting assistance.

Individual health care providers have spoken in support of assisted suicide (Quill, 1991). Those against assisted suicide view participation as a violation of the role of healer. Participation would violate the professions' goal of healing as a societal good (Miller & Brody, 1995; Miles, 1995). Some have suggested resolving this conflict by creating a new profession of persons whose role is to assist with suicides. But would a referral to those persons constitute complicity in the event?

A *rights* perspective views assisted suicide as the ultimate exercise of the right of autonomy. A *duty* perspective views assisted suicide as the ultimate abrogation of the duty to leave the moment of death in the hands of a Supreme Power.

By referendum, Oregon developed legislation supporting assisted suicide that provides safeguards to assure the person requesting assistance has made a carefully considered decision. The person must be suffering from a terminal disease that will end in death within six months. The person must make three requests over a period of time, one in writing and witnessed, in order to put the process in motion. Oregon's law has been challenged and is currently under judicial review for constitutionality in Lee v. Oregon (Meisel, 1995).

Staff and Administrative Concerns

Consent concerns, use of life-sustaining measures, and the issue of assisted suicide place the executive nurse in the bioethics arena. Reproductive interventions, transplants, and soon-to-be more frequent genetic screening and treatment will be of concern. All are issues involving consumer autonomy versus provider obligations for care.

Executive nurses need to assure nurse involvement in the periodic evaluation of policies addressing use of life-sustaining measures. Nurses work closely with dying persons and are likely to be aware of circumstances that might warrant addressing in a policy. For example, in our evolving family culture, does the policy address the role of stepchildren in the decision-making process? Does the policy *need* to address this concern? Nurses might also provide input into resolution of conflict when families request futile treatment. From a goal-oriented ethical perspective, use of scarce or even available but costly resources violates many provider's commitment to cost-effective care.

An emerging concern in the delivery of home health services is the processing of "do not resuscitate" (DNR) orders. Home health personnel can find themselves in the position of calling paramedics for transport to care. When the client arrests while awaiting transport, paramedics view an obligation to resuscitate as their legal responsibility. State legislation will provide comfort to paramedics who view providing resuscitation under all circumstances as their legal obligation. Executive nurses responsible for delivery of home health care services can support legislation that provides for honoring consumer wishes. Agency policies need to be developed to assure that professional, support staff, and volunteers providing services in the home are aware of the client's DNR order.

Nurses exposed continually to death—particularly traumatic deaths and deaths of young persons—need to work in a climate that acknowledges and facilitates the nurse's own grief processes. Not only availability but also active support of grief counseling can be considered an ethical obligation of executive nurses. That obligation is consistent with support provided other human service workers such as firefighters and police.

Both consumers of care and nursing staff deserve access to facility bioethics committees for resolution of ethical concerns. A living will makes the consumer's wishes known. A durable power of attorney permits a designated person to speak for a person in relation to health care. Neither instrument, however, reduces the possibility of disagreement among family members regarding the person's care. When staff efforts fail to resolve conflict, committee access and input broadens the base and the objectivity of the resolution process. Furthermore, nurses executives might view themselves as having a professional ethical obligation to support nurse membership on bioethics committees under the ANA Code. Statement one speaks to respect for human dignity and uniqueness. Statement three speaks to safeguarding clients from unethical practice. Bioethical issues of the future will address genetic screening and genetic treatments. Knowledge of consumer responses to health problems places nurses in a prime position to contribute to ethics committees educational, policymaking, and conflict-resolution processes.

The nature of decision making in this bioethical arena deserves attention equal to clinical decision making. This equality dictates the executive nurse's obligation to keep abreast of bioethical concerns.

LABOR LAW: RESPONSIBILITY TO CONSUMERS AND STAFF

Ethical and legal responsibilities of executive nurses and nurse managers include safeguarding staff and consumer health and employee hiring and termination. Federal and state constitutional law, statutes, case law, and administrative law guide these processes.

Workers' Compensation

Workers' compensation laws provide both medical benefits and compensation for partial and total permanent disability and partial and total temporary disability. The disability must be caused by an illness or injury suffered in the workplace. For the worker, this system affords certain compensation when the causal relationship has been established. The implications for executive nurse response are several.

Policies and procedures requesting reports of needlesticks and other puncture or cutting wounds such as those occurring during surgical procedures should include immediate and subsequent testing for HIV and other bloodborne pathogens. Sound policy and procedure protects both staff and facility. Protection of staff occurs when a negative initial result turns positive. Compensation can then occur for AIDS-related illness. Protection of the facility occurs when a positive result initially indicates a source of infection other than work exposure.

Report and testing for needlesticks is important. Antecedent to reporting, however, is monitoring the use of protective apparel and equipment designed to prevent injury. Threshold levels for compliance need to be established just as for any other quality assurance/improvement indicator. Standards should be set based on both the literature and specific facility characteristics. Threshold levels below literature standards require justification; when reached they should be maintained or improved. In every instance, rationale for these judgments should be documented.

Other policies and procedures are similarly relevant in light of workers' compensation laws. Testing for tuberculosis protects against another biological threat to staff health and consumer safety. Physical and chemical threats to health also deserve attention. Back injuries are the most common work-related injury for nurses. Other injuries may derive from exposure both to radiologic and cytotoxic agents. In relation to handling cytotoxic agents, the Occupation Safety and Health Administration (OSHA) has invoked the "general-duty clause" to enforce use of protective measures. The agency's guidelines do not carry the force of law, but the general-duty clause can be applied when a health hazard is common knowledge in the industry.

Executive nurses have an economic interest in awareness of all workplace illness and injury. Early notification and intervention may permit prevention of permanently disabling consequences. Since awareness creates opportunities for risk-reduction efforts, escalating workers' compensation rates may be avoided. Successfully extending that awareness through nurse managers to staff is a necessary component of any risk-reduction effort.

Civil Rights Laws

The 1960s' Great Society programs included passage of historic civil-rights legislation. Title VII of the 1964 Civil Rights Act provides for equal employment opportunity on the basis of ethnicity, race, and gender. The 1978 Pregnancy Discrimination Act extended that protection to pregnant women. The Civil Rights Act proscribes discrimination that is evident on its face or has discriminatory impact except when that discrimination can be justified as a bona fide occupational qualification or business necessity.

Affirmative-action programs are active efforts to redress past injustices against members of minority groups. Publicly supported institutions, among them health care facilities receiving public funds, must have affirmative action programs. In the Supreme Court's 1994–1995 term, the Court in Adarand Constructors v. Pena added to existing constraints on preferential treatment based on race by requiring that programs of affirmative action serve a compelling state interest and be narrowly tailored to identifiable past discrimination. The decision came in the wake of rising nationwide resistance to the perceived requirements and costs of affirmative action. Racial minority groups are divided. Some support reduced emphasis on affirmative action because programs can generate the impression that racial minorities receive employment simply because of race, not because of qualifications. Those supporting continuation of programs suggest past injustices have not been sufficiently redressed to justify program curtailment. Executive nurses should seek legal guidance on the application of this decision to their hiring and dismissal actions.

In 1991 the Supreme Court examined discriminatory concerns with respect to protective health care measures (U.A.W. v. Johnson Controls). The Court found Johnson Controls' policy, of eliminating all fertile women from a workplace environment that would potentially expose them to high lead levels, overbroad in its provisions. Johnson Controls based its policy on potential hazard to the health of a fetus. The Court found company policy discriminatory because the policy did not extend to men despite evidence that male reproductive systems were also affected by exposure to lead.

Ethical fallout of the Johnson decision is double-edged. From a rights perspective, it clearly favors the woman's rights in employment over the health of the fetus. On the other hand, from a societal, goal-oriented perspective the same decision can be viewed as encouraging industry to increase levels of protection for all workers by enforcing the use of protective measures.

Enforcement of use of protective measures should alleviate concerns about risk of lawsuits. Workers may be unlikely to sue for damages to a child if protective measures are enforced. Although there was no history of such suits, this was precisely the scenario Johnson Controls sought to avoid with its discriminatory policy. Executive nurses should also be familiar with provisions of the Rehabilitation Act of 1973, which places affirmative obligations for employment of qualified handicapped persons where facilities receive federal funds. The 1990 Americans with Disabilities Act (ADA) extends that obligation to private employers with over 15 employees. Reasonable accommodation must be provided for disabled persons. The societal good to be achieved by both acts is employment of the disabled. A corollary to this public policy is reducing dependence of the disabled on public monies for health care and other welfare programs.

Executive nurses must make reasonable accommodations for disabled nurses. Alcoholism and AIDS are generally covered under the 1990 Act. Consultation with attorneys familiar with labor law should occur when considering accommodating the disabled nurse, as case law will inevitably provide further direction on the meaning of "reasonable accommodation."

Special Case: Alcohol and Drug Abuse

Six to twenty percent of nurses currently in practice are estimated to be chemically dependent on alcohol or another drug (Sullivan, Bissell & Williams, 1988). The professional future of the chemically dependent nurse is contingent on many factors, including the policy of the employing institution, the state's nurse practice act, and the involvement of the state's board of nursing and nurses' association (Lippman & Nagle, 1992). In the past, a nurse suspected of addiction may have been fired for reasons relating to poor job performance or poor attendance without addressing the true problem. A nurse with a proven addiction may have had the license permanently revoked. The firing and license revocation has been called the "throw-away nurse syndrome," and resulted in enormous costs both to the individual who failed to get treatment and to the institution who had to replace the fired nurse (Sullivan et al., 1988).

Today, nurse managers are more likely to confront or report nurses suspected of drug or alcohol abuse. This makes it more likely that the nurse will receive treatment for addiction and even continue working with appropriate supervision.

Because the ADA defines recovering alcohol and drug addicts as handicapped, nurses in this category cannot be denied employment as long as they can perform in the work role. Active alcoholics must meet the same performance requirements and may not be dismissed as long as they do not come to work impaired or drink on the job. The same protection is not extended to active users of illicit drugs.

To assist persons with alcohol and drug problems, peer assistance programs may be offered by employers, the state board of nursing, or the state nurses' association. Employer assistance programs may be in house or offered via a contract with another provider. Programs offer assistance with education about alcohol and drug abuse, case finding, treatment, and monitoring (Sullivan et al., 1988).

Peer assistance programs offered by a state board of nursing are made possible by state legislation. Many states now have what is referred to as diversion legislation. This diverts nurses from the disciplinary process to a treatment program. In these states, the chemically dependent nurse is reported to the state board and may be required to submit the professional license until treatment has begun. In contrast, some states offer advocacy programs through the state board. These programs allow the nurse voluntarily to enter a treatment program. The impaired nurse is not reported to the state board of nursing unless treatment fails (Daum, 1990).

The treatment program may last several years and includes strict monitoring once the nurse returns to work. Nurses who fail to continue the treatment program will revert to the disciplinary process. For nurses successfully completing the program, no report of the nurse's substance abuse will appear on the nurse's record. Many diversion programs are also joint effort of the state board of nursing and state nurses association.

Reporting of alcohol and drug abuse by nurses varies from state to state. Some states require reporting even suspected cases of drug abuse. Requirements may include reporting all drug use, with or without addiction, or be limited to cases where the nurse is practicing while impaired.

State law varies when nurses take drugs. Nurses may either be charged criminally or allowed to enter treatment programs. Nurses who reach a point of review by the state board may have action taken against their license. Actions cover the range from probation to revocation. Practice with a limited license is not unusual.

Executive nurses in concert with nurse managers must make determinations, in accord with state law, as to whether the individual nurse's situation warrants a report to the state board. Professionals have a privilege, not a right, to practice. The ethical dilemma experienced by executive nurses and nurse managers is a matter of balancing the right of the consumer to safe treatment with the right of the nurse to treatment for a recognized disability. At issue will be whether the nurse should be removed from the workplace while in recovery. The American Nurses Association (1984) outlined the rights of the addicted nurse to include protection from slander and stigma, knowledge of legal rights in relation to self-incrimination, health care benefits, and modifications of the work setting during recovery.

Early recognition and treatment are always preferable to loss of employment and state board disciplinary action. Covering up for an impaired nurse is never preferable to confrontation.

Staff Hiring and Dismissal

Inevitably the executive nurse will face ambiguous situations in both hiring and firing situations.

At Will versus Contractual Employment

Ordinarily, persons are hired at the will of the employer. This means the employer holds power over the employee's employment status. Exceptions to this employer power include employment contracts. Covered individuals generally include those with personal employment and often those covered under a collective-bargaining agreement. Employee contracts may also be discerned from employee handbooks. This might be the case if, for example, a handbook states persons will continue to be employed while they maintain positive relations with customers. Both federal and state statutes prohibit termination based on race, gender, disability, religion, or age. Persons may not be terminated in retaliation for pursuing a workers' compensation claim or acting as a "whistleblower"(Starr & Mueller, 1995).

Public policy may also be an exception to termination. In Ohio, for example, the Supreme Court has found termination of an employee because a court ordered child-support payments deducted from his paycheck a violation of public policy (Greeley v. Miami Valley Maintenance Contractors, Inc., 1990). In another case the Court found termination for truthfully providing testimony unfavorable to an employer also a violation of public policy (Sabo v. Schott, 1994). The Ohio Supreme court founded its public policy exceptions in state statue, state and federal constitution, administrative rules and regulations, and case law. Executive nurses must seek counsel and nurse managers must seek executive-nurse guidance before initiating termination actions in instances like the examples above.

National Labor Relations Act and Professional versus Supervisor Tension

A nurse cannot be a supervisor and still come under the National Labor Relations Act (NLRA). In National Labor Relations Board v. Health Care & Retirement Corporation of America (1994), four practical nurses brought an unfair labor practice action against their employer for disciplining them for complaints about working conditions. The National Labor Relations Board (NLRB) found the nurses were not acting as "supervisors" and ordered the nurses' reinstatement. Both the Court of Appeals and the Supreme Court found the nurses to be "supervisors." The decision represents a history of tension between the Act's inclusion of professional employees under its protection and its exclusion of supervisors.

The Court, in a 5–4 decision, found the board's test for determining whether nurses are supervisors inconsistent with the statute. The Court held the nurses to be supervisors because their supervision of nursing assistants was "acting in the interest of the employer." In contrast, the administrative law judge for the NLRB found the nurses' focus to be on the well-being of the residents.

Justice Ginsburg, in her dissent, reiterated the tension between Congress' intent to permit coverage of professional employees and its exclusion of supervisors. She notes NLRB decisions have found professionals whose chief responsibility is not management to be professionals implicitly covered under the Act.

Since the NLRA protects not only collective bargaining but also any concerted activity, the decision threatens the status of nurses in two ways. Statutory changes to the National Labor Relation Act have been suggested by the American Nurses Association. One approach would provide for clear statutory coverage of professional employees who, by virtue of their professional responsibilities, necessarily have some authority over other personnel (ANA, 1995).

Executive nurses working with unions need to monitor the impact of the decision closely. The decision is not only a legal challenge; it is an ethical challenge as well. If nurses cannot speak out in favor of quality of care because they are part of management, who will assume the advocacy role? Is there inconsistency between consumer advocacy and nursing management?

Unemployment Compensation

Availability of unemployment compensation reflects in law the societal good and thus societal obligation to individuals for financial support during a period of transition from a lost job to a new job. Like workers' compensation, unemployment compensation rates for a health care facility are also based on experience. Thus, executive nurses seeking to keep those rates within control should educate nurse managers about approaches to termination that will keep rates reasonable. Staff terminated without cause (e.g., because of downsizing or unit closings) will receive unemployment compensation. Persons dismissed for cause (e.g., having a track record of providing unsafe care) cannot collect unemployment compensation.

Dismissed staff can seek administrative review of agency denials of unemployment compensation. Administrative denials can be pursued in court. Similarly, health care facilities can seek administrative and court review of awarding of unemployment compensation. Administrative reviewers will look askance at a 15-year-employee dismissed on the basis of one consumer's complaint. For the long-term employee, documentation of instances of unsafe care, followed by counseling and provision of opportunities for growth with no improvement, are much more likely to be regarded as dismissals for cause. In a situation where employment for a short period is followed by termination for being unable to perform in a job, an administrative reviewer is likely to award unemployment compensation. In this situation, the manager is regarded as having made a poor hire instead of the dismissed employee's being at fault.

Executive nurses should provide workshops for nursing managers that include sample cases illustrating appropriate approaches to staff termination. Many state licensing statutes mandate employers report incompetent practice to the state board of nursing. Thus, legal, professional, and ethical accountability may not end with staff termination.

HANDLING CONSUMER HEALTH CARE DATA

One of the last bastions of privacy is information about individual health. In an age of vast computer networks and virtual universal access to cyberspace, retaining this privacy will be a constant challenge. Laws like the Americans with Disabilities Act can, in the aggregate, address societal goals for reducing bias against employment of persons with various health problems. The law cannot always cover the individual bias that garbs itself in other no-hire rationale. And curiously, despite commitment to hiring the handicapped, health care insurers themselves currently continue to have the privilege of access to all health care information, and the right to exclude certain preexisting conditions completely from coverage or to subject applicants with such conditions to long waits for initiation of coverage.

Increasing use of genetic screening for both presence and risk of genetically influenced illness raises more concern about transmission of information. Even before illness occurs, individuals may be excluded from coverage. If a person is billed for Diagnostic Related Group (DRG) classifications that receive higher levels of reimbursement, insurers may view a person as at greater risk than is congruent with reality. In such a threatening climate, executive nurses need to understand clearly the distinctions between confidentiality, privacy, and privilege, as both legal and ethical concepts.

Confidentiality

Confidentiality addresses information provided within a professional relationship between provider and consumer. Confidentiality is essentially an ethical concept. The ANA Code (1985) notes it derives from the moral principle of respect for persons. The Code admonishes nurses to "safeguard the client's right to privacy by judiciously protecting information of a confidential nature." The Code's interpretive statements note "confidentiality . . . is not absolute when innocent parties are in direct jeopardy." This puts in a quandary the nurse who knows that a provider, not forthcoming about HIV-positive status, continues procedures with potential for commingling of blood. Does the nurse have a right and obligation to share that information, even though the information does not derive from a professional relationship?

No law presently exists that mandates disclosure of health-professional HIV status. Disclosure continues to be a matter of individual's choice and the policy of individual health care facilities. Both state and federal law govern the confidentiality of patient information.

Privilege

Privilege is a legal concept. Privilege protects the health care consumer's right to privacy under state statutes. Privilege applies to court testimony. The consumer holds the privilege and only the consumer can waive the privilege.

State laws vary as to who is legally covered under privilege. Physicians, nurses, counselors, and social workers are examples of persons covered under privilege statutes. In states where nurses are covered by privilege statutes, nurses cannot reveal information obtained within the nurse/client health care relationship. Thus, an emergency room nurse who knows that a consumer engaged in heavy drinking prior to an accident cannot share that knowledge in any subsequent lawsuit without the permission of that consumer of care *unless* state statute overrides the privilege.

Persons bringing malpractice suits against providers automatically waive privilege. In states where nurses are not expressly covered by statute, they may be covered because their close work with physicians brings them under the protection of physician privilege.

Testimonial privilege is limited by many exceptions. In fact, federal law does not generally recognize physician-patient privilege. Therefore, it may not be available for cases brought in a federal court.

Privacy

A person's common-law right to privacy prevents the public disclosure of private or embarrassing facts, regardless of the truth of the facts. Illness falls within the purview of such private information.

The interpretive statements of the ANA Code suggest that access to client data be limited to members of the health care team directly concerned with the client's care. Nurses not involved directly in the care of the person should first obtain that person's permission.

The general consent to care discussed earlier includes consent to sharing necessary information for peer review and other quality-assurance mechanisms as well as third-party payers. Federal law requires patient consent for release of records for treatment of alcohol and drug abuse (42 CFR, Part 2; 42 U.S.C. S 290ee-3(b)(b)(1)). Similarly, state statutes may permit release of mental health records only with consumer consent.

Reporting Statutes

Under certain circumstances, lawmaking bodies have made the decision that individuals and society are best protected by the sharing of information without the consumer's consent. Thus, child, domestic, and senior abuse in both home and institution may require reporting by name. Registries for persons obtaining prescriptions of controlled substances, having diagnoses of cancer, diagnoses of drug abuse, abortions, and birth defects may be maintained for epidemiological study. Death or injury from the use of medical devices, and misadministration of radioactive materials, are also reportable.

HIV-positive findings may be reported anonymously by laboratories. Diagnoses of AIDS and other highly infectious diseases, as well as occupational illness and injury, are also reportable.

Implications for Executive Nurses

Faced with the enormity of available health care data, executive nurses must educate nurse managers and others to the importance of confidentiality. Monitoring and reporting on breaches of confidentiality will serve to raise the consciousness of all staff. This can be done by simply having uninvolved nurses from another unit request a person's record. Lack of questioning as to reason for access is a violation of confidentiality. Elevator conversation breaches of confidentiality deserve review. Everyday occurrences such as these suggest computerized record security may also be casually breached without consistent efforts to enforce confidentiality.

Record security involves protection from unintentional destruction and modification as well as disclosure. Policies for restriction and access should be thoughtful. Drug and alcohol use, mental health problems, and HIV status may require a higher level of staff security clearance. Passwords would be needed for more than one level. Restrictions on downloading records will be analogous to moving paper records out of a facility.

Facilities seeking Joint Commission on Accreditation of Healthcare Organization (JCAHO) review should note that the "Medical Records" section of the 1995 manual has changed to "Management of Information." Manual guidelines include the cautions identified above.

Summary

As new health care paradigms in payment, delivery, and health care facility relationships develop, the executive nurse cannot ignore parallel developments in law. Neither can the executive nurse ignore ethical professional commitments to the patient, professional, and societal beliefs espoused in the profession's code of ethics. If restructured systems of nursing-care delivery result in increased consumer harm, executive nurses will have an ethical obligation to look to revisions. If seamless care does occur across consumer care settings, executive nurses in both care settings and academic institutions will well deserve accolades. At all costs, the face of new paradigms should be respectful of the person, of the consumer in choice and privacy, and of the care-delivering nurse in health and professional satisfaction.

Discussion Questions

1. Identify and describe an ethical issue you face in your health care provider role.

2. How would you resolve the issue in your setting, and what supports are present to assist you?

References

Adarand Constructors v. Pena, 115 S.Ct. 2097 (1995).

American Medical Association. (1992). Code of medical ethics. In *Current opinions of the Council on Ethical and Judicial Affairs.* Chicago, Il: Author.

ANA testifies before workforce commission. (1995). *Capital Update, 12,* 1–2.

American Nurses Association. (1995). *Nursing report card for acute care settings: A tool for protecting our patients, February 2.* Washington: Author.

American Nurses Association. (1995). *Summary of the Lewin-VHI, Inc. report: Nursing report card for acute care settings, February 2.* Washington: Author.

American Nurses Association. (1985). *Code for nurses with interpretive statements.* Washington: Author.

American Nurses Association, Division on Mental Health and Psychiatric Nursing Practice. (1984). *Addictions and psychological dysfunctions in nursing: The profession's response to the problem.* Washington: Author.

American Nurses Association. (1981). *The nursing practice act: Suggested state legislation.* Washington: Author.

Americans with Disabilities Act of 1990, 42 U.S.C.A. S 12101 *et seq.*(West 1993).

Bertholf, C. (1986). Alaska implements new prescriptive regulations for advanced NPs. *Nurse Practitioner, 11,* 10,15–16.

Brophy v. New England Sinai Hospital, Inc., 398 Mass 417, 497 N.E.2d 626 (1986).

Bullough, B. (1980). *The law and the expanding nursing role.* 2nd ed. New York: Appleton-Century-Croft.

Callahan, D. (1987). *Setting limits.* New York: Simon & Schuster.

Civil Rights Act, 28 U.S.C. SS 1971, 1975 (a), 1975 (d), 2000(a), 2000 (b) (6), 78 Stat 241 (1964).

Courting the right: Conservatism reigns supreme in high court's 1994–95 session. (1995, July 2). *The Cincinnati Enquirer,* p. E1.

Darling v. Charleston Community Memorial Hospital, 33 Ill.2d 326, 211 N.E.2d 253 (1965), cert. denied 383 U.S. 246 (1966).

Daum, S. M. (1990). When nurses need help: The Ohio peer assistance program for nurses. *Addiction and Recovery, 10,* 35.

Durable Power of Attorney for Health Care, Ohio Revised Code, S 1337.

Employee Income Retirement Security Act of 1974, Pub. L. No. 93-406, 88 Stat. 829 (1974) (codified in sections of 29 U.S.C.).

42 C.F.R. Part 2; 42 U.S.C. S290ee-3(b) (1). 47 Fed. Reg. 26,027 (1982).

45 C.F.R. S 1340.15 (b) (2) (1985).

Greeley v. Miami Valley Maintenance Contractors, Inc., 49 Ohio St.3d 228, 551 N.E.2d 981 (1990).

General Accounting Office. (1995). *Medicaid restructuring approaches leave many questions* (GAO Publication No. GAO/HEHS-95-103). Washington: U.S. General Accounting Office.

General Accounting Office. (1993). *Managed health care: Effect on employers' costs difficult to measure* (GAO Publication No. GAO/HRD-94-3). Washington: U.S. General Accounting Office.

Hadley, E. H. (1989). Nurses and prescriptive authority: A legal and economic analysis. *American Journal of Law and Medicine, 15,* 245–299.

Himali, U. (1995). More than 25,000 RNs march on Washington, issuing a wake-up call to consumers and lawmakers. *The American Nurse, 27,* 1, 20–21.

Indiana *ex rel.* Infant Doe v. Monroe Circuit Court, No. 482—5140 (Ind. Apr. 16, 1982) *cert.denied*, 464 U.S. 961 (1982).

Inglis, A. B., & Kjervik, D. K. (1993). Empowerment of advanced practice nurses: Regulation reform needed to increase access to care. *The Journal of Law, Medicine, and Ethics, 21*, 193–205.

Joint Commission on Accreditation of Healthcare Organizations. (1995). *Comprehensive Accreditation Manual for Hospitals.* Chicago: Author.

Lippman, H., Nagle, S. (1992). Addicted nurses: Tolerated, tormented, or treated? *RN, 55*, 36.

Marzen, T. J. (1995, Winter). Oregon and the new face of health care: New piece in the health care puzzle. *American Society of Law, Medicine, and Ethics Briefings, 12*, 1, 6–7.

Meisel, A. (1995). Oregon and the new face of health care: Reflections on "Death with Dignity Act." *American Society of Law, Medicine, and Ethics Briefings, 12*, 1, 4–5.

Miles, S. H. (1995). Physician-assisted suicide and the profession's gyrocompass. *Hastings Center Report, 25*, 17–19.

Miller, F. G., Brody, H. (1995). Professional integrity and physician-assisted death. *Hastings Center Report, 25*, 8–17.

National Council of State Boards of Nursing. (1993). *Position paper on the regulation of advanced nursing practice.* Chicago: Author.

National Labor Relations Board v. Health Care & Retirement Corporation of America, 114 S.Ct. 1778 (1994).

Pregnancy Discrimination Act, 42 U.S.C. S 2000 (e) (K), 92 Stat 2076 (1978).

Quill, T. E. (1991). Death and dignity: A case of individualized decision making. *New England Journal of Medicine, 324*, 691–694.

In re Quinlan, 70 N.J. 10, 355 A.2d 647, *cert. denied sub nom Garger v. New Jersey*, 429 U.S. 922 (1976), *overruled in part, In re Conroy*, 98 N.J. 321, 486 A.2d 1209 (1985).

Rehabilitation Act, 29 U.S.C., SS 701,709, 730–732, 740, 741, 750, 760–764, 770–776, 87 Stat 355 (1973).

Sabo v. Schott, 1994 Westlaw 59464, No. C-920941 (Ohio Ct. App. Hamilton Cty. Mar. 2, 1994).

Schloendorff v. Society of New York Hospital, 211 N.Y. 125, 105 N.E. 92 (1914).

Starr, L. F., & Mueller, W. (1995). Employment-at-will doctrine: Public policy exceptions. *Ohio Lawyer, 9*, 12–13, 30.

Sullivan, E., Bissell, L., Williams, E. (1988). *Chemical dependency in nursing: The deadly diversion.* Menlo Park: Addison-Wesley.

U.A.W. v. Johnson Controls, Inc., 111 S.Ct. 1196, 113 L.Ed. 2d 158 (1991).

Sue Fitzsimons
Rita E. Numerof

CHAPTER 14

Educating Nurses for the Future

Introduction

This chapter describes the evolving role of nurses and their educational needs. It is intended to prepare them to function in future health care systems. A developmental model is presented that is based on a curriculum, built over time, and that uses a defined strategy of information sets. The underlying premise of this model is that essential competencies that enable caregivers to manage quality outcomes effectively for patients and families will need to be continually developed.

In addition to discussing the model and its context, we will examine the role of the executive nurse in gaining broad organization support for the strategy.

A FUTURE SCENARIO

It's the year 2006. Mary McCarthy is arriving at work early today for a strategic marketing meeting. Mary is administrative director for cardiopulmonary services at Gotham City Memorial Hospital, a position she has held for seven years. Her world has certainly changed in the last decade. Just ten years ago, she managed a dozen surgical suites. Looking back at those days, she remembers the challenge — what a euphemism *that* was! — of coordinating schedules; arguing to maintain her dedicated specialty nurses for open-heart and vascular procedures; making sure that the floors were ready and able to accept her patients. There was pressure in 1996 to control costs, so Mary and her surgery manager colleagues worked with physicians to reexamine preference cards and introduced standardized products wherever possible. Custom packs were introduced, changed, eliminated, and reintroduced. Materials management worked with surgery managers to store supplies in central stores in an attempt to reduce inventory and lower costs while ensuring timely delivery, particularly of emergency items.

In the early nineties, specialists and technicians were rarely, if ever, asked to do anything outside of their narrow job duties. Housekeepers kept things pretty clean but they did not see themselves as part of the delivery team. It was a stressful, high-pressured, difficult time. In retrospect, the hardest thing was the constant pressure to turn rooms around faster, contain cost, increase staff productivity, and try to maintain staff morale in the face of constant budget justifications to finance.

It was ironic that no one back then had ever asked Mary and her staff about revenue enhancement. That was always left to the reimbursement specialists in finance. Today, ten years later in a capitated environment, Mary's whole world has changed. Her responsibilities have changed; jobs no longer look anything like they did a decade before.

Mary is now head of a full-spectrum service line, addressing the entire range of cardiac services from prevention to rehabilitation across the full range of service settings. The catheterization lab, once under a separate manager, is part of Mary's world in 2006, as are the surgical suites, coronary intensive-care unit, cardiac step-down areas and nursing units, cardiac rehabilitation center, and educational and support services for patients and their families. Mary's world is truly an interdisciplinary world—a world of specialty surgeons, cardiologists, internists, nurses, physiotherapists, respiratory therapists, patient-care assistants, financial analysts, marketers, social workers, dieticians, and support service technicians —all centered on the patient's experience.

Most striking in the last decade has been the dramatic change in the role of the nurse. Effective nursing diagnosis has been more challenging than ever, but the real change has been in the staff nurse's position as coordinator and manager of the patient's care (of course, under the jurisdiction of the primary physician, but more collaborative than anyone in 1996 could have imagined). Nurses are now responsible for managing the process to ensure that appropriate pathways are followed, that financial considerations are appropriately managed, and that discharge planning begins the minute the patient arrives for treatment. The coordination of other service personnel in the specialty is also a major function of this nurse's job, who interacts more and more with patients and family members about lifestyle issues, prevention, and health maintenance across a diverse array of settings.

There are fewer nurses than in 1996, but their jobs are more influential now and they earn more respect. The year 2006 is an exciting time. Who, ten years ago, could have predicted it, Mary thought as she picked up the marketing plans she prepared for today's meeting.

The scenario just outlined, while hypothetical, is a projection of the opportunities and challenges that lie ahead for the nursing profession as health care delivery institutions struggle with cost concerns and patient-focused care amidst discussion of health care reform. Although described as evolving from acute-care settings, similar scenarios could be written from the community, long-term care, home, or occupational-health care arenas.

LOOKING AT CONTEXT

Debate over health care reform has been a major topic of discussion and concern for several years. Financial issues, access for the millions of uninsured, and control of total costs dominate the debates in many legislative arenas. Concern for total quality and focus on outcomes has fueled significant interest in the issues of process engineering, job restructuring, and the changing nature of work.

At the practice level, increasing acuity and shorter length of stay (LOS) have increased daily pressures and job demands. Coupled with continued financial pressure and broader managerial spans of control, morale issues continue to surface. Pressures to ensure continuous improvement, document quality outcomes, and manage cross-functional issues become higher priorities with new accreditation standards. Cost containment processes have eliminated support jobs in environmental-service and related areas. Alternative jobs are designed to off-load nonessential nursing functions to other service extenders, creating career opportunities for previously dead-end positions and modifying the role of nurses. Ambulatory and home health services continue to grow, creating shifts where health services are delivered. Finally, consistent competitive pressures, which put a premium on patient satisfaction, are offering opportunities to design delivery systems around patient needs, as opposed to provider needs. The future will be based on a managed health care delivery system in which informed purchasers contract with providers to deliver the highest-value care. There is now the opportunity—and expectation—that the way in which we design health care delivery and educate our future practitioners will be reexamined as an essential mandate for survival.

Clearly, an increasingly visible revolution in health care delivery is taking place. Underlying this revolution are the concepts of total quality management and continual process improvement that are repositioning American industry. In addition to health care reform, other societal issues are creating major change for the health care system. An increasingly older population, rapid changes in the number and type of new technologies (including information technology), labor shortages as well as oversupplies, increased litigation and regulation, and public dissatisfaction with the health care delivery system have put enormous pressure on health care institutions while simultaneously offering significant opportunities for innovation.

THE NURSE OF THE FUTURE

As we look forward, we can expect that the majority of caregivers are going to be cross-trained to provide more services on the unit, which will increase flexibility and responsiveness in delivering care. At the same time, the number of job categories will shrink dramatically. Previously dead-end support jobs will be redefined as patient-care support through job redesign. These redesigned and titled caregivers will admit patients, perform medical record coding, change linen, pass out meal trays, draw blood, clean rooms, and plan care directly on units with nursing staff. Turnaround times for services will be determined by patients and physicians, not by centralized departments who have traditionally operated out of a "silo" mentality. (See Chapter 8 for a discussion on silos.) We can expect charting will be exception-based whenever feasible, resulting in less documentation time and more service delivery. In turn, personnel levels will be reduced by up to 20 percent. Bedside computer terminals will support decentralized admitting, discharging, billing, and bed control, further supporting the seamless integrated delivery of care. Nonspecific nursing tasks will be off-loaded to other personnel. Staff nurses will be used as coordinators and managers of patient care.

The movement to a patient-focused delivery system is driven by cost and service delivery problems (i.e., poor coordination, and discontinuity). Future changes will be strategic in nature and dramatic. They will cut across traditional departments and challenge the way health care has traditionally been organized and structured. We are looking not only at the reorganization of the way nursing does nursing but at the impact nursing has throughout the health care system. As the years continue, the pressure on health care delivery will increase, and the need for us to make these changes will become even more pressing.

Responsibilities of the Future Nurse

If these scenarios are what we can expect, what will the responsibilities of the nurse of the future entail? Nurses are increasingly being asked, and will continue to be asked, to oversee the financial aspects of patient care. To perform this function well, they are going to need to be sensitive to diagnostic-related group (DRG) and diagnostic appropriateness, consulting with physicians on coding as well as treatment. They will be involved in the management of clinical pathways and more actively involved in discharge planning, which will be implemented at the onset of treatment. They will call in social-work staff for special cases, but they will not wait until the day or two before discharge to determine family status and patient needs. Being more directly involved in assessing the psychosocial factors of current illness, they will look at the impact of illness on the functioning of patients, as well as the functioning of the patient's family unit. The nurse of the future will have to look beyond hospital-based nursing to home care, nursing home, and ambulatory-care settings, and coordinate care given by patient-care technicians and assistants, caregivers, and physicians. Finally, they will be asked to educate patients, perform nursing diagnoses, administer medication, develop care plans, monitor patient status, and perform other roles only licensed RNs can perform.

If emerging jobs will take on these dimensions, then what will the requisite skill sets be for the nurse at the turn of the next century? What do our institutions need to be doing now in order to prepare our nurses for the future?

EVOLVING COMPETENCY REQUIREMENTS

Given the magnitude of these changes, the executive nurse needs to assure that the caregiver staff is prepared to manage these changes effectively while on a learning curve. A more clearly defined, structured plan of continuing education needs to be developed and implemented to educate experts who will lead this change at the staff level.

Traditionally, hospitals have focused on the development of technical/clinical competencies in mandatory and voluntary in-services. Clearly, a real and ongoing concern for the executive nurse is the incidence of errors made by staff that either harm or have the potential to harm patients. Most typically, review organizations, such as each state's federally funded medical peer review organization (PRO), have focused attention on the role of nurses in quality outcomes through identifying "mistakes" and reviewing incidents with the intent to reduce and ultimately eliminate them. Now, the functions of federally mandated peer review organizations are collaborative patient outcome projects, system process improvement, and continuous quality improvement.

Traditional fixes for such error patterns have been focused on the individual nurse, geared to increasing the individual's knowledge of diagnostic tests, medication side effects, and so on. It is now becoming apparent that looking more broadly at system issues and involving staff in managing and analyzing the system deficits will yield greater returns than an emphasis on individual performance.

Critical Competencies

As a result of these changes, the critical competencies for caregivers and for those who will play leadership roles are being redefined. Beyond technical skill, such competencies as information management, financial analysis and synthesis, critical thinking, presentation skills, and systems thinking will have to be developed. In addition, research skills, the ability to ask probing questions, and the willingness to collaborate with peers and across functions will also be critical. In this new, more complex environment, the ability to use influence effectively, manage group process, and resolve conflict will increasingly determine success.

Such a list of advanced skills will not be developed in generic schools of nursing, but will, more than likely, be the expected outcomes for master's-prepared practitioners. It will be critical for the executive nurse to have a strong interface with university programs and be able to influence graduate curricula in order to meet these evolving needs. However, reliance on academe alone will result in an inadequate response. The executive nurse must also lead the institution in developing a vision and related strategies for the development of experts internally.

Clearly, executive nurses must emphasize education beyond technical competence. They are going to have to look at decision-making and problem-solving skills that are used in making clinical judgements and managing care. Sophisticated communication skills need to be emphasized to develop the competencies of the nonnursing staff and ensure that high performance standards are met. These communication skills will be used with more traditional interactions with nurse colleagues, physicians, patients, and families. Nurses will need to master conflict management skills to resolve cross-functional and patient-management issues. Economic and financial analysis will be another skill set necessary to increase awareness of the cost of health care and ensure accountability for cost-effective quality care. The economics of health care do affect decision making. Nursing professionals are going to have to take a leadership role in this arena as well; to ensure that participation among work-group members is high, group process skills will be essential.

Delegation and coaching skills will have to be developed to ensure that each participant on the team contributes up to ability, as well as to secure increasing staff autonomy and assumption of professional accountability. Analytic systems thinking, which enables nurses rapidly to evaluate multiple pieces of information from multiple sources, is another ability that will be needed. Coordination and management skills, to manage and facilitate the work of other caregivers, is essential. Perhaps more important is the ability to exercise great flexibility under conditions of continuous flux.

Today's Executive Nurse

Scenario 14.1

Today, Jayne and Chris met to review the previous month's data on their benchmarked groups. Jayne had completed a monthly and year-to-date financial analysis of utilization data related to DRGs and physician practice patterns. She had met with finance to provide input into the production of a more user-friendly form that was to be shared later in the year with nursing staff on the inpatient units as well as the emergency center staff. She was also preparing a report to share with a number of key physicians to review their specific practice patterns in light of their peers' patterns and results.

Chris shared the quality data that had been concurrently reviewed during the month and had prepared a variance report reflecting where specific patients had not followed the care protocols and critical paths. He also shared some educational interventions that he had prepared for selected nursing units who were having difficulty with specific issues.

Both of these master's-prepared RNs had been in case manager roles for approximately two years and were seen as experts in the institution. Their relationships with hospital administration, finance, and the medical staff were excellent. Their skill in analyzing data had improved with time; both had developed information management skills as a result of continuing education. Jayne had become increasingly expert at managing a cost accounting data-management system and had made numerous contributions to the development of user-friendly tools that could be easily shared with patient-care staff. She was also an expert in explaining their meaning so that staff could see the outcomes of care management. Chris excelled in the area of human relationships and conflict management. He was especially good at involving physicians and nurses in reviewing and improving care, and at intervening to assure compliance with care management protocols when appropriate.

Jayne and Chris usually met weekly to assure movement towards goals; monthly meetings were held to review month and year-to-date data. They then planned interventions and determined strategies for the future. Both Jayne and Chris met annually with hospital and medical staff leadership to evaluate outcome achievement and set future directions. At that time they also planned an annual presentation to the board.

Today's meeting ended on a positive note; compliance with the critical paths was going well and there had been definite improvements in outcomes over the past months.

DEVELOPING THE CURRICULUM

A pivotal issue in these changing roles revolves around how an institution can develop its own resources. It is obvious that in this era of regulation and concern for clinical/technical competency, the majority of acute-care institutions must have programs in place to identify competencies and ensure ongoing competency of staff. However, outside of technical skills and skills related to new technology, institutions have not been so effective in developing their experts.

With health care reform, the role of the advanced practitioner of nursing in acute-care institutions is continually being defined. The executive nurse has to take a clear leadership role in the institution to help shape this definition and to develop resources and programs to meet emerging needs effectively.

One approach to the development of experts within an institution is the development of a curriculum of **information sets**, building from the simple to the complex. To determine the core competencies of such a curriculum, the role of the nurse in the institution should be examined and compared with the institutional values. Strategic redefinition must occur along the lines outlined earlier in this chapter. Suffice it to say that delivery systems must be able to reward and recognize differential competence adequately. While a system of recognition and rewards should be in place surrounding these values and competencies, it is beyond the scope of this chapter to define it. The following section provides a list of information sets and skills around which curricula can be built to develop expert nurses who can manage care at a sophisticated level.

Information Sets: Integrated Curriculum Design

Table 14.1 contains eight content areas, or information sets, that are very amenable to the development of modules that can be delivered as a course or learned in sections, based on individual assessment of need. Whether these are developed in-house or in collaboration with local institutions is a decision based on available resources in local situations. Each information set contains three skills levels: Level I,Core; Level II, Intermediate; and Level III, Advanced; they are discussed within each set.

APPLYING THE CURRICULUM IN PRACTICE

Without question, the performance bar has been raised significantly. Once the curriculum has been successfully communicated to nursing management and to the institution's executive team, curriculum design will need to proceed using either internal or external resources, or a combination of both. Time lines for the introduction of various modules need to be determined and critical communication needs to occur to ensure buy-in from essential constituents within nursing and outside nursing. To the extent that information sets are relevant beyond nursing specialists, it is preferable that these modules be offered more broadly for the development of nonnursing staff within the institution.

The Clinical Ladder

Implicit in the design of this developmental model is the concept of advancing knowledge, skill, and demonstrated competency. An important challenge for the institution will be to ensure that a system is in place to identify experts within the organization and reward them appropriately both monetarily and otherwise. A successful and frequently used approach has been the **clinical ladder**. Common to most clinical ladders, levels are identified (II–IV most often) that recognize increasing expertise in clinical practice. Clinical ladder programs identify specific criteria a nurse needs to meet in order to achieve advancement to the next level. Effective clinical ladders give visible institutional recognition for various domains of practice, linking accountability for more complex competencies with professional development. Additionally, they provide for differential compensation.

The use of a clinical ladder allows an institution to develop appropriate resources for staff development. It provides focus in determining appropriate budgetary needs and allocations that are tied to strategic priorities and institutional goals. Once these determinations are made, information is imparted in a structured and systematic way.

There are numerous strategies to impart this information. Some information will need to be taught formally; other information or education is developed through appropriate coaching of staff by managers and other experts.

For the novice or new graduate nurse, emphasis on the mastery of technical skills is the typical focus. Additionally, the novice needs assistance with decision-making skills and delegation to others. A first job may be the first interaction with interdisciplinary teams; working in groups, therefore, needs to be emphasized.

There need to be expectations for mastery of these areas within the first year. Typically, the manager is in an excellent position to evaluate the skill level of the new nurse and arrange for appropriate mentoring or classes.

Much has been researched and written in the literature about the transition of the new graduate to the work environment. Successful programs prepare staff to deal effectively with expectations that are clear and well documented. Potential leaders can be identified in this early career stage and mentored and encouraged to continue professional development.

As nurses pursue career development and attempt to climb the ladder, the institution needs to be involved with developmental activities. Opportunities abound through formal relationships with schools of nursing for on-site education as well as continuation of formal education. Additionally, in-service programs can be developed by expert staff and offered to staff nurses.

Clinical ladders can be built around the information sets seen in Table 14.1, and can be structured to reflect language desired by the institution. One such system has been developed at a large midwestern teaching hospital. The domains addressed in this particular ladder system include experience, education, citizenship, clinical practice, nurse/patient relations, and collaboration. The expert has mastered the core competencies within each domain as described below.

- Experience: Core competencies may include institution-specific clinical needs, prior positions that include working with people representative of different cultures and religions, foreign language skills, skill in working with individuals with handicaps, and setting-specific expertise at home care or outpatient surgery.

Table 14.1 • *Curriculum Information Sets: Integrated Curriculum Design*

Information Sets	Skill Levels
Set I: *Financial* *Analysis*	**Core** The ability of nurses to understand the care implications of basic financial concepts is critical, as seen in the following examples.

Set I:
Financial
Analysis

Core

The ability of nurses to understand the care implications of basic financial concepts is critical, as seen in the following examples.

- Decisions to toss and replace partially used IV solution bags with full ones contribute to unnecessary delivery costs.

- Actively facilitating the sequential scheduling of procedures to minimize physician and patient "wait time" and facility "down time" requires an understanding of and identification with economic concerns beyond "quality of care."

An understanding of basic financial concepts, unit, and departmental results is included at this level.

Intermediate

The ability to analyze data to discern trends and forecast the impact of these trends is essential at this next level. Clearly, the ability to understand and manage variances and use spread sheets effectively are also important skills. Finally, an understanding of institutional accounting methods rounds out the requisite skills at this level.

Advanced

Projecting costs and forecasting resource needs constitute the advanced curriculum.

Set II:
Quality
Management

Core

A basic understanding of CQI concepts is critical for all nursing staff, as they will increasingly be expected to contribute suggestions for process improvements as a fundamental part of their jobs. At a minimum, staff should be expected to be good consumers of improvement indicators and data collection. Presently, the need to obtain accurate data is seen by too many clinicians as an onerous and irrelevant chore, getting in the way of good patient care rather than facilitating it, or worse, as a means of management control.

Intermediate

Trend analysis requires effective data management and facility with statistical process control, both important skill elements at this level. The ability to translate data into important information from which conclusions can be drawn is an essential component of effective data management. The practitioner at this level should be comfortable with various types of data presentation (e.g., graphs, charts, etc.), and have some ability to determine which presentation format would be most appropriate under certain circumstances.

Advanced

Increased comfort with data management and data presentation is reflected at the advanced level. In addition, practitioners at this level must be able to give feedback to a wide range of other health care providers in order to gain their understanding of the trends and their support for changes based on data. Included in this area, then, must also be effective problem-solving, project management, and change management skills.

Table 14.1 • *Curriculum Information Sets: Integrated Curriculum Design (continued)*

Information Sets	Skill Levels
Set III: *Teaching and Learning Strategies*	**Core** Given that project nurses will be responsible for coordinating and overseeing the work of other care providers as well as for delivering care themselves, nurses of the future will need to understand the basic principles of adult learning. Those responsible for teaching others must be comfortable with a variety of strategies appropriate for different learning needs. Unfortunately, most nurses do not understand that this is a body of knowledge that can be taught, and that teachers are not "born." **Intermediate** While the core level emphasizes the learning needs of individuals, the intermediate level takes this knowledge to the next step—application to groups. **Advanced** Evaluation of learning needs and curriculum design are included at this level.
Set IV: *Computer Skills*	**Core** All nurses require some familiarity with basic computer skills. If the future world of health care includes on-line records and bedside terminals, nurses must be comfortable with accessing and entering data. **Intermediate** The use of computers and relevant software to support trend analysis and the management of patient care is essential at this level. **Advanced** At the advanced level, nurse experts can be expected to give input into the design of appropriate technology to meet the delivery of cost effective quality patient care.
Set V: *Presentation Skills*	**Core** All nurses must be able to communicate ideas clearly and effectively in oral and written formats. **Intermediate** The ability to differentiate and utilize appropriate quantitative and analytic tools for the presentation of ideas to differing audiences is essential at this level. More sophisticated written communication skills would be required, and the ability to present effectively before groups would be essential. **Advanced** At this level, staff would be expected to present to larger audiences effectively, having mastered general effective presentation skills. Additionally, they would be expected to present at increasingly higher levels of the organization.

Table 14.1 • *Curriculum Information Sets: Integrated Curriculum Designs (continued)*

Information Sets	Skill Levels
Set VI: *Evaluation and Research Technology*	**Core** At this level, an appreciation of the need for evaluation and an understanding of its implications are important. For the nurse guiding the development of more junior staff and non-nursing personnel, they must be in a position to structure the effective evaluation of the critical competencies of these staff. Research findings must be utilized and incorporated into practice. **Intermediate** At this level, principles of evaluation research and design are appropriate as these expert nurses will be asked to participate in the evaluation of various treatment approaches, assessing the efficiency and efficacy of one methodology over another. **Advanced** For the advanced practitioner, the actual design of clinical research and/or evaluation research studies becomes important. At this level, writing of grant proposals is important.
Set VII: *Clinical Knowledge in Area of Expertise*	**Core** Demonstrated technical knowledge relevant to an area of practice is essential here—an area generally assessed well by most health care delivery institutions at present. **Intermediate** At this level, practitioners must demonstrate model practice, gaining the respect of their colleagues. **Advanced** At this level, staff introduce new concepts and modes of practice to colleagues, effectively managing change and introducing innovation in patient care.
Set VIII: *Collaboration and Delegation*	**Core** Clearly the ability to contribute to team goals and to work effectively as a team member are basic competencies under this model. The ability to influence others, listen effectively, and communicate essential ideas non-defensively provide a necessary foundation to achieve the anticipated outcomes. Being able to prioritize personal tasks effectively and delegate appropriately to other team members is essential at this level.

- *Education*: Core competencies are dependent on state licensing regulations, need for additional specific clinical knowledge or credentials, the legal environment, the availability of personnel with formal and/or informal education, and the need for continuing education.

- *Citizenship*: Core competencies include working as part of a team, leadership skills, working effectively in groups, change management, presentation of information in written and verbal formats, and systems thinking.

- *Clinical practice*: Core competencies include appropriate technical skills, statistical process-analysis skills, continual process-improvement skills, research and evaluation skills, crisis management, decision-making skills, use of information technology, prioritization skills, financial analysis skills, and care management and coordination skills.

- *Nurse/patient relations*: Core competencies include teaching skills and communication skills; active listening and empathy.

- *Collaboration*: Core competencies include working with others, consultation skills, delegation skills, and conflict management skills.

GAINING ORGANIZATION SUPPORT

In addition to setting the vision and providing the stimulus to evolve such a system of learning, the executive nurse is responsible for gaining the support of the organization in order to implement the programs previously described. In today's era of diminishing resources and attention to returns on investments, programs that develop and reward nursing experts need to be positioned within the overall strategy of an institution.

The ability to articulate and position these programs requires careful planning. In an age where the role of the nurse in health care reform is gaining momentum and interest, the executive nurse can capitalize her strategies within such a context. In a capitated system, expert nurses can play a significant role in facilitating and coordinating care within an institution as well as coordinating effective discharge plans and movement of patients into a continuum of community care settings or the home.

Summary

Expert nurses clearly play a role in utilization management of patient care as well as in the definition of quality. Effectively articulating this role and its relationship to reducing expenses and improving quality can be very important in positioning a clinical ladder, development program, or other reward program.

The development of expert staff can be expensive. However, when tied to strategic priorities, such programs become meaningful. The traditional rationale of recruitment and retention of staff is not nearly as effective as reducing expenses and positioning an institution for survival in tomorrow's health care networks.

Most institutions view nurses as dependent caregivers who cannot effect an institution's future to a significant degree. The executive nurse can strategize and plan to change these perceptions through collection of data related to both DRG reimbursement and institutional costs of those same DRGs. Identifying high-impact DRGs and using techniques such as benchmarking and CQI to identify processes for improvement are strategies that can place nursing in a leadership role during both analysis of opportunity and implementation of change. Identifying the role of the nurse in managing paths or care protocols can establish the rationale for development and the need for reward. Developing staff to case-manage patients, track the impact of shortened LOS, and use fewer resources can be very powerful information.

The executive nurse is in a unique situation in today's environment. As leader of the largest area in any institution and most other health care settings in terms of overall budgetary expense, she can help lead these organizations to successful futures. This can only be done when the organization is positioned and supportive of developing a group of experts who can help lead this change.

Discussion Questions

1. The future of nursing requires that nurses acquire new competencies. What are they, and how will you attain them?

2. What will the health care system look like in 2006? How can nurses and the nursing profession help to shape this future?

References

Becker-Reems, E. D.(1994). *Self-managed work teams in health care organizations.* American Hospital Publishing, Inc.

Block, P. (1993). *Stewardship: Choosing service over self-interest.* San Francisco: Berrett-Koehler.

Bridges, W. (1993). *Managing transitions: Making the most of change.* New York: Addison-Wesley.

Brown, B. E.(1993). *Nursing administration quarterly series: Volumes I, II, III.* Maryland: Aspen.

Byham, W. (1993). *Zapp! Empowerment in health care.* New York: Fawcett Columbine.

Covey, S. R., Merrill, A. R., Merrill, R. R. (1994). *First things first.* New York: Simon & Schuster.

Finkler, S. Kovner, C. (1993). *Financial management for nurse managers and executives.* Philadelphia: WB Saunders.

Gift, R. G., Mosel, D. (1994). *Benchmarking in health care: A collaborative approach.* American Hospital Publishing, Inc.

Gillies, D. A. (1994). *Nursing management: A systems approach.* Philadelphia: WB Saunders.

Hakim, C. (1994). *We are all self-employed.* San Francisco: Berrett-Koehler.

Hamel, G., Prahalad, C. K.(1994). *Competing for the future.* Boston: Harvard Business School Press.

Hammer, M., Champy, J. (1993). *Reengineering the organization.* New York: HarperCollins.

Hein, B. E., Nicholson, M. J. (1994). *Contemporary leadership behavior. 4th ed.* Philadelphia: JB Lippincott.

Herman, S. M. (1994). *The tao at work: On leading and following.* San Francisco: Jossey-Bass.

Huge, E., Collins, B.(1993). *Management by policy: How companies focus their total qualtiy efforts to achieve competitive advantage.* Milwaukee: ASQC Quality Press.

Joiner, B. L. (1994). *Fourth-generation management: The new business consciousness.* New York: McGraw-Hill.

Joint Commission of Accreditation of Healthcare Organizations/ (1993). *The Measurement Mandate: On the Road to Performance Improvement in Health Care.* Oakbrook Terrace, IL: JCAHO.

Katzenback, J. R., Smith, D. K. (1993). *The wisdom of teams: Creating the high-performance organization.* Boston: Harvard Business School Press.

Kline, P., Saunders, B. (1993). *Ten steps to a learning organization.* Virginia: Great Ocean Publishers.

Kohn, A. (1993) *Punished by rewards: The trouble with gold stars, incentive plans, A's, praise, and other bribes.* Boston: Houghton Mifflin.

Kouzes, J. M., Posner, B.Z. (1993). *Credibility: how leaders gain and lose it, why people demand it.* San Francisco: Jossey-Bass.

Lathrop, J. P. (1993) *Restructuring health care: The patient-focused paradigm.* San Francisco: Jossey-Bass.

Lipnack, J., Stamps, J. (1993). *The TeamNet factor.* Essex Junction, VT: Oliver Wight.

Martin, D. (1993). *Team think: Using the sports connection to develop, motivate, and manage a winning business team.* New York: Dutton.

Mintzberg, H. (1993). *Structure in fives: Designing effective organizations.* Englewood Cliffs, NJ: Prentice-Hall.

Murphy, T. B., Hardy, C. T. (1994). *Hospital-physician integration: Strategies for success.* American Hospital Publishing, Inc.

Parsons, M. L., Murdough, C. L. (1994). *Patient-centered care.* Gaithersburg, MD: Aspen.

Senge, P., Roberts, C., Ross, R. B., et al. (1994) *The fifth discipline fieldbook: Strategies and tools for building a learning organization.* New York: Doubleday.

Toffler, A. (1990). *Power shift: Knowledge, wealth, and violence at the edge of the 21st century.* New York: Bantam.

Wheatley, M. J. (1992). *Leadership and the new science: Learning about organization from an orderly universe.* San Francisco: Berrett-Koehler.

Wheeler, D. J. (1993). *Understanding variation: The key to managing chaos.* Knoxville: SPC Press.

APPENDIX

NUCAT–3
Nursing Unit Cultural Assessment Tool

The primary purpose of this tool is to describe and understand your immediate work group in your practice setting. Your work group will likely consist of people who work the same hours on the same unit (section, department) as you do and with whom you have frequent contact. Many members of this work group will be members of the same profession as you are. However, there is no need to limit your work group to members of your profession. Think of your work group as consisting of all those who work closely with you, share your work-related values, and work with you to get the job done. These are the people you would describe as being "part of us."

The tool will describe your work group by picturing your group's culture. Culture has been defined as the set of solutions devised by a group of people to meet specific problems posed by the situations they face in common. In other words, it's "how we get things done around here."

There are no right or wrong answers for this tool. Rather, the primary goal of the tool is to understand how your group functions so that you can make the best decisions for the group.

The answers from all the members of your group will be added together to determine your group picture. In no way will anyone know the individual answers you give. Only group scores will be recorded.

You will notice the behaviors are listed down the center of the page. Please use the ***left-hand column*** to indicate how important or acceptable the behavior is to you personally and the ***right-hand column*** to indicate how important or acceptable the behavior is to your work group. In each case, use the accompanying scale to record your answers.

1 = not at all
2 = slightly
3 = somewhat
4 = quite
5 = extremely

(Copyright © 1991 by Harriet Coeling)

274

Nursing Unit Cultural Assessment Tool

My Preferred Behavior						My Group's Typical Behavior				

1 2 3 4 5   1) How important is it to understand the patient's feelings?   1 2 3 4 5

1 2 3 4 5   2) How acceptable is it to refuse to help your co-workers when they ask for help?   1 2 3 4 5

1 2 3 4 5   3) How important is it to work in an efficient manner?   1 2 3 4 5

1 2 3 4 5   4) How important is it to follow nursing policies and procedures?   1 2 3 4 5

1 2 3 4 5   5) How important is it to be competent?   1 2 3 4 5

1 2 3 4 5   6) How important is it to promote group morale?   1 2 3 4 5

1 2 3 4 5   7) How important is it to follow the organizational chain of command?   1 2 3 4 5

1 2 3 4 5   8) How accceptable is it to tell others how to do something if they haven't asked for advice?   1 2 3 4 5

1 2 3 4 5   9) How important is it to work hard?   1 2 3 4 5

1 2 3 4 5   10) How important is it to attend in-service classes?   1 2 3 4 5

1 2 3 4 5   11) How important is it to be creative in the nursing care you give?   1 2 3 4 5

1 2 3 4 5   12) How acceptable is it to do your work by yourself rather than working together with others?   1 2 3 4 5

1 2 3 4 5   13) How important is it to be comfortable handling emergencies?   1 2 3 4 5

1 2 3 4 5   14) How acceptable is it to question a physician's order?   1 2 3 4 5

1 2 3 4 5   15) How important is it to take on added professional responsibility either on or off the unit?   1 2 3 4 5

1 2 3 4 5   16) How acceptable is it to disagree with your manager?   1 2 3 4 5

1 2 3 4 5   17) How acceptable is it to try to change people's behavior by joking about it?   1 2 3 4 5

1 2 3 4 5   18) How important is it to get together with your co-workers outside the hospital?   1 2 3 4 5

1 2 3 4 5   19) How acceptable is it to call in sick when you are physically ill?   1 2 3 4 5

1 2 3 4 5   20) How important is it to offer help to others even before they ask for help?   1 2 3 4 5

1 2 3 4 5   21) How acceptable is it to tell someone directly, rather than indirectly, that you dislike their behavior?   1 2 3 4 5

1 2 3 4 5   22) How important is it to go along with peer pressure in giving nursing care?   1 2 3 4 5

1 2 3 4 5   23) How important is it to be nonjudgmental of someone else's behavior?   1 2 3 4 5

1 2 3 4 5   24) How acceptable is it to discuss new nursing care ideas you have read or heard about?   1 2 3 4 5

1 2 3 4 5   25) How acceptable is it to compete with your co-workers?   1 2 3 4 5

Nursing Unit Cultural Assessment Tool (continued)

My Preferred Behavior		**My Group's Typical Behavior**
1 2 3 4 5	26) How important is it to have one person, rather than the whole group, decide what nursing care is needed for a particular patient?	1 2 3 4 5
1 2 3 4 5	27) How important is it to act on the latest ideas?	1 2 3 4 5
1 2 3 4 5	28) How important is professional growth and development?	1 2 3 4 5
1 2 3 4 5	29) How important is it to have fun while you are working?	1 2 3 4 5
1 2 3 4 5	30) How acceptable is it to focus on maintaining life, rather than enabling death to be comfortable, when death is inevitable?	1 2 3 4 5
1 2 3 4 5	31) How acceptable is it to use your individual judgement in deciding what nursing care to give?	1 2 3 4 5
1 2 3 4 5	32) How acceptable is it to achieve clinical advancement and promotion?	1 2 3 4 5
1 2 3 4 5	33) How important is it to care for your co-workers?	1 2 3 4 5
1 2 3 4 5	34) How acceptable is it to call in sick when you need a day off to rest up?	1 2 3 4 5
1 2 3 4 5	35) How important is it to provide emotional support for your co-workers?	1 2 3 4 5
1 2 3 4 5	36) How important is it to attend college classes for a degree?	1 2 3 4 5
1 2 3 4 5	37) How important is it to spend a lot of time on paperwork?	1 2 3 4 5
1 2 3 4 5	38) How important is it to meet patient's physical needs before their psychological needs?	1 2 3 4 5
1 2 3 4 5	39) How acceptable is it to ask a co-worker for help directly, rather than indirectly, when you are falling behind?	1 2 3 4 5
1 2 3 4 5	40) How important is it to follow the directions your head nurse (unit manager) gives you regarding patient care?	1 2 3 4 5
1 2 3 4 5	41) How important is it to be comfortable in watching for life-threatening complications?	1 2 3 4 5
1 2 3 4 5	42) How important is it to become involved in the personal lives of patients and families?	1 2 3 4 5
1 2 3 4 5	43) How acceptable is it to be assertive with your co-workers?	1 2 3 4 5
1 2 3 4 5	44) How important is it to teach patients?	1 2 3 4 5
1 2 3 4 5	45) How acceptable is it to tell others directly what to do, rather than give them ideas about what they could do?	1 2 3 4 5
1 2 3 4 5	46) How important is it to make patients comfortable?	1 2 3 4 5
1 2 3 4 5	47) How important is it to learn new technologies?	1 2 3 4 5
1 2 3 4 5	48) How acceptable is it to prefer the old ways of doing things, rather than to look for new ways?	1 2 3 4 5
1 2 3 4 5	49) How acceptable is it to stay angry with someone longer than a day?	1 2 3 4 5
1 2 3 4 5	50) How acceptable is it to share your personal and/or family concerns with your co-workers?	1 2 3 4 5

INDEX